Cardiac Rehabilitation for Older Adults

Editor

DANIEL E. FORMAN

CLINICS IN GERIATRIC MEDICINE

www.geriatric.theclinics.com

November 2019 • Volume 35 • Number 4

ELSEVIER

1600 John F. Kennedy Boulevard • Suite 1800 • Philadelphia, Pennsylvania, 19103-2899

http://www.theclinics.com

CLINICS IN GERIATRIC MEDICINE Volume 35, Number 4
November 2019 ISSN 0749–0690, ISBN-13: 978-0-323-70910-1

Editor: Katerina Heidhausen
Developmental Editor: Laura Fisher

Clinics in Geriatric Medicine (ISSN 0749-0690) is published quarterly by Elsevier Inc., 360 Park Avenue South, New York, NY 10010-1710. Months of issue are February, May, August, and November. Business and Editorial Offices: 1600 John F. Kennedy Blvd., Suite 1800, Philadelphia, PA 191023-2899. Periodicals postage paid at New York, NY, and additional mailing offices. Subscription prices are $286.00 per year (US individuals), $632.00 per year (US institutions), $100.00 per year (US student/resident), $320.00 per year (Canadian individuals), $801.00 per year (Canadian institutions), $195.00 per year (Canadian student/resident), $402.00 per year (international individuals), $801.00 per year (international institutions), and $195.00 per year (international student/resident). Foreign air speed delivery is included in all *Clinics* subscription prices. All prices are subject to change without notice. POSTMASTER: Send address changes to *Clinics in Geriatric Medicine*, Elsevier Health Sciences Division, Subscription Customer Service, 3251 Riverport Lane, Maryland Heights, MO 63043. **Telephone: 1-800-654-2452 (U.S. and Canada); 314-447-8871 (outside U.S. and Canada). Fax: 314-447-8029. E-mail:** journalscustomerservice-usa@elsevier.com **(for print support) or** journalsonlinesupport-usa@elsevier.com **(for online support)**.

Reprints. For copies of 100 or more, of articles in this publication, please contact the Commercial Reprints Department, Elsevier Inc., 360 Park Avenue South, New York, New York 10010-1710. Tel.: 212-633-3874; Fax: 212-633-3820, E-mail: reprints@elsevier.com.

Clinics in Geriatric Medicine is covered in *MEDLINE/PubMed (Index Medicus), EMBASE/Excerpta Medica, Current Contents/Clinical Medicine (CC/CM), and the Cumulative Index to Nursing & Allied Health Literature*.

Contributors

EDITOR

DANIEL E. FORMAN, MD, FAHA, FACC
Professor of Medicine, University of Pittsburgh, Chair, Section of Geriatric Cardiology, Divisions of Geriatrics and Cardiology, University of Pittsburgh Medical Center, University of Pittsburgh, Director, Cardiac Rehabilitation and GeroFit, Physician Scientist, Geriatric Research, Education, and Clinical Center, VA Pittsburgh Healthcare System, Pittsburgh, Pennsylvania, USA

AUTHORS

PHILIP A. ADES, MD
Professor, Department of Medicine, Division of Cardiology, Director, Cardiac Rehabilitation and Prevention, University of Vermont Medical Center, South Burlington, Vermont, USA

JONATHAN AFILALO, MD, MSc, FACC, FRCPC
Director, Geriatric Cardiology Fellowship Program, Division of Cardiology and Centre for Clinical Epidemiology, Associate Professor, McGill University, Jewish General Hospital, Montreal, Quebec, Canada

RAKESH C. ARORA, MD, PhD, FRCSC
Institute of Cardiovascular Sciences, St. Boniface Hospital, Albrechtsen Research Centre, Department of Surgery, Section of Cardiac Surgery, Max Rady College of Medicine, University of Manitoba, Winnipeg, Manitoba, Canada

THERESA M. BECKIE, PhD
Professor, Associate Dean of PhD Program, College of Nursing, University of South Florida, Tampa, Florida, USA

KEVIN F. BORESKIE, MSc
Faculty of Kinesiology and Recreation Management, Health, Leisure & Human Performance Research Institute, University of Manitoba, Institute of Cardiovascular Sciences, St. Boniface Hospital, Albrechtsen Research Centre, Winnipeg, Manitoba, Canada

MARY A. DOLANSKY, RN, PhD, FAAN
Associate Professor, Case Western Reserve University, Frances Payne Bolton School of Nursing, Cleveland, Ohio, USA

TODD A. DUHAMEL, PhD
Faculty of Kinesiology and Recreation Management, Health, Leisure & Human Performance Research Institute, Institute of Cardiovascular Sciences, Albrechtsen Research Centre, Department of Surgery, Section of Cardiac Surgery, Max Rady College of Medicine, University of Manitoba, St. Boniface Hospital, Winnipeg, Manitoba, Canada

YAOSHAN DUN, MD, PhD
Division of Cardiac Rehabilitation, Department of Physical Medicine and Rehabilitation, Xiangya Hospital Central South University, Changsha, Hunan, P.R. China; Division of Preventive Cardiology, Department of Cardiovascular Medicine, Mayo Clinic, Rochester, Minnesota, USA

MARIA ANTOINETTE FIATARONE SINGH, MD, FRACP
John Sutton Chair of Exercise and Sport Science, Faculty of Medicine and Health, Professor, Sydney Medical School, University of Sydney, Sydney, Australia; Senior Research Associate, Hebrew SeniorLife, Hinda and Arthur Marcus Institute for Aging Research, Boston, Massachusetts, USA

KELSEY M. FLINT, MD, MSCS
Assistant Professor, Division of Cardiology, Rocky Mountain Regional VA Medical Center, University of Colorado School of Medicine, Aurora, Colorado, USA

DANIEL E. FORMAN, MD, FAHA, FACC
Professor of Medicine, University of Pittsburgh, Chair, Section of Geriatric Cardiology, Divisions of Geriatrics and Cardiology, University of Pittsburgh Medical Center, University of Pittsburgh, Director, Cardiac Rehabilitation and GeroFit, Physician Scientist, Geriatric Research, Education, and Clinical Center, VA Pittsburgh Healthcare System, Pittsburgh, Pennsylvania, USA

EIRAN Z. GORODESKI, MD, MPH
Department of Cardiovascular Medicine, Heart and Vascular Institute, Cleveland Clinic, Cleveland, Ohio, USA

PARAG GOYAL, MD, MSc
Divisions of Cardiology and General Internal Medicine, Assistant Professor, Department of Medicine, Weill Cornell Medicine, New York, New York, USA

JACQUELINE L. HAY, MSc
Faculty of Kinesiology and Recreation Management, Health, Leisure & Human Performance Research Institute, University of Manitoba, Institute of Cardiovascular Sciences, St. Boniface Hospital, Albrechtsen Research Centre, Winnipeg, Manitoba, Canada

NICOLE M. JOHNSTON, BKin
Faculty of Kinesiology and Recreation Management, Health, Leisure & Human Performance Research Institute, University of Manitoba, Institute of Cardiovascular Sciences, St. Boniface Hospital, Albrechtsen Research Centre, Winnipeg, Manitoba, Canada

D. SCOTT KEHLER, PhD
Division of Geriatric Medicine, Dalhousie University, QEII Health Sciences Center, Halifax, Nova Scotia, Canada

SHERRIE KHADANGA, MD
Assistant Professor, Department of Medicine, Division of Cardiology, Cardiac Rehabilitation and Prevention, University of Vermont Medical Center, South Burlington, Vermont, USA

KANWAL KUMAR, MD
Department of Surgery, Section of Cardiac Surgery, Max Rady College of Medicine, University of Manitoba, St. Boniface Hospital, Winnipeg, Manitoba, Canada

EDWARD LIN, MSc
Department of Exercise Sciences, Faculty of Kinesiology and Physical Education, University of Toronto, Toronto, Canada

SUIXIN LIU, MD, PhD
Division of Cardiac Rehabilitation, Department of Physical Medicine and Rehabilitation, Xiangya Hospital Central South University, Changsha, Hunan, P.R. China

ZACHARY A. MARCUM, PharmD, PhD
Department of Pharmacy, School of Pharmacy, University of Washington, Seattle, Washington, USA

SUSAN MARZOLINI, PhD
R. Kinesiologist, Scientist, Cardiovascular Prevention and Rehabilitation Program, KITE, University Health Network, Toronto, Canada

CINDY H. NGUYEN, MSc
Department of Exercise Sciences, Faculty of Kinesiology and Physical Education, University of Toronto, Toronto, Canada

DEIRDRE O'NEILL, MD, MSc, FRCPC
Department of Medicine and Mazankowski Heart Institute, Division of Cardiology, University of Alberta Hospital, Alberta, Canada

PAUL OH, MD
Medical Director and Scientist, Cardiovascular Prevention and Rehabilitation Program, KITE, University Health Network, Toronto, Canada

CHRISTOPHER J. OLDFIELD, BKin
Faculty of Kinesiology and Recreation Management, Health, Leisure & Human Performance Research Institute, University of Manitoba, Institute of Cardiovascular Sciences, St. Boniface Hospital, Albrechtsen Research Centre, Winnipeg, Manitoba, Canada

THOMAS P. OLSON, PhD
Division of Preventive Cardiology, Department of Cardiovascular Medicine, Mayo Clinic, Rochester, Minnesota, USA

AMY M. PASTVA, PT, PhD
Assistant Professor, Departments of Medicine, Orthopedic Surgery, and Population Health Sciences, Duke University School of Medicine, Duke Claude D. Pepper Older American Independence Center, Durham, North Carolina, USA

MARY ANN C. PODLOGAR, BSN, MAEd
Nursing PhD Student, Robert Wood Johnson Future of Nursing Scholar, Case Western Reserve University, Frances Payne Bolton School of Nursing, Cleveland, Ohio, USA

JULIE REDFERN, PhD, BAppSc (Physiotherapy Hons 1), BSc
Professor, University of Sydney, Westmead Applied Research Centre, Faculty of Medicine and Health; The George Institute for Global Health, UNSW Medicine, Sydney, Australia

GORDON R. REEVES, MD, MPT
Department of Medicine, Division of Cardiology, Thomas Jefferson University, Philadelphia, Pennsylvania, USA; Director of Advanced Heart Failure for the Greater Charlotte Market, Novant Health Heart and Vascular Institute, Charlotte, North Carolina, USA

ALEXANDRA V. ROSE, BSc
Faculty of Kinesiology and Recreation Management, Health, Leisure & Human Performance Research Institute, University of Manitoba, Institute of Cardiovascular Sciences, St. Boniface Hospital, Albrechtsen Research Centre, Winnipeg, Manitoba, Canada

PATRICK D. SAVAGE, MS
Department of Medicine, Division of Cardiology, Senior Exercise Physiologist, Cardiac Rehabilitation and Prevention, University of Vermont Medical Center, South Burlington, Vermont, USA

JOSHUA R. SMITH, PhD
Division of Preventive Cardiology, Department of Cardiovascular Medicine, Mayo Clinic, Rochester, Minnesota, USA

FRANCO TARRO GENTA, MD
Department of Cardiology, Istituti Clinici Scientifici Maugeri SpA SB, Torino, Italy

SCOTT G. THOMAS, PhD
R. Kinesiologist, Professor, Faculty of Kinesiology and Physical Education, University of Toronto, Toronto, Canada

OLGA TOLEVA, MD, MPH, CCFP, FRCPC
Department of Medicine, Section of Cardiology, Max Rady College of Medicine, University of Manitoba, Bergen Cardiac Centre, Winnipeg, Manitoba, Canada

NANETTE K. WENGER, MD
Professor, Division of Cardiology, Department of Medicine, Emory University School of Medicine, Atlanta, Georgia, USA

BIANCA W. YOO, MD
Fellow, Division of Cardiology, Department of Medicine, Emory University School of Medicine, Atlanta, Georgia, USA

Contents

CLINICS IN GERIATRIC MEDICINE

FORTHCOMING ISSUES

February 2020
Parkinson Disease
Carlos Singer and Stephen G. Reich, *Editors*

May 2020
Diabetes in Older Adults
S. Sethu K. Reddy, *Editor*

RECENT ISSUES

August 2019
Anemia in Older Adults
William B. Ershler, *Editor*

May 2019
Falls Prevention
Steven C. Castle, *Editor*

SERIES OF RELATED INTEREST

Cardiology Clinics
Heart Failure Clinics
Medical Clinics of North America
Primary Care: Clinics in Office Practice

Preface

Cardiac Rehabilitation for Older Adults: Vital Opportunity to Improve Patient-Centered Cardiovascular Disease Care amid Worldwide Patient Aging

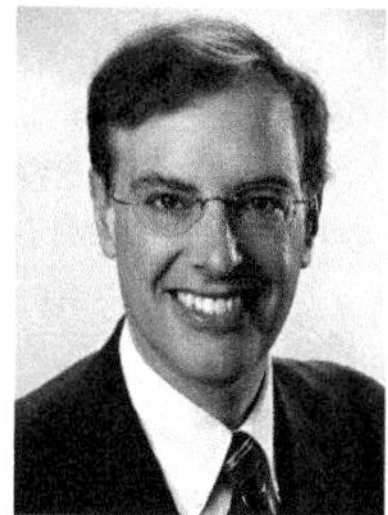

Daniel E. Forman, MD, FAHA, FACC
Editor

Cardiac rehabilitation (CR) has particular value for contemporary patients with cardiovascular disease (CVD) as it provides a unique opportunity to evaluate and address the distinctive needs of adults who are, on average, much older and complex than patients of years past. People are living longer in the United States and in much of the world, and aging is the number 1 risk factor for CVD as well as to its presentation in a context of multimorbidity, frailty, polypharmacy, and other geriatric complexities of care (also commonly including cognitive decline, sensory impairments, and increased falls). Thus, even if their incident CVD is treated flawlessly, older CVD patients are more susceptible to death as well as to high morbidity, functional decline, and worse quality of life. Approaches to CVD oriented exclusively to traditional disease management precepts of procedures and medications are rarely sufficient for older patients as their efficacy is often less reliable amid confounding geriatric intricacies. Overall, non-CVD factors become relatively more determinant of outcomes and patient-perceived value of care. CR affords opportunities for broader assessments and novel approaches that address such challenges and which can also monitor recovery over time.

This special issue of the *Clinics in Geriatric Medicine* provides an expansive overview of pertinent perspectives. Articles by O'Neill and colleagues and Fiatarone Singh provide orientation to the geriatric domains impacting older CVD patients. Afilalo focuses particularly on frailty, and articles by Khadanga and colleagues, Dun and colleagues, Redfern, and Beckie focus more specifically on distinctive approaches in CR with

Clin Geriatr Med 35 (2019) xiii–xiv
https://doi.org/10.1016/j.cger.2019.08.001

resistance training, high-intensity interval training, smart devices and wearables, and home-based strategies, respectively. Similarly, Flint and colleagues, Thomas and colleagues, and Tarro Genta and colleagues focus on CR for older adults in respect to its application to diseases/procedures that are most likely to occur in adults who are older, including heart failure, peripheral arterial disease, and transcatheter aortic valve replacement. Subsequent articles focus on novel applications of CR: Goyal and colleagues describe a novel strategy to expand CR to also deprescribe pills from older patients with heart failure who may be overmedicated, Podlogar and colleagues describe the value of CR in postacute care, and Boreskie and colleagues describe utility of prehabilitation in older adults before CVD procedures. Finally, Yoo and colleagues focus on pertinent sex-related issues in CR as women outlive men and benefit from approaches that address sex-related underpinnings to CVD and non-CVD in older patients.

This collection from authors throughout the world showcases the value of CR as a way to improve care amid health care challenges that are very distinctive for older populations. The articles do not promote CR as it has been, but rather they highlight the potential to expand and enrich CR to address contemporary needs. We hope many readers will be inspired to champion efforts that advance this approach for their own communities and patients.

Daniel E. Forman, MD, FAHA, FACC
Section of Geriatric Cardiology
Divisions of Geriatrics and Cardiology
University of Pittsburgh
University of Pittsburgh Medical Center
3471 Fifth Avenue, Suite 500
Pittsburgh, PA 15213, USA

E-mail address:
formand@pitt.edu

Never Too Old for Cardiac Rehabilitation

Deirdre O'Neill, MD, MSc, FRCPC[a], Daniel E. Forman, MD[b,c,*]

KEYWORDS

- Cardiac rehabilitation • Cardiorespiratory fitness • Cardiovascular disease
- Exercise • Older adult

KEY POINTS

- Cardiovascular disease is a chronic illness for which age is a risk factor.
- As our population ages, the associated burden of cardiovascular morbidity, mortality, and disability is expected to increase, with associated cost burden and despair.
- Cardiac rehabilitation is a cost-effective intervention that can improve function and quality of life, reducing disability and age-related deconditioning and contributing favorably to improved health outcomes in an aged population.

THE AGING POPULATION AND ASSOCIATED CARDIOVASCULAR DISEASE

Longevity in the United States has been increasing dramatically since the 1900s, when average life expectancy was approximately 50 years, to the current average life expectancy of close to 80 years.[1,2] As a result, by the year 2050, it is estimated that 1 in 4 Americans will be older than 65 years old, with close to 5% of the population being older than 85 years.[3,4] This exponential increase in the population of older adults, colloquially termed the "silver tsunami," presents a challenge to the health care system, as their medical complexities and age-related decline can lead to clinical outcomes that are less well aligned to standards established for younger adults, as well as associated increases in health care utilization and costs.[5]

Cardiovascular disease (CVD) is a chronic illness for which age is a risk factor. In addition, advancing technology within cardiology and cardiac surgery has contributed

Disclosure: The authors have nothing to disclose.
Funding: Dr D.E. Forman is supported by NIA R01 AG060499-01, R01AG058883, R01AG053952, P30AG024827 and NIH UO1AR071130.

[a] Department of Medicine and Mazankowski Heart Institute, Division of Cardiology, University of Alberta Hospital, 11220 83 Avenue, Edmonton, AB T6G 2J2, Canada; [b] Section of Geriatric Cardiology, Divisions of Geriatrics and Cardiology, University of Pittsburgh, Pittsburgh, PA, USA; [c] Geriatric Research, Education, and Clinical Center (GRECC), VA Pittsburgh Healthcare System, Pittsburgh, PA, USA
* Corresponding author. Section of Geriatric Cardiology, Division of Geriatric Medicine, University of Pittsburgh Medical Center, 3471 Fifth Avenue, Suite 500, Pittsburgh, PA 15213.
E-mail address: formand@pitt.edu

Clin Geriatr Med 35 (2019) 407–421
https://doi.org/10.1016/j.cger.2019.07.001
geriatric.theclinics.com

to patterns wherein more adults with CVD are surviving into old age, when chronic cardiovascular conditions and associated debility commonly accrue.[6] CVD is the most common primary diagnosis at admission to nursing home and the most common cause of death in those older than or equal to 65 years.[7] As our population ages, the associated burden of cardiovascular morbidity, mortality, and disability is expected to increase, with associated cost burden and despair. Therefore, an important public health goal is not only increased life expectancy but also preserved functional capacity, well-being, and confidence among older adults with CVD, such that a larger number live well and enjoy preserved independence and life value.[8] Cardiac rehabilitation (CR) is a cost-effective intervention that can improve function and quality of life, reducing disability and age-related deconditioning and contributing favorably to improved health outcomes in an aged population.[7,9]

CARDIAC REHABILITATION

CR is a multidimensional and comprehensive treatment program, typically involving medical evaluation, exercise training, cardiac risk factor modification, and education, aimed to promote lifelong health and wellness in those with CVD.[10,11] One of the aims of CR is to help patients transition from hospital, with supervised physical activity to reduce illness- and hospital-associated deconditioning and provide valuable support and education.[12] CR programs are individualized to the needs of each patient and provide many benefits to the growing population of older adults with CVD (**Table 1**).[13]

Table 1
Cardiac rehabilitation benefits

Improvement	Functional Benefit
Improved exercise capacity	Increased ability to perform activities of daily living
Improved strength	Increased ability to perform activities of daily living Increased muscle strength, mass, and power Reduced sarcopenia
Improved balance	Reduced risk of falls
Improved cognition	Reduced or delayed cognitive dysfunction
Improved frailty	Improved morbidity and mortality Improved gait velocity
Improved sarcopenia	Increased muscle mass, muscle strength, and protein synthesis Reduced dependence on wheelchairs and walkers
Improved depression	Reduced morbidity Reduced health care utilization Improved quality of life
Improved self-efficacy	Improved self-esteem Improved quality of life Improved physical function
Improved socialization	Reduced risks associated with social isolation—cognitive decline, negative physical and mental health Improved emotional support
Improved medication monitoring	Reduced polypharmacy and associated adverse drug reactions, falls, mortality Hemodynamic monitoring and assessment of patient tolerance of medications Improved medication adherence

Referral to outpatient phase II CR is a class I recommendation from the American Heart Association and American College of Cardiology after myocardial infarction (MI), coronary revascularization, valvular heart surgery, heart or heart-lung transplant, and in stable heart failure with reduced ejection fraction.[14] Despite this, literature suggests that only between 13% and 34% of eligible patients attend CR, and older adults, particularly older women, are among the least likely to attend.[15,16]

IMPROVING THE FUNCTION OF OLDER ADULTS WITH CARDIAC REHABILITATION

Older adults commonly have more numerous accumulated comorbidities and are more vulnerable to becoming sedentary, thus having poorer baseline function and less reserve if hospitalization is to occur. This also results in a higher likelihood of development of disability, dependency, and frailty.[16] CR has been shown to improve the function of older adults, enabling individuals to perform activities of daily living at a lower percentage of overall fitness and with a greater self-efficacy.[5] Thus, an important opportunity of CR is to expand its application to older adults, enabling more to preserve mobility, independence, and function and to better restore independence after an acute CVD event.[17,18]

Exercise Capacity

A common primary outcome in CR literature is that of cardiorespiratory fitness (CRF), measured by cardiopulmonary exercise test as peak oxygen uptake (Vo_2). It is known that peak Vo_2 declines with age, declining by 8% to 10% per decade.[19] In younger patients, CRF is primarily determined by cardiovascular and pulmonary components, but with age, other factors influence CRF, including changes in muscle atrophy, the interrelated effects of comorbidity (eg, chronic obstructive pulmonary disease, chronic kidney disease, depression), cognitive impairment, musculoskeletal limitations, deconditioning, and even changes in sensation (vision, hearing, proprioception).[16] Although measurements of peak Vo_2 may not be as physiologically robust in older adults due to the many factors that influence exercise decline, exercise capacity remains vitally relevant as a fundamental metric of health. Adults with poor CRF are at significantly greater prognostic risk. Moreover, a decline in CRF implies that everyday submaximal activities become relatively more difficult to perform, leading to increasing avoidance of activities that have become tantamount to more work and further exacerbating a cycle of progressive inactivity and functional decline. Sedentary behavior predisposes to disability and dependence that can be particularly aggravated by a CVD illness, especially among those hospitalized and/or after enduring prolonged bed rest. CR is an important intervention to interrupt this vicious cycle of progressive disability.[20,21] Thus, the overall clinical benefit of CR in the deconditioned older adult may be even greater than that of a younger patient who has a greater exercise capacity at baseline, because it results in a greater improvement in overall functional capacity and potentially helps to preserve independence.[22]

Several studies have compared the efficacy of CR in older patients. These studies have consistently shown that older adults derive similar or greater improvements in exercise capacity as younger patients.[23–25] Balady and colleagues[25] studied 778 consecutive patients enrolled in a phase II CR program and categorized them into 3 age groups: younger than 65 years, 65 to 75 years, and older than 75 years. At baseline, exercise tolerance was significantly lower with age. However, after CR, all age groups achieved similar relative improvements in exercise tolerance, with multivariate analysis showing that the greatest change in exercise tolerance was in those with the lowest baseline exercise capacity (<5 metabolic equivalents). This was again demonstrated by Lavie and Milani, who found patients older than or equal to 75 years achieved similar or greater benefits in exercise tolerance compared with those younger than 60 years, with a 39% increase in exercise tolerance in those older than or equal to 75 years, compared with 31% in those younger than 60 years.[24] Physical function improved similarly, with an increase by 27% in those older than or equal to 75 years, compared with 20% in those younger than 60 years. Baldasseroni and colleagues[26] showed the same trend when they studied 160 patients older than 75 years, after percutaneous coronary intervention, coronary bypass surgery, or valve replacement surgery, and found that CR resulted in clinically relevant improvements in all indices of physical function, with the poorest functioning individuals achieving the greatest relative benefit. Thus, current literature supports the idea that patients with limited physical function (or exercise capacity) can still benefit significantly from CR and that poor baseline function is certainly not a reason for exclusion.

STRENGTH AND BALANCE TRAINING

Whereas improved CRF in younger adults stems primarily form aerobic training, for many older adults who have less muscle mass and greater malnourishment, strengthening is of relatively greater importance. Strength training enhances not only muscle strength and mass but also muscle power and maximal neuromuscular activity in the older adult, at a magnitude similar to that of untrained younger subjects.[27] Age-related declines in muscle power output have been shown to be a predictor of functional limitation in older adults; therefore, the improvement in neuromuscular adaptations with strength training is important to maintain the older adults' ability to perform activities of daily living.[27]

Balance is rarely a concern for younger adults. However, for many older adults, imbalance is common, affected by muscle weakening, and further exacerbated by vasoactive meds, reduced thirst sensation, neuropathy, and impaired vision. Poor balance is significant in the older adult as it affects gait, thereby potentially compromising independence, and it increases the risk of fall and injury. It is estimated that one in every 3 adults older than or equal to 65 years and close to half of those older than or equal to 80 years suffer at least 1 fall annually.[28] Sustaining a fall, even without serious injury, has been shown to result in function decline, poorer self-rated health, and fear of falling that can impair activities of daily living (ADL) ability and negatively affect one's quality of life.[29,30] Low-intensity exercise has been shown to improve postural control and improve maintenance of upright stance, improve balance and lower limb strength, and reduce the incidence of falls.[31,32]

Barnett and colleagues[31] studied 163 adults older than or equal to 65 years, who after screening, were deemed to be at risk of falling. Patients were randomized to an exercise intervention or control. At baseline, groups were similar in terms of physical performance, health, and activity level. The exercise group was found to have a 40% lower rate of falling than that of the control group (relative risk 0.60, 95% confidence interval [CI] 0.36–0.99). Weerdensteyn and colleagues[32] studied 113 older adults with a history of falls, finding that exercise decreased falls by 46% (incidence rate ratio 0.54, 95% CI 0.34–0.86) compared with the control group, and balance confidence scores were improved by 6% in the exercise group.

Busch and colleagues[33] randomly assigned individuals aged older than or equal to 75 years to usual CR versus CR with additional resistance and balance training intervention. Exercise capacity, strength, and health-related quality of life improved in both groups, but the intervention group had significantly better functional capacity, as measured by 6MWT, TUG, and relative workload; this suggests that CR programs specialized for older adults have the potential to achieve an even greater benefit in this vulnerable population.

Tai Chi has been widely adopted as a form of low-intensity exercise with integrated components of strength, balance, and aerobic training that can be integrated in CR and that may particularly help achieve fall prevention. A study of Tai Chi compared with a 6-month stretching program found that Tai Chi resulted in fewer falls, fewer injurious falls, improved balance, and reduced fear of falling, as compared with those in the stretching group.[34] In addition, Lai and colleagues[35] have shown that older adults who regularly participated in Tai Chi over a period of 2 years had improvements in CRF, with less decline in their maximal oxygen uptake ($\dot{V}O_2$) over the 2 years, compared with their sedentary counterparts.

Therefore, low-intensity exercise has been shown to have a myriad of benefits in the older adult, including balance training, fall reduction, and delay in the decline of CRF with age. Although these benefits are generally presumed to occur with exercise training in younger adults, they need to be addressed more specifically in older adults and in a more individualized manner, based on an individual's current level of function and their accumulated functional deficits. These deficits can be improved on when strategies targeting specific deficits are integrated into the preexisting CR model, tailoring the program to the individuals' needs.

COGNITION

Cognitive impairment is common in older adults, with its prevalence increasing with age. The US Preventative Services Task Force estimates that 2.4 to 5.5 million Americans have dementia; 5% of those aged 71 to 79 years, 24% of those aged 80 to 89 years, and 37% of those older than or equal to 90 years. The prevalence of mild cognitive impairment is more difficult to estimate, with stated prevalence of 3% to 42% of those older than or equal to 65 years.[36] CVD worsens this burden, with chronic heart failure, coronary artery disease, cerebrovascular disease, and atrial fibrillation all known to be risk factors for cognitive impairment.[37,38] There is suggestion that exercise interventions and CR may improve cognitive function in older adults with CVD, potentially lessening this burden.

Lifelong exercise is preferred, but becoming more physically active at any age has been shown to be beneficial to delay or reverse cognitive impairment. The optimal intensity and duration of exercise has not been determined, but generally, higher levels of exercise have been associated with better cognitive outcomes.[39] Improvements in multiple cognitive domains, including that of attention, executive function, psychomotor function, and memory were seen after a short 12-week CR program, suggesting global cognitive function may be modified by exercise.[40] A systematic review and meta-analysis of 39 randomized controlled trials on exercise interventions in community dwelling adults older than or equal to 50 years found that exercise significantly improved cognitive function ($P<.01$), with aerobic training, resistance training, multicomponent training, and tai chi all having significant point estimates.[41] They found that 45 to 60 minutes of at least moderate intensity exercise was most beneficial to cognitive function and that the effect was independent of baseline cognitive status.

FRAILTY

Frailty is a syndrome of decreased reserve and vulnerability to stressors, resulting from cumulative declines across various physiologic systems. There is an increased incidence of frailty in those with CVD, thought potentially to be due to the similar pathophysiologic mechanisms of inflammation.[42,43] In addition, frailty is known to accelerate with the onset of CVD and with hospitalization, likely due to rapid loss of muscle mass and strength associated with hospitalization and bed rest.[16,44,45] It has been shown that 1% to 5% of muscle strength is lost per day while in hospital and up to one-third of older adults will develop a new disability in ADL with hospitalization, with half of those individuals never retaining the ability to perform that function,[46,47] showing the tremendously detrimental effects of hospitalization in older individuals.

Those who are frail have a significantly worse prognosis, with more than twice the morbidity and mortality than age-matched individuals without frailty.[48] Oftentimes frail patients are thought to be inappropriate for physical rehabilitation. However, in the last decade, an increasing number of frail patients have been enrolled in CR, further increased by cardiac innovations such as transcatheter aortic valve replacement. Despite this, there still remains a large gap in the literature on the CR of frail individuals.

There is a growing body of evidence suggesting exercise in itself is effective in improving or reversing frailty, even in the frailest population. In a seminal study, Fiatarone and colleagues[49] published a randomized controlled trial randomizing 100 frail nursing home residents, mean age 87 years, to a progressive resistance exercise training program, multinutrient supplementation, both or neither intervention, over a 10-week period. They found those randomized to an exercise intervention had increased muscle strength, gait velocity, stair climbing power, and cross-sectional thigh muscle area, as compared with those who did not exercise, showing that even in oldest old, frail, nursing home residents, a short 10-week exercise program can result in significant improvement in physical function and frailty. Another study randomized 115 older adults, mean age 83 years, with mild to moderate frailty, to a low-intensity flexibility-focused home exercise program or a progressive exercise training program. The exercise training group improved significantly in 3 of 4 measures of physical function, showing that intensive exercise training can improve physical function in the oldest old patients with baseline frailty and disability.[50] Therefore, although the literature supporting CR in frailty is limited, exercise interventions are some of the only consistently supported interventions affecting frailty in literature today. Furthermore, the utility of associated nutritional enhancement, particularly protein supplementation for patients with muscle atrophy, remains a dynamic area of investigation.[51]

SARCOPENIA

Sarcopenia is defined as the age-related loss of muscle mass, strength, and function.[52] Evidence has shown that older adults lose approximately 0.5% of their total skeletal muscle mass per day and 0.3% to 4.2% of their muscle strength per day.[53] Furthermore, sarcopenic loss of muscle strength progresses independently of muscle atrophy. The cause is multifactorial, often related to reduced exercise, insufficient dietary intake, reduction in type II skeletal muscle fibers, and reduction of insulin-like growth factor 1.[54] Muscle strength is an important determinant of overall function (aerobic and balance), particularly in older adults, with low muscle strength being predicting future functional decline and higher incidence of disability and mortality.[55,56]

Exercise has been shown to prevent and treat sarcopenia—increasing muscle mass, muscle strength, and protein synthesis.[54] This may be best done with resistance training. A study by Chen and colleagues[54] randomly assigned older adults aged 65 to 75 years with sarcopenic obesity to resistance training, aerobic training, combination training, or no intervention, over an 8-week period. Muscle strength was found to be higher in the resistance training group compared with all other groups at 8 and 12 weeks. Resistance training was compared with control intervention of yoga or breathing exercises in women older than or equal to 65 year with CVD, finding that a 6-month resistance training program resulted in statistically significant improvement in physical work capacity, balance coordination, and 6MWT performance, when compared with the control intervention.[57] Even very old patients with poorer baseline function can benefit from strength training, with Fiatarone and colleagues[58] showing that introducing a strength training program in institutionalized octogenarians and nonagenarians can increase strength by 100% after several weeks, with many individuals being able to reduce their dependence on wheelchairs and walkers. Therefore, resistance training can help prevent and treat sarcopenia as well as promote beneficial effects in strength and endurance, enhancing each individual's ability to perform ADLs.

QUALITY OF LIFE

The literature on CR suggests benefit not only in terms of hard outcomes, such as morbidity and mortality, but also in outcome measures such as quality of life, which are equally, if not more, important to older patients. Lavie and Milani compared adults aged 70 years and older with patients younger than 55 years, participating in CR. The older patients had significant improvement in quality of life scores, with improvements even greater than that of younger patients (20% vs 15%, $P = .03$).[23] Another study by Lavie and Milani found quality of life, pain, energy, physical function, well-being, general health, and mental health scores were all significantly improved in cardiac patients who participated in CR and that this improvement was as significant in patients older than or equal to 65 years as it was in younger individuals.[24]

DEPRESSION

Depression is prevalent in older adults, with an estimated 34 million Americans older than or equal to 65 years suffering from depression.[59] It is also prevalent in patients with CVD, with estimates that depression in those with CVD occurs 2 to 3 times more often than in the general public.[60] Recognizing and treating depression in CVD is important, as its presence has been shown to result in a greater than 4-fold increase in death post-MI, as well as increased health care utilization and decreased perceived quality of life.[61,62] In addition, treatment of depression can lead to improved physical function, with Callahan and colleagues[63] showing that older patients with depression randomized to a collaborative treatment intervention for depression not only had improved depression but experienced significantly better physical function at 1 year than those patients receiving usual care.

CR has been reported to improve the prevalence of and symptoms of depression by 50% to 70%, similar to that of antidepressant medications.[18] Milani and Lavie[18] studied 522 consecutive patients with CVD enrolled in CR, with a mean age of 64 years. They found that the prevalence of depression decreased 63% after CR completion, from 17% to 6% ($P<.0001$). Those who remained depressed after CR had a greater than 4-fold higher mortality than those who were no longer depressed (22% vs 5%, $P = .0004$). In addition, those who were depressed but completed CR had a 73% lower mortality than control patients who were depressed and did not complete a rehabilitation program (8% vs 30%, $P = .0005$). Even mild improvements in fitness level were associated with decreased depression and mortality reduction. Milani and colleagues[64] also investigated 189 patients with stage C heart failure, mean left ventricular ejection fraction of 35%, enrolled in CR, following them for a mean of 5 years. The prevalence of depression decreased by 40% after CR, from 22% to

13%, $P<.0001$. Again, those who remained depressed despite CR had close to a 4-fold increased mortality compared with those whose depression resolved post-CR (43% vs 11%, $P = .005$), and those who remained depressed but completed CR had lower mortality than those who were depressed and dropped out of CR (44% vs 11%, $P<.05$).

A meta-analysis of 18 randomized controlled trials assessed the effect of CR on depression in older adults, aged more than 64 years. They found that exercise therapy combined with psychological interventions was more effective in decreasing depression than usual care.[65] Therefore, the addition of cognitive behavioral therapy to the current multidisciplinary CR program may improve both depression and mortality in individuals with depression, and a reduction in depression can improve physical function and quality of life in these patients.

SELF-EFFICACY

Self-efficacy is defined by Bandura as a "patient's belief that they have the ability to influence their lives via self-imposed actions."[66] Higher self-efficacy has been related to higher self-esteem, increased quality of life, increased ADL participation, reduced depression and anxiety, and better disease management.[16,67] Research suggests that physical exercise is beneficial to positive self-efficacy. A randomized controlled trial of 174 older adults, aged 60 to 75 years, compared a 12-month exercise program with a stretching/toning control program. There were significant increases in all levels of self-esteem in the intervention group.[68] Another trial included more than 400 older adults, ages 70 to 89 years, who were deemed to be at elevated risk for disability and randomized them to a physical activity intervention or a successful aging educational control group for 12 months. The physical activity group had more favorable changes in self-efficacy and physical functioning than those in the control group, even in this group of very old adults with baseline impairment in function.[69]

SOCIALIZATION

Social isolation is widespread in older adults, with estimates that one-third to one-half of the older adult population experience social isolation and loneliness.[70] Social isolation is known to have a negative impact on physical and mental health, is associated with cognitive decline and dementia, and has been identified as a risk factor for all-cause morbidity and mortality.[70–72] In addition, socialization with patients who have similar disease processes and are at various stages in recovery and CR is thought to be beneficial, especially to older patients who are at higher risk of social isolation. A survey of older adults aged 65 years or more found that the socialization aspect of CR was very important and they would prefer to have an even larger socialization component,[73] suggesting CR serves as a means to counteract yet another vulnerability in older adults.

POLYPHARMACY

Polypharmacy is the use of numerous drugs by a single individual, commonly defined in the literature as greater than or equal to 5 medications.[74] It is common in older adults, who often have multimorbidity and is associated with adverse outcomes such as increased mortality, falls, and adverse drug reactions.[74] Population-based survey and cross-sectional study results have suggested that polypharmacy affects 40% to 50% of older adults.[75] It has been suggested that certain medications may be detrimental to physical activity and rehabilitation in older adults.[76] Thus, CR can provide a unique opportunity to review medications in all participants, particularly older adults, potentially reducing polypharmacy. In addition, for older patients with cardiac disease, many beneficial medications are counterbalanced by age-related compromises, such as incontinence with diuretics and hypotension and falls with beta blockers.[5] CR allows a longitudinal hemodynamic monitoring and assessment of individual patient tolerance of medications. This can ensure that cardiovascular management is well-coordinated and more patient-centered.

In addition to addressing polypharmacy and assessing individual patients' tolerance of mediations, CR has also been shown to be beneficial in terms of patient medication adherence. It is known that up to 50% of patients will stop medications for chronic conditions such as diabetes, hypertension, and dyslipidemia in the first year.[77] CR may also promote medication adherence, by providing education and access to health care professionals to which patients can direct medication-related inquiries. The ACTION-Registry-GWTG was used to study close to 12,000 adults, older than or equal to 65 years, participating in CR after MI.[78] It was found that participation in an increased number of CR sessions was associated with improved adherence to secondary prevention medications and each 5-session increase in participation was associated with both lower mortality (adjusted hazard ratio [HR] 0.87, 95% CI 0.83–0.92) and lower risk of major adverse cardiac events (adjusted HR 0.69, 95% CI 0.65–0.73). Therefore, medication management is another valuable and often undervalued service provided through CR.

BARRIERS TO CARDIAC REHABILITATION IN OLDER ADULTS

Despite the evidence described earlier, participation in CR is poor, with overall participation rate of less than 30%.[11] Suaya and colleagues[79] found that of Medicare beneficiaries older than or equal to 65 years, CR was only used in 13.9% of those after MI and 31% of those after coronary bypass surgery. Literature suggests older adults are 1.5 to 2 times less likely to participate in CR compared with younger adults,[22] with participation rate of only 13% in those older than or equal to 80 years ,[79] discouraging in light of evidence supporting its use.

Lack of referral to CR is a multifactorial, with physician recommendation playing a key role.[80] Firstly, a physician's lack of knowledge of programs in the area and of the potential benefits of CR can lead to lower referral rates. Patients under the care of a cardiologist or cardiac surgeon are more likely to participate in CR compared with those cared for by a primary care physician, potentially because of a greater knowledge of the presence and benefits of CR.[81] Secondly, some physicians believe lifestyle interventions are of less benefit in older adults, as life expectancy is limited.[44,82] However, an average 65-year-old has an anticipated life expectancy of 15 to 17 years, remaining functionally independent for two-thirds of this time. People aged 75 and 85 years have an average life expectancy of 10 to 11 years and 6 years, respectively and will remain independent for one-half of this time.[22,83]

Thirdly, physicians are concerned about the safety of CR in older adults.[44,82] There is a risk of cardiac complications with CR; however, this risk is low, with a statement from the American Heart Association regarding the risk of cardiovascular events during CR, estimating the risk of death, cardiac arrest, or MI as 1/60,000 to 80,000 hours of exercise.[84] There is no reported higher incidence of cardiac events among older adults undergoing CR compared with the general population.[23,64,85] There is also a concern regarding older patients sustaining a fall during CR; however, this is inconsistent with the literature, which shows exercise reduces the risk of fall-related injuries.[30,86] Nonetheless, it is prudent to take additional precautions when older adults are participating in CR, including longer warm-ups to improve flexibility and blood flow to large muscle groups and longer cool-down periods, to allow for exercise-related vasodilation to recover, reducing the risk of postexercise hypotension.[5]

Lastly, it is thought that physicians do not refer due to the lack of well-conducted, high-quality studies on CR in older adults.[44,82] Much of what is currently published is observational or substudies of randomized controlled trials. In addition, there is lack of evidence on participation and outcome of patients with heart failure with preserved ejection fraction in CR, one of the most common cardiac diagnoses in the older population. There is a desperate need for the development of novel interdisciplinary CR programs, developed by geriatricians and cardiologists, to improve the utility for older adults. This should focus on issues important to older adults, such as improving coordination, balance, and physical and cognitive functioning, in order to improve the older adult's ability to perform ADLs independently and retain independence. There is also a great need for high-quality research on CR in older adults and broad dissemination of this research, in order to reassure physicians and patients of the safety and benefits of participation in CR.

In addition, patient-related factors influence the lack of participation of older adults in CR. They often no longer drive, making transportation to facility-based programs difficult.[87,88] Older adults, particularly women, are often caregivers for sick spouses, thus they are unable to easily participate in activities outside of the home. Older individuals often have more numerous medical comorbidities, contributing to their becoming more sedentary, and this can result in anxiety about their ability to participate. Home-based CR aims to bridge the gap between patients who are interested in participating in CR but are limited by logistics. There has been a proliferation of literature on home-based CR within the past few years, providing data on beneficial outcomes and safety of this method of CR, with suggestion that it may provide longer lasting physical function benefits, as it teaches patients skills they can use in the long term, potentially creating a more permanent change in lifestyle than hospital-based CR.[89] However, the safety and efficacy of home-based CR has not been assessed in the oldest, most frail individuals. A trial recently initiated by National Institute of Aging, Modified Approach to CR in Older adults (MACRO), will further investigate hybrid- and home-based CR models in older adults (ClinicalTrials.gov Identifier: NCT03922529). CR will be tailored to the individual's needs throughout, using hybrid- and home-based options to best meet these challenges. This study will pioneer novel CR approaches for vulnerable older adults.

SUMMARY

In conclusion, cardiac disease is extremely prevalent in older adults, a population that is expanding rapidly. Age-related decline and multimorbidity can lead to decreased function, further exacerbated by cardiac disease and hospitalization. CR provides an effective means of reintroducing these patients to exercise in a safe and monitored setting, where they can regain confidence and physical ability that can allow them to continue to function and live independently for as long as possible. In addition, CR provides an opportunity to treat other geriatric-specific issues that commonly arise in this population, such as deconditioning, frailty, balance retraining and fall reduction, sarcopenia, polypharmacy, depression, and cognitive decline. Despite these important functional improvements with CR, older adults remain one of the most infrequently enrolled. This is multifactorial, but largely led by the fact that there is a need for the development of novel CR programs individualized to this population and a lack of high-quality literature supporting outcomes in older adults, both of which could improve physician referral patterns and patient participation in CR in future.

REFERENCES

1. Roger VL, Go AS, Lloyd-Jones DM, et al. Heart disease and stroke statistics - 2012 update: a report from the American Heart Association. Circulation 2012; 125:e2–220.
2. Felg JL. Aerobic exercise in the elderly: a key to successful aging. Discov Med 2012;13:223–8.
3. Centers for Disease Control/National Center for Health Statistics. Table 22. Life expectancy at birth, at 65 years of age, and at 75 years of age, by race and sex: United States, selected years 1900-2007. 2010. Available at: http://www.cdc.gov/nchs/data/hus/2010/022.pdf. Accessed February 10, 2019.
4. Ortman JM, Velkoff VA, Hogan H. An aging nation: the older population in the United States. Population estimates and projections. 2014. US Department of Commerce. Economics and Statistics Administration. US Census Bureau. Available at: https://www.census.gov/prod/2014pubs/p25-1140.pdf. Accessed July 26, 2019.
5. Schopper DW, Forman DE. Growing relevance of cardiac rehabilitation for an older population with heart failure. J Card Fail 2016;22:1015–22.
6. Kleipool EEF, Hoogendijk EO, Trappenburg MC, et al. Frailty in older adults with cardiovascular disease: cause, effect or both? Aging Dis 2018;9:489–97.
7. Audelin MC, Savag PD, Ades PA. Exercise-based cardiac rehabilitation for very old patients (>75 years). Focus on physical function. J Cardiopulm Rehabil Prev 2008;28:163–73.
8. Schopfer DW, Forman DE. Cardiac rehabilitation in older adults. Can J Cardiol 2016;32:1088–96.
9. Shepherd CW, While AE. Cardiac rehabilitation and quality of life. A systematic review. Int J Nurs Stud 2012;49:755–71.
10. Balady GJ, Williams MA, Ades PA, et al. Core components of cardiac rehabilitation/secondary prevention programs: 2007 update: a scientific statement from the American Heart Association Exercise, Cardiac Rehabilitation, and Prevention Committee, the Council on Clinical Cardiology; the Councils on Cardiovascular Nursing, Epidemiology and Prevention, and Nutrition, Physical Activity, and Metabolism; and the American Association of Cardiovascular and Pulmonary Rehabilitation. Circulation 2007;115:2675–82.
11. Thomas RJ, King M, Lui K, et al. ACC/AHA Task Force Members. AACVPR/ACC/AHA 2007 performance measures on cardiac rehabilitation for referral to and delivery of cardiac rehabilitation/secondary prevention services. J Am Coll Cardiol 2007;50:1400–33.
12. Deer RR, Dickinson JM, Fisher SR, et al. Identifying effective and feasible interventions to accelerate functional recovery from hospitalization in older adults: a randomized controlled pilot trial. Contemp Clin Trials 2016;49:6–14.
13. Matata BM, Williamson SA. A review of interventions to improve enrolment and adherence to cardiac rehabilitation among patients aged 65 years or above. Curr Cardiol Rev 2017;13:252–62.
14. Anbe DT, Armstrong PW, Bates ER, et al. ACC/AHA guidelines for the management of patients with ST - elevation myocardial infarction: executive summary: a report of the American College of Cardiology/American Heart Association Task Force on Practice Guideline. J Am Coll Cardiol 2004;44:671–719.

15. Suaya JA, Stason WB, Ades PA, et al. Cardiac rehabilitation and survival in older coronary patients. J Am Coll Cardiol 2009;54:25–33.
16. Forman DE, Arena R, Boxer R, et al. Prioritizing functional capacity as a principal end point for therapies oriented to older adults with cardiovascular disease. A scientific statement for healthcare professionals from the American Heart Association. Circulation 2017;135:e894–918.
17. Piepoli MF, Corra U, Benzer W, et al. Secondary prevention through cardiac rehabilitation: from knowledge to implementation. A position paper from the cardiac rehabilitation Sectin of the European Association of Cardiovascular Prevention and Rehabilitation. Eur J Cardiovasc Prev Rehabil 2010;17:1–17.
18. Milani RV, Lavie CJ. Prevalence and effects of cardiac rehabilitation on depression in the elderly with coronary heart disease. Am J Cardiol 1998;81:1233–6.
19. Fleg JL, Morrell CH, Bos AG, et al. Accelerated longitudinal decline of aerobic capacity in healthy older adults. Circulation 2005;112:674–82.
20. Greysen SR, Srijacic Cenzer I, Auerbach AD, et al. Functional impairment and hospital readmission in Medicare seniors. JAMA Intern Med 2015;175:559–65.
21. Ferrante LE, Pisani MA, Murphy TE, et al. Functional trajectories among older persons before and after critical illness. JAMA Intern Med 2015;175:523–9.
22. Lavie CJ, Milani RV, Littman AB. Benefits of cardiac rehabilitation and exercise training in secondary coronary prevention in the elderly. J Am Coll Cardiol 1993;22:678–83.
23. Lavie CJ, Milani RV. Disparate effects of improving aerobic exercise capacity and quality and quality of life after cardiac rehabilitation in young and elderly coronary patients. J Cardiopulm Rehabil 2000;20:235–40.
24. Lavie CJ, Milani RV. Effects of cardiac rehabilitation and exercise training programs in patients > or = 75 years of age. Am J Cardiol 1995;76:177–9.
25. Balady GJ, Jette D, Scheer J, et al. Changes in exercise capacity following cardiac rehabilitation in patients stratified according to age and gender. Results of the Massachusetts Association of Cardiovascular and Pulmonary Rehabilitation Multicenter Database. J Cardiopulm Rehabil 1996;16:38–46.
26. Baldasseroni S, Pratesi A, Francini S, et al. Cardiac rehabilitation in very old adults: effects of baseline functional capacity on treatment effectiveness. J Am Geriatr Soc 2016;64:1640–5.
27. Cadore EL, Pinto RS, Bottaro M, et al. Strength and endurance training prescription in healthy and frail elderly. Aging Dis 2014;5:183–95.
28. Karlsson MK, Magnusson H, von Schewelov T, et al. Prevention of falls in the elderly: a review. Osteoporos Int 2013;24:747–62.
29. Biderman A, Cwikel J, Galinsky D. Depression and falls among community dwelling elderly people: a search for common risk factors. J Epidemiol Community Health 2002;56:631–6.
30. Vellas BJ, Wayne SJ, Romero LJ, et al. Fear of falling and restriction of mobility in elderly falls. Age Ageing 1997;26:189–93.
31. Barnett A, Smith B, Lord SR, et al. Community=based group exercise improves balance and reduces falls in at-risk older people: a randomized controlled trial. Age Ageing 2003;32:407–14.
32. Weerdesteyn V, Rijken H, Geurts AC, et al. A five-week exercise program can reduce falls and improve obstacle avoidance in the elderly. Gerontology 2006; 52:131–41.
33. Busch JC, Lillou D, Wittig G, et al. Resistance and balance training improves functional capacity in very old participants attending cardiac rehabilitation after coronary bypass surgery. J Am Geriatr Soc 2012;60:2270–6.

34. Li F, Harmer P, Fisher KJ, et al. Tai Chi and fall reductions in older adults: a randomized controlled trial. J Gerontol A Biol Sci Med Sci 2005;60:187–94.
35. Lai JS, Lan C, Wong MK, et al. Two-year trends in cardiorespiratory function among older tai chi chuan practitioners and sedentary subjects. J Am Geriatr Soc 1995;43:1222–7.
36. Moyer VA on behalf of the U.S Preventative Services Task Force. Screening for cognitive impairment in older adults: U.S Preventative services task force recommendation statement. Ann Intern Med 2014;160(11):791–7.
37. Albabtain M, Brenner MJ, Nicklas JM, et al. Hyponatremia, cognitive function and mobility in an outpatient heart failure population. Med Sci Monit 2016;22:4978–85.
38. Singh-Manoux A, Fayosse A, Sabia S, et al. Atrial fibrillation as a risk factor for cognitive decline and dementia. Eur Heart J 2017;38:2612–8.
39. Hammer M, Chida Y. Physical activity and risk of neurodegenerative disease: a systemic review of prospective evidence. Psychol Med 2009;39:3–11.
40. Stanek KM, Gunstad J, Spitznagel MB, et al. Improvements in cognitive function following cardiac rehabilitation for older adults with cardiovascular disease. Int J Neurosci 2011;121:86–93.
41. Northey JM, Cherbuin N, Pumpa KL, et al. Exercise interventions for cognitive function in adults older than 50: a systematic review with meta-analysis. Br J Sports Med 2018;52:154–60.
42. Walston J, Hadley EC, Ferrucci L, et al. Research agenda for frailty in older adults: toward a better understanding of physiology and etiology: summary from the American Geriatrics Society/National Institute on Aging Research Conference on frailty in older adults. J Am Geriatr Soc 2006;54:991–1001.
43. Woods JA, Wilund KR, Martin SA, et al. Exercise, inflammation and aging. Aging Dis 2012;3:130–40.
44. Brown TM, Hernandez AF, Bittner V, et al. Predictors of cardiac rehabilitation referral in coronary artery disease patients: findings from the American Heart Association's Get with the Guidelines Program. J Am Coll Cardiol 2009;54:515–21.
45. Kortebein P, Ferrando A, Lombeida J. Effect of 10 days of bed rest on skeletal muscle in healthy older adults. JAMA 2007;297:1772–4.
46. Creditor MC. Hazards of hospitalization in the elderly. Ann Intern Med 1993;118: 219–23.
47. Covinsky KE, Palmer RM, Fortinsky RH, et al. Loss of independence in activities of daily living older adults hospitalized with medical illnesses: increased vulnerbility with age. J Am Geriatr Soc 2003;51:451–8.
48. Afilalo J, Karunananthan S, Eisenberg MJ, et al. Role of frailty in patients with cardiovascular disease. Am J Cardiol 2009;103:1616–21.
49. Fiatarone MA, O'Neill EF, Ryan ND, et al. Exercise training and nutritional supplementation for physical frailty in very elderly people. N Engl J Med 1994;330: 1769–75.
50. Binder EF, Schechtman KB, Ehsani AA, et al. Effects of exercise training on frailty in community-dwelling older adults: results of a randomized, controlled trial. J Am Geriatr Soc 2008;50:1921–8.
51. Strasser B, Volaklis K, Fuchs D, et al. Role of dietary protein and muscular fitness on longevity and aging. Aging Dis 2018;9:119–32.
52. Malafarina V, Uriz-Otano F, Iniesta R, et al. Sarcopenia in the elderly: diagnosis, pathophysiology and treatment. Maturitas 2012;2:109–14.
53. Wall BT, van Loon LJ. Nutritional strategies to attenuate muscle disuse atrophy. Nutr Rev 2013;71:195–208.

54. Chen HT, Chung YC, Chen YJ, et al. Effects of difference types of exercise on body composition, muscle strength, and IGF-1 in the elderly with sarcopenic obesity. J Am Geriatr Soc 2017;65:827–32.
55. Legrand D, Vaes B, Mathei C, et al. Muscle strength and physical performance as predictors of mortality, hospitalization and disability in the oldest old. J Am Geriatr Soc 2004;62:1030–8.
56. Newman AB, Kupelian V, Visser M, et al. Strength, but no muscle mass, is associated with mortality in the health, aging and body composition study cohort. J Gerontol A Biol Sci Med Sci 2006;61:72–7.
57. Ades PA, Savage P, Cress ME, et al. Resistance training on physical performance in disabled older female cardiac patients. Med Sci Sports Exerc 2003;92: 1265–70.
58. Fiatarone MA, Marks EC, Ryan ND, et al. High-intensity strength training in nonagenarians: effect on skeletal muscle. JAMA 1990;263:3029–34.
59. Mental Health America. Depression in older adults: more facts. Mental Health America; 2018. ©Copyright Mental Health America. Available at: http://www.mentalhealthamerica.net/conditions/depression-older-adults-more-facts. Accessed February 10, 2019.
60. Rutledge T, Reis VA, Linke SE, et al. Depression in heart failure: a meta-analytic review of prevalence, intervention effects and associations with clinical outcomes. J Am Coll Cardiol 2006;48:1527–37.
61. Milani RV, Lavie CJ. Impact of cardiac rehabilitation on depression and its associated mortality. Am J Med 2007;120:799–806.
62. Sherwood A, Blumenthal JA, Trivedi R, et al. Relationship of depression to death or hospitalization in patients with heart failure. Arch Intern Med 2007;167:367–73.
63. Callahan CM, Kroenke K, Counsell SR, et al. Treatment of depression improves physical functioning in older adults. J Am Geriatr Soc 2005;53:367–73.
64. Milani RV, Lavie CJ, Mehra MR, et al. Impact of exercise training and depression on survival in heart failure due to coronary heart disease. Am J Cardiol 2011; 107:64–8.
65. Gellis ZD, Kang-Yi C. Meta-analysis of the effect of cardiac rehabilitation interventions on depression outcomes in adults 64 years of age and older. AM J Cardiol 2012;110:1219–24.
66. Bandura A. Self-efficacy: toward a unifying theory of behavioral change. Psychol Rev 1977;84:191–215.
67. Elavsky S, McAuley E, Motl RW, et al. Physical activity enhances long-term quality of life in older adults: efficacy, esteem, and affective influences. Ann Behav Med 2005;30:138–45.
68. McAuley E, Blissmer B, Katula J, et al. Physical activity, self-esteem, and self-efficacy relationships in older adults: a randomized controlled trial. Ann Behav Med 2000;22:131–9.
69. Rejeski WJ, King AC, Katula JA, et al. Physical activity in prefrail older adults: confidence and satisfaction related to physical function. J Gerontol B Psychol Sci Soc Sci 2015;63:P19–26.
70. Tomaka J, Thompson S, Palacios R. The relation of social isolation, loneliness, and social support to disease outcomes among the elderly. J Aging Health 2006;18:359–84.
71. Cacioppo JT, Hawkley LC, Norman GJ, et al. Social isolation. Ann N Y Acad Sci 2011;1231:17–22.
72. Landeiro F, Barrows P, Musson EN, et al. Reducing social isolation and loneliness in older people: a systematic review protocol. BMJ Open 2017;7:e013778.

73. Dolansky MA, Moore SM, Visovsky C. Older adults' views of cardiac rehabilitation program: is it time to reinvent? J Gerontol Nurs 2006;32:37–44.
74. Masnoon N, Shakib S, Kalisch-Ellett L, et al. What is polypharmacy? A systematic review of definitions. BMC Geriatr 2017;17:230–9.
75. Morin L, Johnell K, Laroche ML, et al. The epidemioloy of polypharmacy in older adults: register-based prospective cohort study. Clin Epidemiol 2018;10:289–98.
76. Clarke CL, Witham MD. The effects of medication on activity and rehabilitation of older people – opportunities and risks. Rehabilitation Process and Outcome 2017;6:1–7.
77. Cramer JA, Benedict A, Muszbek N, et al. The significance of compliance and persistence in the treatment of diabetes, hypertension and dyslipidemia: a review. Int J Clin Pract 2008;62:76–87.
78. Doll J, Hellkamp A, Thomas L, et al. Effectiveness of cardiac rehabilitation among older patients after acute myocardial infarction. Am Heart J 2015;170:855–64.
79. Suaya JA, Shepard DS, Normand SLT, et al. Use of cardiac rehabilitation by Medicare beneficiaries after myocardial infarction or coronary bypass surgery. Circulation 2007;116:1653–62.
80. Servey JT, Stephens M. Cardiac rehabilitation: improving function and reducing risk. Am Fam Physician 2016;94:37–43.
81. Ghisi GLM, Polyzotis P, Oh P, et al. Physician factors affecting cardiac rehabilitation referral and patient enrollment: a systematic review. Clin Cardiol 2013;36:323–35.
82. Grace SL, Gravely-Witte S, Brual J, et al. Contribution of patient and physician factors to cardiac rehabilitation enrollment: a prospective multilevel study. Eur J Cardiovasc Prev Rehabil 2008;15:548–56.
83. Yusef S, Furberg CD. Are we biased in our approach to treating elderly patietns with heart disease? Am J Cardiol 1991;68:843–7.
84. Thompson PD, Franklin BA, Balady GJ, et al. Exercise and acute cardiovascular events placing the risks into perspective: a scientific statement from the American Heart Association Council on Nutrition, Physical Activity and Metabolism and the Council on Clinical Cardiology. Circulation 2007;115:2358–68.
85. Miiani RV, Lavie CJ, Spiva H. Limitations of estimating metabolic equivalents in exercise assessment in patients with coronary artery disease. Am J Cardiol 1995;75:940–2.
86. Kim S, Lockhart T. Effects of 8 weeks of balance or weight training for the independently living elderly on the outcomes of induced slips. Int J Rehabil Res 2010;33:49–55.
87. King KM, Humen DP, Smith HL, et al. Predicting and explaining cardiac rehabilitation attendance. Can J Cardiol 2001;17:291–6.
88. Grace SL, Shanmugasegaram S, Gravely-Witte S, et al. Barriers to cardiac rehabilitation: does age make a difference? J Cardiopulm Rehabil Prev 2009;29:183–7.
89. Marchionni N, Fattirolli F, Furnagalli S, et al. Improved exercise tolerance and quality of life with cardiac rehabilitation of older patients after myocardial infarction. Results of a randomized, controlled trial. Circulation 2003;107:2201–6.

Tailoring Assessments and Prescription in Cardiac Rehabilitation for Older Adults

The Relevance of Geriatric Domains

Maria Antoinette Fiatarone Singh, MD, FRACP[a,b,*]

KEYWORDS

• Sarcopenia • Polypharmacy • Cognitive impairment • Depression
• Resistance training • Mobility impairment

KEY POINTS

- Cardiac rehabilitation in older adults can address remediable comorbidities contributing to cardiovascular morbidity and mortality.
- Cardiovascular assessment in older adults is complemented by evaluation of body composition, functional status, mobility and falls risk, musculoskeletal impairments/capacity, neuropsychological function, nutritional status, and polypharmacy.
- Understanding the interactions of exercise, medications, and nutritional intake/status is critical to safe and effective exercise prescription, monitoring, and adaptation.
- Frailty and sarcopenia are not contraindications to robust anabolic exercise prescription in cardiac rehabilitation but conversely represent the most important reasons to promote it.

INTRODUCTION

Exercise-related therapeutic objectives for middle-aged and older adults have traditionally focused on physical activities designed to improve cardiorespiratory fitness and thus potentially prolong life[1] as well as to prevent and treat cardiovascular and other chronic diseases. Cardiac rehabilitation is one of the most well-established models of utilizing exercise as medicine, with robust evidence that it improves survival and disease expression and progression in this cohort.[2,3] It is increasingly recognized, however, that older adults with cardiovascular diseases (CVDs) also can benefit

Disclosure Statement: The author has nothing to disclose.
[a] Faculty of Medicine and Health, Sydney Medical School, University of Sydney, Sydney, Australia; [b] Hebrew SeniorLife, Hinda and Arthur Marcus Institute for Aging Research, Boston, MA, USA
* University of Sydney, Cumberland Campus, Room K 221, 75 East Street, Lidcombe, New South Wales 2041, Australia.
E-mail address: maria.fiataronesingh@sydney.edu.au

Clin Geriatr Med 35 (2019) 423–443
https://doi.org/10.1016/j.cger.2019.07.013
geriatric.theclinics.com

substantially from physical activities designed to maintain or improve functional independence[4] by addressing age-related changes in physiology and syndromes related to disuse and neuropsychological function, thus enhancing quality of life.[5] The poor referral to, and uptake of, the exercise component of cardiac rehabilitation programs in older adults globally[6] may reflect an inaccurate understanding of the perceived risks and potential benefits of exercise, even in the oldest old, among both patients and health care professionals. Therefore, the approach to cardiac rehabilitation in older adults, and its successful adoption by this cohort, is integrally linked to a greater understanding of the inter-relatedness of all of these domains in the context of cardiometabolic disease as well as better dissemination of the evidence about safety gathered from both clinical trials and epidemiologic data.

The specific physical fitness components that optimize physical function as individuals age include muscle strength and power, cardiovascular and muscular endurance, balance, and, to a lesser extent, flexibility.[7,8] The prevalent problems of mobility impairment, falls, arthritis, osteoporotic fractures, and functional status are clearly related in part to sarcopenia (loss of muscle strength, mass, and function), a feature of aging that is amenable to intervention even in the frailest elders.[9] Additionally, the metabolic benefits of retention and activation of muscle mass are now increasingly recognized as an important facet of the epidemic of age and obesity-related insulin resistance and type 2 diabetes mellitus,[10,11] which are some of the most important risk factors and comorbidities relevant to CVD and rehabilitation.[12]

Current general US guidelines for general fitness[13] or physical activity for older adults[7,8] are essentially similar to cardiac rehabilitation exercise guidelines,[14,15] although there is variable emphasis on resistance exercise across the rehabilitation guidelines from the United States, Europe, and Australia. The general physical activity guidelines have been examined for their relationship to mortality in the National Health Interview Survey cohort of 242,397 adults,[16] demonstrating that adherence to the aerobic or combined aerobic and strength training guidelines significantly reduced mortality, with the greatest benefits in older adults with at least 1 chronic condition, in whom adherence reduced adjusted mortality risk by 48%. Other large longitudinal studies now provide epidemiologic evidence that specific engagement in resistance/strength training substantially reduces mortality risk independently of any aerobic activity.[17] Unfortunately, US survey and other data indicate that women in general (who are at higher risk of sarcopenia-related morbidity) report lower than average adult participation levels, particularly for strength training (11% vs 16%).[18] Despite the evidence for more than 3 decades on its safety and efficacy in even frail elders,[19,20] however, the engagement rate for resistance exercise is even lower among the old (6% at ages 65–74) and the very old (4% above age 75). Individuals in this latter age group, particularly over the age of 85, are primarily women, making an understanding of the risks and benefits of exercise in this population a priority.[21] The statistics in cardiac rehabilitation settings are similar, with a disproportionately higher uptake among younger men compared with older men and women. Thus, the group of patients with CVD who are least likely to be referred for cardiac rehabilitation (older adults) are in fact harmed by this practice of nonreferral, because not exercising substantially increases their risk of mortality from cardiovascular and other causes.

ASSESSMENT OF THE OLDER ADULT FOR CARDIAC REHABILITATION

Most older adults, despite the presence of chronic diseases and disabilities, are able to undertake and benefit from an exercise prescription that is tailored to their physiologic capacities, comorbidities, and neuropsychological and behavioral needs. The relatively few permanent exclusions to any structured exercise generally are severe irreversible conditions that are obvious exclusions because of the nature of the specific exercise prescription under consideration or the risk the exercise would impose on the health status of the individual (**Box 1**). There may be some forms of exercise that even permanently bed-bound patients, or those with severe behavioral problems, may engage in, but they are not able to participate in the usual aerobic, resistive, or balance exercises prescribed in cardiac rehabilitation. For some older adults, such as those with critical aortic stenosis, cardiac or peripheral vascular ischemia at rest, or an enlarging aortic aneurysm or known cerebral aneurysm (when surgery is not an option due to other medical considerations or very advanced age), any exercise that significantly elevates cardiac workload or blood pressure is considered high risk and, therefore, not recommended.[10,21] It is anticipated that relatively few older adults would be excluded from cardiac rehabilitation programs based on items in this list outside of those with severe forms of dementia or terminal illness.

Importantly, a vast majority of chronic illnesses, including those in **Box 2**, are indications for, rather than contraindications to, regular exercise.[6] For example, if a patient with osteoporosis, chronic renal failure, osteoarthritis, and depression is not exercising, the medical management can be seen as suboptimal, because regular exercise is in fact additive to the benefits of usual medical care in these and most other chronic conditions. Therefore, screening a patient for exercise should be seen as an opportunity to "screen in" those sedentary adults who have exercise-responsive diseases, rather than primarily a task of "screening out" those few adults with conditions that absolutely preclude exercise of any kind. This is particularly important for conditions for which there either is no medical treatment (eg, sarcopenia, frailty, falls risk, and dementia) or for which pharmacologic treatment is less effective or more has a lower risk:benefit ratio than exercise (eg, antidepressants, insomniacs, and anxiolytics).[22,23]

SPECIFIC SCREENING AND ASSESSMENT RECOMMENDATIONS FOR OLDER ADULTS BEFORE CARDIAC REHABILITATION

Although exercise is safe for the vast majority of older adults, using it like a medication for cardiovascular morbidity and mortality requires knowledge about a wide array of conditions prevalent in this cohort, which may determine exactly how it is implemented, choices of specific modalities or intensities of exercise, and the need to assess impact on potential areas of both risk and benefit. The domains that are relevant extend far beyond cardiovascular/pulmonary disease, the most common focus of cardiac rehabilitation programs, and include assessments of frailty, sarcopenia, nutrition,

Box 1
Screening older adults for a cardiac rehabilitation exercise program: permanent exclusions to exercise prescription

STOP! Permanent exclusion

If any conditions below apply, the individual is ineligible for any progressive exercise prescription at this time other than simple range of motion or incidental ambulation:

- End-stage, progressive congestive heart failure or respiratory failure/hypoxemia
- Permanent bed-bound status/contractures
- Severe cognitive impairment or behavioral disturbance precluding mimicking movements or understanding instructions
- Untreated severe aortic stenosis
- Rapidly terminal illness

STOP, don't initiate exercise.

Box 2
Screening older adults for a cardiac rehabilitation exercise program: temporary exclusions requiring evaluation prior to initiating or continuing exercise

WAIT! Temporary exclusion

- Active suicidality/attempt or suicidal ideation
- Acute change in mental status, confusion or delirium, psychosis
- Balance and gait disorder, recurrent falls/injuries
- Cerebral hemorrhage within the past 1 month to 2 months
- Chronic obstructive pulmonary disease or asthma exacerbation until cleared
- Exacerbation of chronic inflammatory musculoskeletal disease or osteoarthritis
- Eye surgery within the past 2 weeks
- Fracture/surgery in healing stage, less than 6 weeks postoperative, until cleared
- Hernia, symptomatic (abdominal or inguinal) or significant bleeding hemorrhoids
- Myocardial infarction or cardiac surgery until cleared by cardiologist
- New significant neurologic sign or symptom, central or peripheral
- Orthostatic hypotension, symptomatic
- Proliferative diabetic retinopathy or severe nonproliferative retinopathy, until cleared
- Pulmonary embolism or deep venous thrombosis within 3 months
- Seizure disorder uncontrolled or recent, until cleared
- Soft tissue injury until healed
- Systemic infection, sepsis, fever
- Uncontrolled blood pressure (>160/100 mm Hg)
- Uncontrolled diabetes mellitus (fasting blood sugar >200 mg/dL)
- Uncontrolled malignant cardiac arrhythmia (ventricular tachycardia, complete heart block, atrial flutter, symptomatic bradycardia) until controlled
- Unstable angina (at rest or crescendo pattern, new ischemic electrocardiogram changes)
- Visual disturbance, sudden or rapidly progressive

WAIT, need to hold exercise temporarily.

psychological well-being, cognition, and special senses, among others. The well-validated tools suggested in **Table 1** are important for both the safety and efficacy of cardiac rehabilitation programs in older adults. It is likely that the low rates of referral and adoption in this cohort would be improved if a better integration of these primary tools of geriatric assessment were incorporated into cardiac rehabilitation assessment protocols. They also assist with prioritization and choice of cardiac rehabilitation modalities so that a prescription with the broadest range of benefits and safety is selected. For example, although both aerobic and resistance training improve cardiovascular risk profile,[24] as well as having independent contributions to cardiovascular, cancer, or overall mortality,[17] resistance training would be recommended as the initial exercise approach to an older patient with sarcopenia and high falls risk as well as CVD.[24]

The usual assessment for cardiovascular and pulmonary function/disease stability is similar to the considerations required in younger cohorts, but it is far more likely that older adults have multiple cardiovascular comorbidities influencing cardiac rehabilitation treatment. In addition, there are many issues in other domains that may not appear commonly among younger patients but may become the primary determinant of what kinds of programming can and should be implemented. Areas of particular importance are musculoskeletal conditions (**Table 2**), neuropsychological function, and other geriatric syndromes/conditions, such as hemorrhoids, hernias, falls, incontinence, loss of special senses, cognitive impairment, polypharmacy, and frailty. None of these conditions or syndromes preclude exercise but they do influence how likely it is that adoption and adherence will be optimal, what specific modalities of exercise are offered, what co-interventions are needed, and how progression and adverse events should be monitored over time, as discussed later.

Table 1
Pre-exercise assessments to assess treatable risk factors for mobility impairment and falls

Domain of Assessment	Validated Tools and Protocols in Older Adults
Frailty	Fatigue, resistance, ambulation, illnesses, and loss of weight (FRAIL) scale[51] Fried index[52]
Functional mobility	Short Physical Performance Battery[53,54] Maximal and habitual gait speed 6-minute walk test[29] 400-m walk test[55]
Dynamic balance	Tandem walk time, errors
Muscle function	Chair stand time One-repetition maximum testing Stair climb power Isometric handgrip, knee extensor, hip abductor strength
Autonomic nervous system dysfunction	Resting tachycardia Orthostatic hypotension Postprandial hypotension Nocturnal reverse dipping or nondipping pattern on ambulatory blood pressure monitoring
Fear of falling	Falls Efficacy Scale[56] Falls Efficacy Scale–International[57]
Vision	Visual acuity Contrast sensitivity Use of multifocal lenses Cataracts Macular degeneration
Polypharmacy	Complete inventory of prescribed, over-the-counter, and prn medications, nutraceuticals, and supplements Beers criteria, STOPP/START criteria[49] Deprescribing pathways
Peripheral neuropathy	Light touch, vibration, proprioception, pain sensation
Sarcopenia	SARC-F[58] Midarm and calf circumferences Dual-energy x-ray absorptiometry scan–appendicular skeletal muscle mass estimates Bioelectrical impedance analysis fat-free mass or skeletal muscle mass index estimates
Nutritional status	Mini-nutritional Assessment[59] Body mass index Waist circumference Food frequency questionnaires; food diary Serum albumin, lymphocyte count, 25-OH vitamin D level
Cognition	Montreal Cognitive Assessment[60] Mini-mental State Exam[61,62] Dual-tasking (simultaneous cognitive and physical task performance)
Depression	Geriatric Depression Scale[63] Patient Health Questionnaire-9[64] *Diagnostic and Statistical Manual of Mental Disorders* (Fifth Edition) depression checklist[65]
Podiatric abnormalities	Fallen arches Ankle instability Ulcerations Arthritis
Environmental hazards	Home safety checklist Review of ambulatory assistive device use

Table 2
Approach to musculoskeletal conditions during exercise prescription and implementation

Condition/Finding	Exercise-Related Recommendations
Achilles tendonitis	• Watch for heel pain, swelling, tenderness, and stiffness • Check for previous Achilles tendonitis • No exercise without adequate footwear or ankle support if prescribed • Ensure hamstring and calf stretching is completed after exercise sessions • Reduce range of motion if pain is present • Avoid high-risk falls situations
Ankle osteoarthritis Ankle sprain history	• Watch for ankle pain, swelling, or stiffness • Ankle instability, especially in single-leg stance • No exercise without adequate footwear or support if needed • Limit exercise to onset of significant pain • If pain is present, add seated rest between exercises, to limit force through the ankle • Standing exercises may be modified to be seated • Provide additional support during unilateral exercise and machine mount/dismount
Back pain	• Watch for lower back pain, aching, reduced range of motion, and loss of function • Check for pain at rest or with unloaded exercise • Ensure the full back support for all seated exercises • For unilateral exercises, provide additional upper limb support and avoid truncal rotation to aid stability • Include core/postural control muscle training • If pain is still present, hip abduction may be performed seated with back support
Baker's cyst	• Watch for swelling, pain, aching, or pressure at the popliteal fossa • Restriction in knee flexion range of motion needed • Leg press: adjust seat position further back from the foot plates to reduce the angle at the hip so as to not aggravate or apply pressure on the back of the knee joint • Knee extension/flexion: adjust the seat position to move the back rest further forward
Carpal tunnel syndrome	• Watch that wrists are maintained in neutral position during all exercises • Affected exercises include chest press, seated row, triceps pushdown, rowing machine, stair climber, and treadmill • Use weight lifting gloves if needed • Advise use of splints at night, if already prescribed, or in daytime if severe • Watch for progression of sensory loss or atrophy of hand muscles; refer as needed
Femorotibial osteoarthritis/ varus or valgus malalignment	• Watch for knee joint pain, stiffness, poor range of motion, crepitus, swelling, and instability • Check for knee malalignment on standing • Check for pain at rest or with unloaded exercise • Cue knee-toe alignment and foot positioning for lower extremity exercises • Limit exercises to onset of significant pain • If pain on weight-bearing limits ambulation, start with resistance training and add aerobic exercise once symptoms have improved • If no pain-free arc of motion is possible, start with isometric resistance exercises

(*continued on next page*)

Table 2
(continued)

Condition/Finding	Exercise-Related Recommendations
Heel spur	• Watch for heel pain on weight-bearing or closed chain resistance exercises • No exercise without adequate footwear or insert to relieve pressure on spur • Limit exercises to onset of significant pain; refer to podiatry as needed • Perform calf stretching to alleviate tight Achilles, as required • Exercises affected: leg press and hip abduction and all weight-bearing aerobic exercises
Hip bursitis	• Question about lateral hip pain or swelling, pain lying on side at night over greater trochanter • Check for pain at rest or with unloaded exercise before proceeding • Limit exercises range of motion to onset of significant pain • Standing hip abduction may be modified to be performed seated or may not be tolerable • If pain severe and not responsive to conservative treatment and topical analgesics consider possibility of gluteus medius tear/ tendinosis, refer as needed
Hip osteoarthritis, hip replacement	• Question regarding hip joint stiffness in the morning, when sitting for extended periods, walking • Pain in groin on flexion/abduction/external rotation and limited internal rotation on testing may be present; check for pain at rest or with unloaded exercise • Cue knee-toe alignment and foot positioning for each repetition • Limit exercises and range of motion to onset of significant pain • If extended seated travel to venue, perform light warm-up prior to exercise • Affected exercises: leg press and hip abduction, stair climbing, and treadmill walking • If total hip replacement, avoid extreme internal rotation, abduction, and flexion
Lateral epicondylitis	• Watch for pain on the outside of the elbow when gripping or extending elbow • Extensor tendon is tender to touch near olecranon • Alter the hand grip to place force through the palm of the hand and reduce finger flexion • If pain persists, modify the movement or eliminate the exercise • Triceps pushdown: use standing triceps pulldown with a straight bar on a cable machine; the straight bar can allow a flat, pronated hand position • Exercises affected: triceps pushdown, chest press, and seated row
Medial meniscal tear/degeneration	• Watch for localized medial knee pain with movement or after prolonged sitting, localized swelling, locking, giving way, and falls • May or may not be a history of acute event, such as torsion or fall prior to symptoms • Check for pain at rest or with unloaded exercise and other signs of osteoarthritis • Refer if needed for persistent and severe symptoms; no exercise until diagnosis confirmed if acute symptoms do not resolve • Limit range of motion to the pain-free range of motion, isometric initially if needed when exercise is started/resumed • If extended travel to training session, perform light warm up prior to exercise

(*continued on next page*)

Table 2
(*continued*)

Condition/Finding	Exercise-Related Recommendations
Neck osteoarthritis	• Watch for neck stiffness, pain, reduced range of motion, and headaches • Neck support should be used on all machines where provided • All communication is face-to-face, requiring no rotational head movements • Both stretching and strengthening of neck muscles are beneficial • Sitting posture is significant contributor; avoid slouching by sitting with feet slightly off the floor and chin tucked in both at home and while using exercise machines
Osteoarthritis of hands	• Watch for pain, tenderness, reduced range of motion, stiffness, and swelling at the base of the thumb • Check for pain at rest or with unloaded exercise • Add padding to handgrip of all aerobic and resistance machines (e.g., a towel or foam) to reduce impact • Alter grip to midhand placement to change the line of force away from the thumb • Alternate upper body and lower body exercises for increased rest of hands • Affected exercises: triceps pushdown, chest press, seated row, all aerobic exercise machines
Osteoarthritis of feet	• Watch for toe stiffness, pain, reduced range of motion, of pain when walking • Check for pain at rest or with unloaded exercise • No exercise without adequate footwear • Limit exercises to onset of significant pain • Standing hip abduction may be modified to be performed seated for reduced force through the feet • Affected exercises: leg press and hip abduction, all weight-bearing aerobic exercise
Osteopenia/osteoporosis History of a minimal trauma fracture or a T score at the hip (total/trochanter/ femoral neck or Ward triangle) in osteopenic/ osteoporotic range (< -1.0) on dual-energy x-ray absorptiometry	• Check 25-OH vitamin D level, if not on vitamin D currently (or is noncompliant) • If vitamin D is <50, advise treatment with 3000 IU vitamin D/d × 3 mo, then 1000 IU vitamin D continuously. • Ask about pain over any skeletal sites during assessment and training • Resistance and balance training recommended; isolated walking exercise increases risk of osteoporotic fracture; add once strength and balance have improved • High-impact exercise (jumping/plyometrics) increases bone density but is not recommended if lower extremity or back osteoarthritis is also present
Patellofemoral pain/osteoarthritis	• Watch for patella pain in knee flexion, for example, when squatting, kneeling, walking stairs, or sitting for an extended time • Watch for knee stiffness • Check for pain at rest or with unloaded exercise • If extended travel to training session, perform light warm up prior to exercise • If pain is present, reduce the range of motion to a pain-free range of motion or isometric • Modify the movement to be unilateral; reduce the load of the affected side • Leg press: perform an isometric contraction against a static resistance, holding for 10 seconds per repetition; avoid Valsalva and breath holding • If pain is still present, perform submaximal isometric contractions

(*continued on next page*)

Table 2
(continued)

Condition/Finding	Exercise-Related Recommendations
Plantar fasciitis	• Watch for pain and stiffness in the bottom of the heel or midfoot • Pain is worse in the morning; perform exercise later in the day to reduce pain • Check for pain at rest or with unloaded exercise; monitor pain post-exercise • Perform calf stretching to alleviate tight Achilles, as required • No exercise without adequate footwear or orthotics, if needed • Exercises affected: leg press and hip abduction, all weight-bearing aerobic exercise, and balance exercises
Rotator cuff tear, tendinosis	• Watch for pain, weakness, reduced range of motion, and atrophy of shoulder girdle • If pathology not diagnosed, refer for evaluation before initiating exercise • Limit exercises to onset of significant pain, follow recommendations of surgeon or physiotherapist depending on pathology present or surgical intervention performed • Avoid overhead movements, such as latissimus dorsi pulldown and military press • Perform exercises unilaterally until resolved • Scapular retraction and depression needed for prevention of tendinosis, recovery • Avoid forward flexion and poor posture which will aggravate tendinosis/inflammation • Affected exercises: chest press, seated row, triceps pushdown, high handles on any machines • Once acute symptoms resolved, resistance exercises to strengthen all rotator cuff muscles indicated, in particular external rotation, scapular retraction and depression, and back extension
Sciatica	• Question regarding pain, paresthesia, loss of sensation, or weakness • Refer for evaluation if new or progressive neurologic signs present prior to initiating exercise • Check for pain at rest or with unloaded exercise, during straight leg raising/dorsiflexion • Ensure the full back support for all seated exercises • Perform gluteus stretching to alleviate tight piriformis, as required • Do not continue exercise after onset of sciatic symptoms during a session • Exercises affected: leg press, knee flexion, knee extension, hip abduction, and walking
Thoracic osteoporosis/ fracture Severe kyphosis	• Evaluation of risk factors for osteoporosis; check vitamin D level/ compliance • Avoid back flexion activities during household or exercise regimens • Back extension exercises indicated for prevention of future fractures • Emphasize scapular retraction/depression while seated; feet off floor to improve posture • Watch for acute onset of back pain on all exercises; rule out acute fracture if indicated • Avoid high-risk falls situations • Cue eyes forward and chin tucked for neck support • Balance exercises needed for falls prevention

MONITORING PROGRESSION IN THE EXERCISE PROGRAM

Many health outcomes seem related to the accumulated volume and/or intensity of exercise; so simply monitoring adherence to the physical activity recommendations theoretically provides evidence that the targeted benefits are occurring, and such monitoring is an important part of behavioral change theory.[25] There is even greater benefit, however, in also monitoring the actual physiologic/functional improvements from training. For example, aerobic capacity itself has an even stronger relationship to mortality than level of physical activity,[26] and an increase in muscle mass after resistance training is directly linked to improved metabolic and inflammatory profile in older adults with type 2 diabetes mellitus,[11,27] as is increase in strength with cognitive improvement after resistance training in mild cognitive impairment.[28] Documenting improvements in fitness, function, or body composition may have a reinforcing effect on long-term behavioral adaptations as well. Improved fitness/function across the multiple domains of exercise capacity may be shown, for example, by:

- Improved measurements of peak aerobic capacity
- Decreased heart rate and blood pressure response to a fixed submaximal workload
- Decreased rating of perceived exertion for a fixed submaximal workload
- Improved muscle strength, endurance, or power
- Ability to lift a submaximal load more times
- Ability to withstand postural stress or negotiate obstacles without losing balance
- Improved joint range of motion
- Improved functional mobility performance (eg, gait speed, chair stand time, stair climbing, and 6-minute walk distance).

Assessing Overall Exercise Capacity and Adaptation to Aerobic and Resistance Training in Cardiac Rehabilitation

One of the most common ways to measure improvement in rehabilitation settings that requires minimal equipment is the 6-minute walk test.[29] This test has been used as an index of rehabilitation in cardiac, pulmonary, and other patients, and is known to predict outcomes and improve with effective interventions. With training, pulse and blood pressure at 6 minutes should decrease and distance covered should increase by at least 25 m to 50 m after either aerobic or resistance training. Alternatives to the 6-minute walk are walking a fixed distance (eg, 400 m) climbing multiple flights of stairs as rapidly as possible, or stepping up and down a single step for several minutes, followed by the measurements discussed previously. Availability of stairs and the potential for musculoskeletal injury due to balance, hip and knee arthritis, or vision problems make rapid stepping tests less desirable in the older adult, however. The 6-minute walk test reflects not only aerobic capacity but also contributions from factors, such as pulmonary function, orthostasis, gait stability, muscle strength, pain, body composition, osteoarthritis, vision, cognition, depression, fear of falling, and self-efficacy, among others, and thus is a good overall index of exercise capacity (not simply aerobic capacity) and has direct clinical relevance to ambulatory function in daily life.[30]

In order to continue to adapt to aerobic exercise, increases in intensity of training or needed. In older adults, this can be difficult when gait and balance disorders or osteoarthritis preclude typical progression to more intensive activities, such as jogging or running. Examples of feasible ways of increasing aerobic intensity without increasing impact on joints with arthritic changes or osteoporotic fragility fracture risk include:

- Walking—add small weights around wrists, swing arms; use race walking style; add inclines, hills, or stairs; carry weighted backpack or waist belt; push a wheelchair or stroller (with someone in it)
- Cycling—increase pedaling speed, increase resistance to pedals, add hills
- Water activities—use arms and legs in strokes, add resistive equipment for water, increase pace
- Tennis—convert from doubles to singles game
- Golf—carry clubs, eliminate golf cart
- Dance—increase pace of movements, add more arm and leg movements.

Assessing Adaptation to Resistance Training

The primary goal of resistance training is to increase muscle strength, and this can only occur if the load is uncustomary/novel and is progressively increased so as to remain uncustomary.[13] This is why unless someone is nonambulatory, simply opposing the force of gravity by walking, even at a brisk pace, is not a stimulus for robust muscle adaptation in terms of higher force-generating capacity. Thus, measurement of strength over time serves as an excellent index that the exercise protocol used in fact conforms to these well-known principles. If maximal strength itself cannot be measured due to lack of equipment or is not considered feasible in a particular older adult, there is an option that is commonly used to rate effort during a lift, using a scale of perceived exertion, such as the Borg Rating of Perceived Exertion scale.[31] On this scale, from 6 to 20, a rating of 15 to 18 (hard to very hard) is equivalent to 70% to 80% of maximum lifting capacity in studies conducted in young and older adults and, therefore, is an appropriate training goal for a robust and safe resistance training prescription.[10,21] In addition, functional tests that may be used as an index of muscle strength and power include multiple chair stand time and stair climb time, although lower extremity arthritis or poor balance may distort the relationship between muscle capacity and performance on these tests. Although grip strength often is used as a general index of muscle function or nutritional status in older adults in epidemiologic studies and does predict mortality, morbidity, and disability,[32,33] measures of lower extremity muscle strength and power, if obtainable, are preferred and are far more directly applicable to mobility impairment, fall risk, and specific exercise recommendations for relevant muscle groups of the hip, knee, and ankle.[4,34]

The safety of resistance training and strength testing in older adults with cardiometabolic and other diseases is well established. In the largest series of maximum strength tests reported, in 26,000 individuals undergoing testing, not a single cardiovascular event occurred.[35] Additionally, the literature suggests a reduction in ischemic signs and symptoms after progressive resistance training (PRT) in cardiac patients, attesting to the safety of this form of exercise even in individuals with heart disease.[24] Techniques that attenuate hemodynamic excursions in response to weight lifting, and thereby maximize safety in a cardiac rehabilitation setting, are the same principles used in all healthy and clinical cohorts of all ages for safety and continuous progression and include:

- Keeping relative intensity of load lifted no greater than 80% to 85% of maximal measured strength for each exercise (15–18 on the Borg Rating of Perceived Exertion scale)
- Avoiding prolonged static contractions (more than 10 seconds)
- Avoiding Valsalva maneuver/breath holding during lifts: breathe out during concentric phase and then breathe in slowly during eccentric phase

- Keeping number of repetitions in a set to 8 to 10 only, then resting
- Using rest intervals of 1 second to 2 seconds between repetitions and 1 minute to 2 minutes between sets; taking an additional breath in and out during the rest interval between repetitions if needed
- Not allowing overfatigue of muscles (performing a set "to failure")
- Using perfect form; not allowing use of accessory muscles to complete a lift
- Sitting after leg exercise for a few seconds before standing to go to the next exercise

Assessing and Improving Balance

Although not generally conceptualized as part of cardiac rehabilitation, many conditions in older adults require balance training before aerobic exercise can be adequately undertaken in ways that are both robust enough to improve cardiovascular outcomes and safe. Although beyond the scope of this article, in general the principles of balance training that are most effective are:

- Narrowing the base of support
- Perturbation of ground support
- Decrease in proprioceptive sensation
- Diminished or misleading visual inputs
- Movement of the center of mass of the body away from the vertical or stationary position
- Dual tasking: addition of a cognitive distractor or secondary physical task while practicing balance task.

Balance training must be challenging to decrease fall risk[36]; therefore, the general approach is to practice the most difficult posture or movement without falling in a safe environment (eg, standing on 1 leg without hand support) and then moving to the next harder level (eg, closing eyes) as soon as the exercise level is mastered. This is essentially the same principle that is applied to PRT is—as soon as a load no longer feels "hard" to lift on the Borg scale, it should be increased to ensure continued adaptation.

Balance training does not generally result in increased strength or aerobic capacity by itself, whereas resistance training in some cases may improve balance.[37] There may be some maintenance of muscle strength, however, from the isometric contractions that occur during many of the balance-enhancing and 1-legged postures and the bent knee stance during tai chi.[38] In addition, to the extent that balance training results in increased overall physical activity and mobility, these other activities may lead to improvements in strength and endurance. Generally, mobility impairment and falls risk mandate prescription of both balance and strength training, not either in isolation, whereas simple walking programs have not been show to enhance falls prevention outcomes[39] and in fact increase the rate of injurious falls and fractures in osteoporotic women.[40]

There might be exacerbation of preexisting arthritic pain or inflammation of the knee during prolonged 1-legged standing or tai chi or yoga postures requiring a semi-crouched stance. These positions may have to be adapted or avoided entirely in those with significant weight-bearing pain in the joint. Once quadriceps muscle strength improves with appropriate resistive exercises (discussed previously), however, these kinds of movements may be tolerable. Impaired flexibility also may limit some tai chi or yoga postures initially and may lead to injury if range of motion is forced in the beginning. Gradual progression over time in the complexity of postures should prevent most injuries to soft tissues.

CHOOSING THE SPECIFIC EXERCISE PRESCRIPTION IN OLDER ADULTS IN CARDIAC REHABILITATION

It is likely that after initial screening, many barriers and difficulties with adherence will be identified in the typically sedentary older individual with cardiometabolic disease. Therefore, it becomes important to know how to deliver the prescription in logical stages that are palatable and feasible and have some likelihood of successful implementation. Current position stands and consensus guidelines for physical activity in older adults[7,8,41] generally recommend a multimodal exercise prescription, including aerobic, strengthening, balance, and flexibility training, via a combination of structured and incidental (lifestyle integrated) activities. It is usually best to start, however, with only 1 mode of exercise and let the older adult get used to the new routine of exercise before adding other components, or optimal adherence and adaptation may be compromised.[42] This approach obviously requires attention to risk factors, medical history, and physical examination findings as well as personal preferences, in order to prioritize prescriptive elements, and is different for each individual. There are a few generalizations, however, that can be made:

- If significant deficits in muscle strength or balance are identified, these should be addressed prior to the initiation of aerobic training. Prescribing progressive aerobic training in the absence of sufficient balance or strength is likely to result in knee pain, fear of falling, falls, and limited ability to progress aerobically and is not recommended. Attempting to ambulate those who cannot lift their body weight out of a chair or maintain standing balance is likely to fail.
- Paying attention to the physiologic determinants of transfer ability and ambulation, and targeting these specifically with the appropriate exercise prescription when reversible deficits are uncovered, is most likely to succeed.
- In some cases, a chronic health condition may benefit equally from resistance or aerobic training (as in the treatment of depression for example[23]), but the decision is made based on ability to tolerate one form of exercise over another. Severe osteoarthritis of the knee, recurrent falls, and a low threshold for ischemia may make resistance training safer than aerobic training as an antidepressant treatment in this case, for example.
- Prioritization requires careful consideration of the risks and benefits of each mode of activity as well as the current health status and physical fitness level.
- Patient preference for group versus individual exercise, structured versus lifestyle physical activity, level of supervision desired, and attraction or aversion to specific modalities of exercise must be considered to optimize behavioral change and long-term adherence.

MONITORING THE RISKS OF EXERCISE

The major potential categories of risk related to exercise are listed in **Table 3**. Most of these adverse events are preventable with attention to the underlying medical conditions present, appropriate choices regarding the modality of exercise used, avoiding exercise during extreme environmental conditions, wearing proper footwear and clothing, and minimizing or avoiding exercise during acute illness or in the presence of new, undefined symptoms. Most fluid balance problems can be handled by exercising in reasonable temperature and humidity only and drinking extra fluid on exercise days.

All older adults should have yearly ophthalmologic examinations for glaucoma and retinal changes, and the initiation of an exercise regimen is a good time to reinforce

Table 3
The risks of exercise in older adults

Musculoskeletal	Cardiovascular/pulmonary	Metabolic/systemic
• Falls, soft tissue injury, hemorrhage	• Aortic stenosis symptoms • Arrhythmias, tachycardia	• Confusion • Dehydration
• Foot ulceration or laceration	• Cardiac failure decompensation • Claudication • Dyspnea, bronchospasm	• Electrolyte imbalance
• Fracture, osteoporotic or traumatic	• Hypertension	• Energy imbalance, weight loss • Fatigue
• Hemorrhoids[a]	• Hypotension	• Heat stroke
• Hernia[a]	• Ischemia	• Hyperglycemia
• Joint or bursa inflammation, exacerbation of arthritis	• Pulmonary/cerebral embolism from preexisting thrombosis	• Hypoglycemia
• Ligament or tendon strain or rupture	• Retinal hemorrhage or detachment, lens detachment	• Hypothermia
• Muscle soreness or tear • Podiatric problem exacerbation; heel spur, plantar fasciitis, callouses, etc.	• Ruptured cerebral, aortic, or other aneurysm • Stroke, transient ischemic attack	• Seizures
• Stress incontinence	• Syncope or presyncope	

[a] Primarily associated with increased intra-abdominal pressure during resistive exercise but may occur if Valsalva maneuver occurs during aerobic activities.

this preventive health measure, particularly in those with hypertension or diabetes. Retinopathy is not a contraindication to exercise, except in cases of proliferative retinopathy or an acute bleed or retinal tear/detachment until stabilized. If someone has had recent ophthalmologic surgery, exercise is contraindicated for several weeks to avoid raising intraocular pressure, and the exact recommendations should be obtained from the ophthalmologist in these cases.

Metabolic complications are rare unless diabetes is out of control at the time exercise is initiated or dehydration, fever, or acute illnesses are present. The improvement in insulin sensitivity at the initiation of regular exercise may require modification of insulin and oral hypoglycemic medications to prevent hypoglycemia. Exercising in the 1 hour to 2 hours after meals should both prevent hypoglycemia and minimize the postprandial rise in serum glucose, which is an independent risk factor for cardiovascular events, even in those without diabetes.[43] This cardiovascular toxicity is mediated by oxidant stress, which triggers inflammation, endothelial dysfunction, hypercoagulability, sympathetic hyperactivity, and other atherogenic changes. Exercise has been shown to attenuate this postprandial dysmetabolism, which may mediate some of the cardioprotective effects of exercise.[43,44]

Cardiovascular complications are most likely if ischemic heart disease is not well controlled medically or surgically prior to exercise initiation, if warning signs are ignored, or if sudden, vigorous exercise is tried in a previously completely sedentary individual. When properly prescribed and monitored, both aerobic training and resistance training have been shown to reduce the incidence of angina and medication use in cardiac rehabilitation settings and are indicated as part of standard medical management of coronary artery disease.[21] Although claudication is a possible adverse side effect of exercise in those with peripheral vascular disease, it has been shown that aerobic exercise (even arm ergometry) significantly increases exercise tolerance in patients with peripheral vascular disease (ie, time to claudication), and resistance training has significant benefit as well.[45] Exercise has been intentionally continued for approximately 30 seconds to 90 seconds if possible after the onset of claudication in some trials (exercise to maximal pain). This remains the recommendation of the Trans-Atlantic Inter-Society consensus document on management of peripheral arterial disease,[46] although the most recent meta-analysis suggests that inducing moderate-to-severe claudication may attenuate fitness benefits in this cohort.[47] Recommendations to continue exercise in the face of peripheral ischemic pain stands in contrast to other cardiovascular symptoms or ischemia or cardiovascular instability, for which exercise should be stopped immediately if they occur.

Musculoskeletal problems are more common than any other risk of aerobic or resistive exercise, particularly in the novice exerciser or very frail adult and those with underlying joint disease (see **Table 2**). Often if significant weakness or balance impairment is present, it is best to avoid aerobic exercise altogether until strength and balance have been improved sufficiently with specific training, so as to allow safe weight-bearing exercise, such as walking. If this is not done, falls, arthritis pain, fear of falling, and muscle fatigue will be so limiting that effective aerobic training is precluded. Warming up muscles gently with slow movements prior to aerobic routines is important to avoid soft tissue injury. The most important point is to avoid high-impact activities (such as jumping, step aerobics, and jogging) in those with preexisting arthritis or weak muscles and ligaments, because this is a principle cause of sports-related injury.

Peripheral neuropathy requires careful assessment in the setting of cardiac rehabilitation and is a good example of the need to integrate care across medical specialties and consider how the effects of treatment by 1 specialist (eg, neuroleptics or opioids for pain relief) on sedation, falls, cognitive impairment, or CVD treatment goals are also relevant for that individual. Awareness of prescribing cascades and their potential for iatrogenesis in older adults is now widespread since initial descriptions in 1995,[48] and application of standardized criteria to identify and intervene in both hazardous polypharmacy or underprescribing, such as screening tool of older people's prescriptions (STOPP)"/screening tool to alert to right treatment (START) criteria,[49] hopefully will improve outcomes in complicated scenarios, such as in older individuals with cardiac disease and multiple comorbidities.[49]

Finally, an important area to consider is that of exercise-medication interactions in cardiac rehabilitation cohorts. No drugs preclude exercise engagement, but many are relevant to the ability of a patient to engage in exercise or adapt to it in some cases, or may influence how it should be implemented and monitored over time. Anticholinergic drug burden is particularly important in relation to cognitive impairment, sedation, and orthostatic hypotension, which may increase the risk of exercise or preclude adoption in older adults. Additionally, given that many older patients are prescribed 1 or more anticoagulants/platelet inhibitors for both cardiovascular and musculoskeletal conditions, the likelihood of bleeding is accentuated due to age-related changes in drug metabolism, changes in body composition influencing pharmacokinetics, nutritional deficiencies or changes over time, and risk of cerebrovascular disease and fall-related injuries. Relevant factors that increase the risk of hemorrhagic complications during exercise in this cohort include poor compliance, female gender, advanced age, polypharmacy, malnutrition, weight loss, recent surgery, liver or renal dysfunction, confusion/delirium, dementia, and elevated falls risk from any etiology. Suggestions for mitigation of this risk during cardiac rehabilitation include supervision of exercise, no prescription of aerobic exercise prior to adequate improvements in strength and balance from resistance and balance/mobility exercises, and monitoring for changes in nutritional intake or medication usage with known interactions with coagulation profile or pharmacokinetics of relevant anticoagulants/antiplatelet agents.

SUMMARY

Exercise is integral to the prevention, treatment, and rehabilitation strategies necessary for the care of the older adult with CVD. Exercise should be prescribed, as is all other medical treatment, with consideration of patient risks and benefits, knowledge of appropriate modality and dose (intensity, frequency, and volume), monitoring for drug interactions, benefits and adverse events, and utilization of the strongest possible behavioral medicine techniques known to optimize adoption and adherence. The emerging recommendations to reduce overall sitting time or length of uninterrupted sitting bouts[50] likely will not be sufficient to oppose the significant changes in physiology and function that have already occurred in this cohort who have had a cardiovascular event or surgical intervention and now require rehabilitation and lifelong promotion of healthful physical activity levels. Given the dose-response relationships demonstrated between the volume and intensity of physical activity engagement

Table 4
Overview of prescriptive elements most relevant to older adults in cardiac rehabilitation

Target	Aerobic Exercise	Resistance Exercise	Comments
Glucose control, insulin resistance	X	X	Combine if possible
Cardiovascular disease, stroke, cardiovascular disease risk profile	X	X	Combine if possible
Obesity	XX	X	Lean tissue loss occurs if dieting without PRT; high volumes needed High intensity best
Sarcopenia	Not beneficial	XXX	High intensity best Add balance training for falls risk
Osteoporosis	Not beneficial	XX	Power training offers additional benefit Add high impact if no arthritis
Osteoarthritis	X low impact	XX	Degenerative tears common; rotator cuff and knees
Retinopathy	X	X	Exercise reduces risk Not used in proliferative or acute disease
Nephropathy	X	XX	PRT needed to combat sarcopenia
Depression	X	X	Adequate dose and intensity Supervision initially
PVD, neuropathy	X low impact	X	PRT for minimally ambulatory Balance exercise for falls risk
Cognitive impairment	X	X	Supervision if advanced

Number of Xs indicate the relative magnitude of the benefits of each modality of exercise for the condition listed.

and cardiometabolic disease treatment and mortality, recommendations focusing on simply reducing sedentary behavior are insufficient as a robust treatment of CVD and many other common diseases/syndromes in this cohort, including depression, diabetes, peripheral vascular disease, sarcopenia/wasting syndromes, falls, osteoporosis, arthritis, chronic lung disease, Parkinson's disease, stroke, cognitive impairment, functional decline, and frailty, for example, By contrast, the evidence for the benefits of a targeted exercise prescription and high levels of adherence as treatment of these and many other conditions is strong. Because most patients present with more than 1 disease, an efficient prescription to optimize both safety and efficacy needs to be carefully constructed, as suggested in **Table 4**. The broad and overlapping spectrum of benefits for aerobic and resistance training are notable and important, because they can substitute for each other for some outcomes, including most manifestations of cardiometabolic disease. For some goals, however, such as sarcopenia and falls risk, it is clear that aerobic exercise is not effective, and so the most economical prescription should be sought to optimize engagement.

Finally, cardiac rehabilitation would be better defined as cardiac optimization, because withdrawal of exercise is swiftly followed by a return to the pathophysiology of aging and disuse, which largely dictates the fate and the function of such individuals. It is no more appropriate than is withdrawal of insulin in type 1 diabetes mellitus. There is no age above which physical activity ceases to have benefits across a wide range of diseases and disabilities, and CVD is a prime example of this paradigm. Insufficient physical activity and excess sedentary behavior are lethal conditions; physical activity is the antidote, and cardiologists and other health care practitioners can serve as well-educated leaders and role models in the effort to enhance functional independence, psychological well-being, and quality of life through promotion of exercise for the aged patient with CVD, whether fit or frail.

REFERENCES

1. Sui X, LaMonte MJ, Laditka JN, et al. Cardiorespiratory fitness and adiposity as mortality predictors in older adults. JAMA 2007;298(21):2507–16.
2. Anderson L, Oldridge N, Thompson DR, et al. Exercise-based cardiac rehabilitation for coronary heart disease: cochrane systematic review and meta-analysis. J Am Coll Cardiol 2016;67(1):1–12.
3. Menezes AR, Lavie CJ, Forman DE, et al. Cardiac rehabilitation in the elderly. Prog Cardiovasc Dis 2014;57(2):152–9.
4. Pahor M, Guralnik JM, Ambrosius WT, et al. Effect of structured physical activity on prevention of major mobility disability in older adults: the LIFE study randomized clinical trial. JAMA 2014;311(23):2387–96.
5. Kim DH, Rich MW. Patient-centred care of older adults with cardiovascular disease and multiple chronic conditions. Can J Cardiol 2016;32(9):1097–107.
6. Schopfer DW, Forman DE. Cardiac rehabilitation in older adults. Can J Cardiol 2016;32(9):1088–96.
7. Nelson ME, Rejeski WJ, Blair SN, et al. Physical activity and public health in older adults: recommendation from the American College of Sports Medicine and the American Heart Association. Med Sci Sports Exerc 2007;39(8):1435–45.
8. Chodzko-Zajko W, Proctor D, Fiatarone Singh M, et al. American College of Sports Medicine position stand. Exercise and physical activity for older adults. Med Sci Sports Exerc 2009;41(7):1510–30.
9. Fiatarone MA, Marks EC, Ryan ND, et al. High-intensity strength training in nonagenarians: effects on skeletal muscle. JAMA 1990;263(22):3029–34.

10. Haskell WL, Lee IM, Pate RR, et al. Physical activity and public health: updated recommendation for adults from the American College of Sports Medicine and the American Heart Association. Med Sci Sports Exerc 2007;39(8):1423–34.
11. Mavros Y, Kay S, Anderberg KA, et al. Changes in insulin resistance and HbA1c are related to exercise-mediated changes in body composition in older adults with type 2 diabetes: interim outcomes from the GREAT2DO trial. Diabetes Care 2013;36(8):2372–9.
12. McLeod JC, Stokes T, Phillips SM. Resistance exercise training as a primary countermeasure to age-related chronic disease. Front Physiol 2019;10:645.
13. Garber CE, Blissmer B, Deschenes MR, et al. American College of Sports Medicine position stand. Quantity and quality of exercise for developing and maintaining cardiorespiratory, musculoskeletal, and neuromotor fitness in apparently healthy adults: guidance for prescribing exercise. Med Sci Sports Exerc 2011; 43(7):1334–59.
14. Price KJ, Gordon BA, Bird SR, et al. A review of guidelines for cardiac rehabilitation exercise programmes: is there an international consensus? Eur J Prev Cardiol 2016;23(16):1715–33.
15. Woodruffe S, Neubeck L, Clark RA, et al. Australian Cardiovascular Health and Rehabilitation Association (ACRA) core components of cardiovascular disease secondary prevention and cardiac rehabilitation 2014. Heart Lung Circ 2015; 24(5):430–41.
16. Schoenborn CA, Stommel M. Adherence to the 2008 adult physical activity guidelines and mortality risk. Am J Prev Med 2011;40(5):514–21.
17. Stamatakis E, Lee I-M, Bennie J, et al. Does strength-promoting exercise confer unique health benefits? A pooled analysis of data on 11 population cohorts with all-cause, cancer, and cardiovascular mortality endpoints. Am J Epidemiol 2017; 187(5):1102–12.
18. Azevedo MR, Araujo CL, Reichert FF, et al. Gender differences in leisure-time physical activity. Int J Public Health 2007;52(1):8–15.
19. Fiatarone MA, O'Neill EF, Ryan ND, et al. Exercise training and nutritional supplementation for physical frailty in very elderly people. N Engl J Med 1994;330(25): 1769–75.
20. Morris J, Fiatarone M, Kiely D, et al. Nursing rehabilitation and exercise strategies in the nursing home. J Gerontol A Biol Sci Med Sci 1999;54(10):M494–500.
21. Williams MA, Haskell WL, Ades PA, et al. Resistance exercise in individuals with and without cardiovascular disease: 2007 update: a scientific statement from the American Heart Association Council on Clinical Cardiology and Council on Nutrition, Physical Activity, and Metabolism. Circulation 2007;116(5): 572–84.
22. Blumenthal JA, Babyak MA, Moore KA, et al. Effects of exercise training on older patients with major depression. JAMA Intern Med 1999;159(19):2349–56.
23. Singh NA, Stavrinos TM, Scarbek Y, et al. A randomized controlled trial of high versus low intensity weight training versus general practitioner care for clinical depression in older adults. J Gerontol A Biol Sci Med Sci 2005;60(6):768–76.
24. Hollings M, Mavros Y, Freeston J, et al. The effect of progressive resistance training on aerobic fitness and strength in adults with coronary heart disease: a systematic review and meta-analysis of randomised controlled trials. Eur J Prev Cardiol 2017;24(12):1242–59.
25. Ainsworth B, Cahalin L, Buman M, et al. The current state of physical activity assessment tools. Prog Cardiovasc Dis 2015;57(4):387–95.

26. Blair SN, Kampert JB, Kohn HW, et al. Influences of cardiovascular fitness and other precursors on cardiolvascular disease and all-cause mortality in men and women. JAMA 1996;276(3):205–10.
27. Mavros Y, Kay S, Simpson KA, et al. Reductions in C-reactive protein in older adults with type 2 diabetes are related to improvements in body composition following a randomized controlled trial of resistance training. J Cachexia Sarcopenia Muscle 2014;5(2):111–20.
28. Mavros Y, Gates N, Wilson GC, et al. Mediation of cognitive function improvements by strength gains after resistance training in older adults with mild cognitive impairment: outcomes of the study of mental and resistance training. J Am Geriatr Soc 2017;65(3):550–9.
29. Guyatt GH, Sullivan MJ, Thompson PJ, et al. The 6-minute walk: a new measure of exercise capacity in patients with chronic heart failure. Can Med Assoc J 1985; 132(8):919–23.
30. Boxer RS, Wang Z, Walsh SJ, et al. The utility of the 6-minute walk test as a measure of frailty in older adults with heart failure. Am J Geriatr Cardiol 2008; 17(1):7–12.
31. Borg G, Linderholm H. Perceived exertion and pulse rate during graded exercise in various age group. Acta Med Scand 1970;472(Suppl):194–206.
32. Yorke AM, Curtis AB, Shoemaker M, et al. Grip strength values stratified by age, gender, and chronic disease status in adults aged 50 years and older. J Geriatr Phys Ther 2015;38(3):115–21.
33. Legrand D, Vaes B, Mathei C, et al. Muscle strength and physical performance as predictors of mortality, hospitalization, and disability in the oldest old. J Am Geriatr Soc 2014;62(6):1030–8.
34. Reid KF, Fielding RA. Skeletal muscle power: a critical determinant of physical functioning in older adults. Exerc Sport Sci Rev 2012;40(1):4–12.
35. Gordon N, Kohl H, Pollock M, et al. Cardiovascular safety of maximal strength testing in healthy adults. Am J Cardiol 1995;76:851–3.
36. Sherrington C, Michaleff ZA, Fairhall N, et al. Exercise to prevent falls in older adults: an updated systematic review and meta-analysis. Br J Sports Med 2017;51(24):1750–8.
37. Orr R, Raymond J, Fiatarone Singh M. Efficacy of progressive resistance training on balance performance in older adults: a systematic review of randomized controlled trials. Sports Med 2008;38(3):1–51.
38. Tsang WW, Hui-Chan CW. Comparison of muscle torque, balance, and confidence in older tai chi and healthy adults. Med Sci Sports Exerc 2005;37(2): 280–9.
39. Sherrington C, Tiedemann A, Fairhall N, et al. Exercise to prevent falls in older adults: an updated meta-analysis and best practice recommendations. N S W Public Health Bull 2011;22(3–4):78–83.
40. Sherrington C, Fairhall NJ, Wallbank GK, et al. Exercise for preventing falls in older people living in the community. Cochrane Database Syst Rev 2019;(1):CD012424.
41. Physical activity guidelines advisory Committee report, 2008. To the secretary of health and human services. Part A: executive summary. Nutr Rev 2009;67(2): 114–20.
42. Baker MK, Atlantis E, Fiatarone Singh MA. Multi-modal exercise programs for older adults. Age Ageing 2007;36(4):375–81.

43. O'Keefe JH, Bell DS. Postprandial hyperglycemia/hyperlipidemia (postprandial dysmetabolism) is a cardiovascular risk factor. Am J Cardiol 2007;100(5): 899–904.
44. Rizvi AA. Management of diabetes in older adults. Am J Med Sci 2007;333(1): 35–47.
45. Parmenter B, Raymond J, Dinnen P, et al. A systematic review of randomized controlled trials: walking versus alternative exercise prescription as treatment for intermittent claudication. Atherosclerosis 2011;218(1):1–12.
46. Norgren L, Hiatt WR, Dormandy JA, et al. Inter-society consensus for the management of peripheral arterial disease (TASC II). J Vasc Surg 2007;45(Suppl S):S5–67.
47. Parmenter BJ, Dieberg G, Smart NA. Exercise training for management of peripheral arterial disease: a systematic review and meta-analysis. Sports Med 2015; 45(2):231–44.
48. Rochon PA, Gurwitz JH. The prescribing cascade revisited. Lancet 2017; 389(10081):1778–80.
49. O'Mahony D, O'Sullivan D, Byrne S, et al. STOPP/START criteria for potentially inappropriate prescribing in older people: version 2. Age Ageing 2015;44(2): 213–8.
50. Thorp AA, Owen N, Neuhaus M, et al. Sedentary behaviors and subsequent health outcomes in adults a systematic review of longitudinal studies, 1996-2011. Am J Prev Med 2011;41(2):207–15.
51. Morley JE, Malmstrom TK, Miller DK. A simple frailty questionnaire (FRAIL) predicts outcomes in middle aged AFRICAN Americans. J Nutr Health Aging 2012;16:601–8.
52. Bieniek J, Wilczyński K, Szewieczek J. Fried frailty phenotype assessment components as applied to geriatric inpatients. Clin Interv Aging 2016;11:453–9.
53. Guralnik JM, Simonsick E, Ferrucci L, et al. A short physical performance battery assessing lower extremity function: association with self-reported disability and prediction of mortality and nursing home admission. J Gerontol 1994;49:M85–94.
54. Pavasini R, Guralnik J, Brown JC, et al. Short physical performance battery and all-cause mortality: systematic review and meta-analysis. BMC Med 2016; 14(1):215.
55. Rolland YM, Cesari M, Miller ME, et al. Reliability of the 400-M usual-pace walk test as an assessment of mobility limitation in older adults. J Am Geriatr Soc 2004;52(6):972–6.
56. Tinetti ME, Richman D, Powell L. Falls efficacy as a measure of fear of falling. J Gerontol 1990;45(6):P239–43.
57. Delbaere K, Close JCT, Mikolaizak AS, et al. The Falls Efficacy Scale International (FES-I). A comprehensive longitudinal validation study. Age Ageing 2010;39(2): 210–6.
58. Malmstrom TK, Miller DK, Simonsick EM, et al. SARC-F: a symptom score to predict persons with sarcopenia at risk for poor functional outcomes. J Cachexia Sarcopenia Muscle 2016;7(1):28–36.
59. Guigoz Y, Vellas B, Garry PJ. Assessing the nutritional status of the elderly: the mini nutritional assessment as part of the geriatric evaluation. Nutr Rev 1996; 54(1):S59–65.
60. Nasreddine ZS, Phillips NA, Bédirian V, et al. The montreal cognitive assessment, MoCA: a brief screening tool for mild cognitive impairment. J Am Geriatr Soc 2005;53(4):695–9.

61. Folstein MF, Folstein SE, McHugh PR. "Mini-mental state": a practical method for grading the cognitive state of patients for the clinician. J Psychiatr Res 1975; 12(3):189–98.
62. Tombaugh TN, McIntyre NJ. The mini-mental state examination: a comprehensive review. J Am Geriatr Soc 1992;40(9):922–35.
63. Yesavage JA, Brink TL, Rose TL, et al. Development and validation of a geriatric depression screening scale: a preliminary report. J Psychiatr Res 1982;17(1): 37–49.
64. Levis B, Benedetti A, Thombs BD. Accuracy of Patient Health Questionnaire-9 (PHQ-9) for screening to detect major depression: individual participant data meta-analysis. BMJ 2019;365:l1476.
65. Tolentino JC, Schmidt SL. DSM-5 criteria and depression severity: implications for clinical practice. Front Psychiatry 2018;9:450.

Evaluating and Treating Frailty in Cardiac Rehabilitation

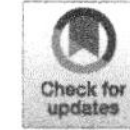

Jonathan Afilalo, MD, MSc, FRCPC

KEYWORDS

- Cardiac rehabilitation • 6-Minute walk test • Short physical performance battery
- Frail elderly

KEY POINTS

- Frailty is a multidimensional syndrome characterized by a variable combination of muscle weakness, mobility impairment, physical inactivity, social isolation, cognitive impairment, mood disturbance, and fatigue.
- Cardiac rehabilitation is a multidimensional therapy with proven beneficial effects on muscle mass and strength, mobility, habitual physical activity, social interaction, cognitive performance, mood, and vitality.
- Opportunities for measuring and treating frailty in the setting of cardiac rehabilitation are reviewed, with practical suggestions to guide clinicians and researchers in addressing frailty using validated tools.

INTRODUCTION

Frailty is a multidimensional syndrome characterized by a variable combination of muscle weakness, mobility impairment, physical inactivity, social isolation, cognitive impairment, mood disturbance, and fatigue.[1] After an acute cardiac event or procedure, frailty has negative effects on older adults' self-efficacy, quality of life (QOL), and risk of fatal and nonfatal adverse events.[2]

Cardiac rehabilitation (CR) is a multidimensional therapy with proven beneficial effects on muscle mass and strength, mobility, habitual physical activity, social interaction, cognitive performance, mood, and vitality.[3] CR has been shown to empower older adults' self-care, avoid unnecessary hospitalizations, and meaningfully improve QOL.

Disclosure: Dr. Afilalo is supported by grants from the Canadian Institutes of Health Research, the Heart and Stroke Foundation of Canada, and the Fonds de recherche du Québec en Santé.
Geriatric Cardiology Fellowship Program, Division of Cardiology & Centre for Clinical Epidemiology, McGill University, Jewish General Hospital, 3755 Cote Ste, Catherine Road, E-222, Montreal, Quebec H3T 1E2, Canada
E-mail address: jonathan.afilalo@mcgill.ca

Clin Geriatr Med 35 (2019) 445–457
https://doi.org/10.1016/j.cger.2019.07.002

CR transcends diagnostic silos, benefitting diverse populations of patients with heart failure,[4] coronary artery disease and bypass surgery,[5] and heart valve surgery.[6] CR also transcends age, benefitting well-selected octogenarians and nonagenarians, with similar relative risk reductions but greater absolute risk reductions observed for all-cause mortality in older adults.[7]

Thus, the benefits of CR are diametrically opposed to the perils of frailty (**Fig. 1**). CR may be considered as (one of the only) comprehensive antidotes available in clinical practice with the potential to counteract frailty and its downstream consequences. Because frailty is prevalent in 20% to 60% of older adults with heart disease,[8] a vast number of patients stand to gain.

Despite this strong rationale, frail older adults are less likely to participate in CR and frailty is seldom measured in this setting. Opportunities for measuring and treating frailty in CR are reviewed, with practical suggestions (**Fig. 2**) to guide clinicians and researchers in addressing frailty using objective tools that have been validated in cardiovascular medicine.

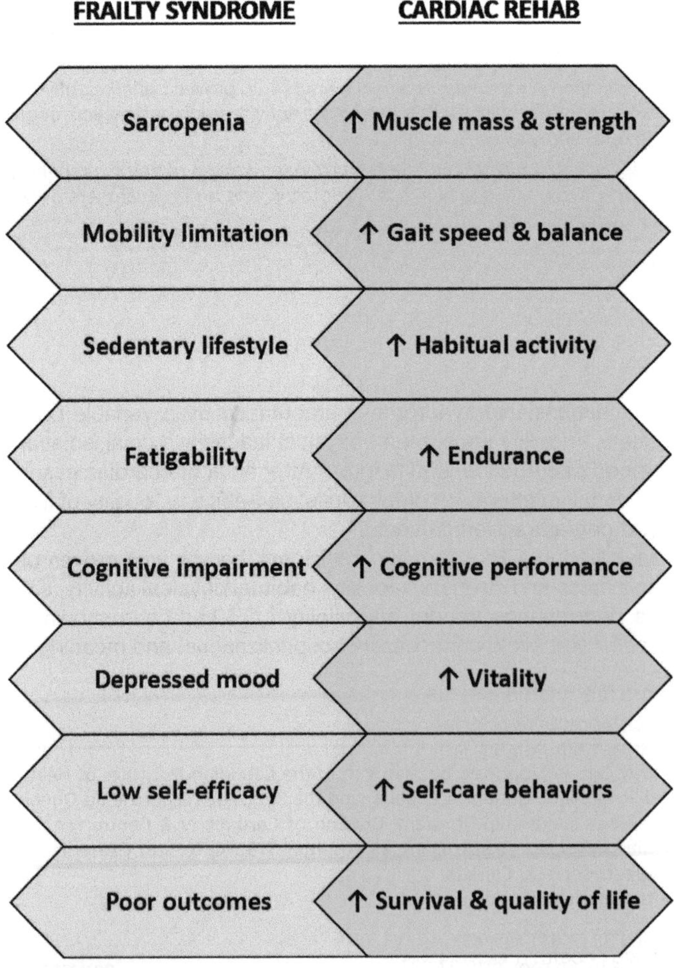

Fig. 1. Perils of frailty versus benefits of CR.

1. Frailty should be objectively measured during the index hospitalization, before initiation of CR, and if possible (optionally), after completion of CR
2. While hospitalized, frail patients should be targeted for early mobilization and protein-dense nutritional support
3. Frail patients should be prioritized for referral and early initiation of CR
4. Patients should be counselled about the person-centered benefits of CR by their treating physician
5. Patients that have difficulty attending a center-based CR facility should be referred to a home-based CR program
6. At the inaugural CR visit, older patients should be screened with a multi-domain frailty scale (such as the Intrinsic Capacity Screener or Edmonton Frailty Scale) to identify and address impairments in locomotion, cognition, mood, vision, hearing, and nutrition
7. At the inaugural CR visit, older patients should be stratified with a 6MWT and SPPB
8. Significant limitations in the 6MWT and SPPB should be addressed before beginning an aerobic exercise program and before transitioning to an unsupervised program
9. Frail patients, particularly those with sarcopenia, should receive lower-extremity strength and balance training as well as protein-dense nutritional supplementation
10. The post-CR care plan should address the patient's needs for physical therapy, occupational therapy, home help services, mental health services, and geriatric follow-up

Fig. 2. Recommendations for measurement and treatment of frailty in CR.

BEFORE CARDIAC REHABILITATION BEGINS

Target Frail Patients for Early Cardiac Rehabilitation Referral

Frailty should be assessed during the index hospitalization (after medical stabilization) to identify frail patients and prioritize their referral to CR. Frail older patients, owing to their physical and nonphysical impairments, have heightened needs for CR compared with their more robust younger counterparts. Nonphysical impairments include reductions in psychological well-being, external support, health literacy, and a greater burden of comorbidities and polypharmacy. Physical impairments include decreases in muscle mass, strength, mobility, balance, exercise capacity, and energy, all of which may be further decreased—and dramatically so—after an acute hospitalization.

The physiologic stress imparted by an acute cardiac event or surgery triggers a brisk catabolic response—breaking down protein in muscle to mobilize amino acids for immune cells and wound healing. This catabolic response is compounded by bedrest and undernutrition, leading to a vicious cycle of deconditioning.[9] In seminal experiments involving (healthy) older adults, 10 days of bedrest caused a loss of −8% in appendicular muscle mass, −13% in knee extensor strength, and −12% in

Vo_{2max}.[10,11] These losses can persist or progress well after apparent medical stabilization and discharge home, contributing to the vulnerable state that has become known as the "post-hospital syndrome."[12]

Early initiation of CR can break the cycle of deconditioning and mitigate the post-hospital syndrome. Emphasis on early initiation is counterculture to the traditional practice of waiting at least 2 to 4 weeks after an acute hospitalization to begin CR. This practice is based on the antiquated belief that exercise is hazardous and should be avoided soon after a cardiovascular event, and in certain countries, on restrictions imposed by health care payers. Beyond the physiologic reasons for early initiation of CR, a randomized, controlled trial (RCT) by Pack and colleagues[13] showed that scheduling CR 10 days after discharge (instead of the usual 35 days) improved attendance rates by 18%, amounting to 1 additional attendee for every 6 patients referred.

Before the initiation of out-of-hospital CR, frail patients should be targeted in the hospital for early mobilization along with physical and nutritional therapy to minimize their losses of muscle mass and strength. An RCT by Martínez-Velilla and colleagues[14] showed that, in 370 hospitalized older adults, simple strength and mobility exercises performed twice daily improved physical performance and ability to perform activities of daily living (ADL) at the time of discharge. A study by Goldfarb and colleagues[15] showed that early mobilization in the cardiac intensive care unit was feasible and effective, regardless of the patient's level of frailty. When mobilized early and often in the hospital, frail patients become more engaged and physically prepared to begin CR soon after discharge.

A systematic review by Doyle and colleagues[16] identified 18 RCTs and prospective studies that tested earlier initiation of CR after cardiac surgery, defined as starting in the hospital ("immediate") or within less than 2 weeks after discharge ("early"). Notably, inpatient initiation of CR was safe and associated with an improved 6-minute walk time (6MWT) at the time of hospital discharge (+79 m compared with usual care), and early outpatient initiation of CR was associated with an improved Vo_{2max}.

Target Frail Patients for Prehabilitation

The rationale and benefits of early CR have been extrapolated to the growing field of cardiac prehabilitation ("prehab"). Interest in prehab has been driven by an unmet need to address the impairments of frail patients awaiting cardiac surgery,[17] sometimes referred to as "de-frailing." Depending on the patient, prehab typically includes aerobic exercise training at 50% to 60% Vo_{2max}, respiratory muscle training, optimization of nutritional status, correction of iron deficiency, engagement of social support resources, and counseling for anxiety and sleep. Certain patients may not be candidates for the exercise component of prehab if they have severe symptoms such as low threshold angina, exertional syncope, or malignant or uncontrolled arrhythmia.

Although the evidence base is still in its infancy, there have been at least 6 RCTs with sample sizes ranging from 17 to 275 patients.[17] In most of these RCTs, prehab tended to decrease intensive care unit and total length of stay, increase 6MWT, and increase QOL. Larger studies are underway, including the Pre-operative Rehabilitation for reduction of Hospitalization After coronary Bypass and valvular surgery (PREHAB) RCT.[18] Prehab exercise interventions are generally administered in-hospital for closer observation in case of adverse events; however, Waite and colleagues[19] suggested that a hybrid approach with home-based exercises could be used safely.

Enable Frail Patients for Participation in Cardiac Rehabilitation

Numerous surveys and reports have reaffirmed that CR is underused, particularly in frail older patients. Flint and colleagues[20] analyzed data from the Translational Research Investigating Underlying Disparities in Acute Myocardial Infarction Patients' Health Status (TRIUMPH) Registry and found that frailty as defined by slow gait speed was associated with a lower likelihood of being encouraged to participate in CR by the treating physician and, in turn, a lower likelihood of attending CR after a hospitalization for myocardial infarction. Both slow gait speed and not attending CR were associated with a 1-year risk of death or functional decline. Kimber and colleagues[21] similarly found that frailty as defined by various scales was associated with a lower likelihood of attending CR after a hospitalization for cardiac surgery.

The barriers to CR participation in frail patients are cultural and contextual in nature. Clinicians and researchers frequently dismiss frail patients as "too unfit for CR"[22] or "inappropriate (for CR) due to frailty,"[23] concerned about their inability to complete a standard exercise program, their risk of adverse events, and a lack of perceived benefit given the paucity of evidence in this demographic. The risk of falls is a common concern, despite evidence showing that exercise training can help to prevent future falls and fall-related injuries.[24] Patients are concerned about their competing priorities for time- and cost-intensive health care visits, their transportation to CR appointments multiple times per week, and their own lack of perceived benefit or motivation when not adequately informed about the importance of CR as a treatment for their underlying heart disease.

One of the most impactful strategies to increase participation in CR is for the treating physician to explain and strongly recommend CR to the patient and family. A survey by Dedeyne and colleagues[25] found that the patients were most responsive and incentivized when the benefits of CR were framed as "helping to perform ADLs as long as possible" and "contributing to healthy aging" (rather than as decreasing reinfarction or mortality rates). Additional strategies, enumerated in a Presidential Advisory from the American Heart Association,[26] include (1) bedside visits by a CR liaison, (2) automated referral to CR in the discharge plan, (3) scheduling a CR appointment at the time of discharge, (4) transportation or parking assistance, and (5) repeated contact with patients who are referred but not yet enrolled.

If difficulties with transportation or mobility are elicited as major barriers to attend a center-based facility, home-based CR should be considered as a viable alternative. A Cochrane systematic review concluded from 17 RCTs encompassing 2172 patients that there was no difference between home-based and center-based CR in terms of participant survival, exercise capacity, and QOL, with home-based programs offering marginal improvements in adherence.[27] The EUropean study on effectiveness and sustainability of current Cardiac Rehabilitation programmes in the Elderly (EU-CaRE) is using a home-based CR program enhanced by telemonitoring to promote attendance and adherence in older patients.[28] Notwithstanding these attractive features, drawbacks of home-based CR include less standardization for quality and safety, less reimbursement by payers, and less opportunity for socialization—one of the most appreciated aspects of CR among older adults.

IMPLEMENTATION IN SUPERVISED CARDIAC REHABILITATION

Treat Frailty First to Maximize the Benefits of Cardiac Rehabilitation

To derive the stated benefits of CR, a participant must have the intrinsic capacity to progress through their exercise program and uphold their behavioral changes. Intrinsic capacity is a construct endorsed by the World Health Organization to reflect the physical and mental frailty domains that can lead to impaired functioning in older age.[29] The domains of intrinsic capacity are (1) locomotion (including muscle strength, mobility, balance), (2) vitality, (3) cognition, (4) psychology, and (5) sensory functions. Impairments in any of these domains can significantly undermine the success of any CR intervention.

Consider the prohibitive effect of an undiagnosed visual impairment or balance problem on an individual's ability to safely exercise on a treadmill, or alternatively an indolent cognitive disorder or untreated depression on their ability to adhere to recommended lifestyle changes. Such impairments are pervasive and often undiagnosed in older adults. Although an in-depth evaluation of these domains is beyond the mandate of most CR professionals, a 10-question intrinsic capacity screening tool has been developed to facilitate screening. Foreseeably, the intrinsic capacity of this screening tool could be an attractive addition to the baseline CR intake for older adults.

If an impairment is suspected or confirmed, it could trigger a referral to the appropriate health care professional for further evaluation and treatment. These evaluations may be outsourced or integrated into the CR framework. One example of successful integration is systematically screening for balance problems at the initial intake and referring impaired patients to a physiotherapist on the CR team before commencing aerobic exercise training. If multiple geriatric impairments are elicited, or if there are multiple interacting comorbidities, it could trigger a referral to a geriatrician for a comprehensive geriatric assessment.

Another example of integration is the Geriatric Rehab Cardio Programme model combining the core elements of CR alongside geriatric rehabilitation. In a feasibility study, van Dam van Isselt and colleagues[30] recruited 58 older adults with significant functional decline during an acute cardiovascular hospitalization in whom multidisciplinary needs were identified. Participants received aerobic and strength training, nutritional intervention, cardiac and noncardiac comorbidity optimization, self-care education, and ADL training. After a mean of 38 days, participants achieved promising gains in ADL functioning, 6MWT, and QOL.

Consider Frailty to Adapt Assessments of Cardiac Rehabilitation

The habitual practice of performing a treadmill exercise stress test at the inaugural CR visit is not universally feasible for frail older patients. Eichler and colleagues[31] showed that 43% of patients referred for CR after transcatheter aortic valve replacement (mean, 81 years of age) were unable to complete an exercise stress test. Even with modified protocols, older adults may be unfamiliar or uncomfortable walking on a treadmill or pedaling on a stationary bicycle. Conversely, 100% of patients in this study were able to perform a 6MWT and a timed-up-and-go test.

Forman and colleagues[32] analyzed data from the Participants in Heart Failure A Controlled Trial Investigating Outcomes of Exercise Training (HF-ACTION) Trial and put forth that the 6MWT was moderately well correlated with Vo_{2max}, similarly predictive of 1-year mortality, more convenient to administer, and more clinically relevant to real-life activities. The 6MWT is also moderately well correlated with the Fried frailty scale[33] and the short distance gait speed test,[34] although it is important the remember the fundamental difference between these tests. Whereas the 6MWT is determined by the functioning of the cardiac, vascular, pulmonary, and musculoskeletal systems, 5-m gait speed is mostly determined by the latter. Otherwise said, walking 5 m does not test or reflect the individual's cardiopulmonary reserves.

In a call to action, the European Association of Preventive Cardiology CR Section advocated for a 6MWT and short physical performance battery (SPPB) to supersede the exercise stress test as the first assessments to stratify older patients at the inaugural CR visit.[35] The SPPB consists of a gait speed test (4 or 5 m at a comfortable pace), a timed chair rise test (5 sit-to-stands at a rapid pace without the use of arms), and a balance test (10 seconds in side-by-side, semi-tandem, and tandem positions).[36,37] Each test is scored from 0 to 4 and summed for a composite SPPB score of 0 to 12, with lower scores indicating greater physical frailty. SPPB scores of 10 to 12 are considered robust, 7 to 9 mildly frail, 4 to 6 moderately frail, and 0 to 3 severely frail. Longitudinal SPPB improvements of 1 or more points are considered clinically meaningful.[38] The SPPB was designed to measure lower extremity function and has been validated extensively as a predictor of disability and mortality in various fields, including cardiovascular medicine.[39–41]

Consider Frailty to Tailor Cardiac Rehabilitation Interventions

Sarcopenia is the age-related loss of muscle mass, strength, and quality that has been dubbed the biological substrate of frailty.[42] There is ongoing debate about whether sarcopenia is the root cause of frailty or one of its many determinants[43,44]; however, there is agreement about the far-reaching prevalence and prognostic impact of sarcopenia in aging populations.[45,46] The diagnostic criteria for sarcopenia have been outlined by the European Working Group of Sarcopenia in Older People,[47] requiring (1) low muscle strength as measured by a chair rise test (part of the SPPB), and (2) low muscle mass as measured by a bioimpedance device, a dual x-ray absorptiometry scan, a computed tomography scan, or an MRI. Dual x-ray absorptiometry scans are most commonly used in clinical practice, but if a computed tomography scan has been acquired for another clinical indication, it can be leveraged to quantify muscle area using web-based software (www.coreslicer.com)[48] with high prognostic value.[49–52]

The most effective strategies to prevent or treat sarcopenia revolve around exercise and nutrition,[53] both core components of CR. Specifically, resistance exercise training and protein-rich nutritional intake have been proven to improve sarcopenia and frailty in older adults[54,55] and should be preferentially integrated into CR programs for frail patients. By integrating functional resistance exercises such as chair rises in addition to usual aerobic exercises, an RCT by Busch and colleagues[56] showed a greater improvement in 6MWT, Vo_{2max}, mobility, and lower extremity strength among 173 patients 75 years of age or older attending CR after cardiac surgery. By integrating a protein-rich diet to ideally achieve an intake of 1.2 to 1.5 g/kg/d of protein,[57] improvements in muscle mass and strength are amplified. These amounts of protein intake may not be obtained from food alone, in which case patients should be encouraged to consume commercially-available oral nutritional supplements that contain 20 to 30 g of protein per serving (unless otherwise contraindicated).

Measure Frailty to Evaluate Outcomes in Cardiac Rehabilitation

Frailty is a dynamic state that may evolve favorably or unfavorably depending on a person's lifestyle behaviors and health status. An epidemiologic study by Gill and colleagues[58] showed that 58% of community-dwelling older adults experienced at least 1 transition between the states of robust, pre-frail, and frail over a period of 5 years. CR, in particular, has the potential to catalyze these transitions from pre-frailty or frailty to more robust states. Rengo and colleagues[59] showed a clinically meaningful improvement of +1.6 points in the SPPB for frail participants after successful completion of CR. Eichler and colleagues[31] similarly showed improvements in physical and nonphysical indices of frailty after CR.

Should frailty be measured before and after CR to gauge its effects? The European Association of Preventive Cardiology CR Section addressed this question and concluded that "frailty scales were developed as prognostic tools but their ability to capture intervention-induced changes over time is unclear."[35] This is because the clinimetric properties (accuracy, reliability, responsiveness, interpretability, content and construct validity) of frailty scales are understudied.[60]

If frailty is to be measured before and after CR, some argue that a multidomain scale should be used to capture the diverse benefits of CR, whereas others argue that these scales lack granularity to detect changes in any given domain.[61] For example, the Fried and Edmonton frailty scales are widely used but their domains are classified as binary subscores that are not sensitive to detect serial changes. The Clinical Frailty Scale is also widely used, but not sensitive to detect serial changes given its subjective and semiquantitative scoring.

Physical performance tests such as the SPPB and 5-m gait speed test are more objective and quantitative, and thus suited to evaluate the longitudinal effects of CR on physical frailty. The SPPB combines essential measures of functional mobility (gait speed), lower extremity strength (chair rises), and balance. However, the SPPB suffers from a ceiling effect in fitter individuals, and Hardy and colleagues[62] have suggested that the gait speed test alone may be preferable to overcome this limitation. In this study of 439 community-dwelling older adults, a change of 0.1 m/s in gait speed was more predictive of 8-year survival than a 1-point change in the SPPB.

In selected cases, or for research purposes, cognitive performance tests such as the Montreal Cognitive Assessment[63] can be added to monitor the longitudinal effects of CR on cognitive frailty. The Montreal Cognitive Assessment is preferred over other instruments for this indication because it has been shown to be responsive to change over time,[64] and several versions are available to obviate learning bias. At the present time, limited evidence suggests that CR has the potential to slow down cognitive decline.[65]

TRANSITIONING TO UNSUPERVISED CARDIAC REHABILITATION

Consider Frailty to Determine Readiness of Unsupervised Cardiac Rehabilitation

At the completion of a supervised CR program, assessment of physical and cognitive frailty can be informative to determine whether an individual is safely capable of transitioning to an unsupervised program. From a physical standpoint, an individual with a global SPPB score of less than 4 or a balance SPPB subscore of less than 2 may be unable to exercise without help or may be at risk of failing. From a cognitive standpoint, an individual with moderate to severe dementia may have difficulty adhering to prescribed exercises or lifestyle changes without additional support.

Therefore, barriers relating to the individual's intrinsic capacity or their environmental milieu should be readdressed before transitioning to an unsupervised CR program. Education relating to the person-centered benefits of habitual physical activity, healthy nutrition, and self-care should be reemphasized. In successful programs, periodic contact by telephone or follow-up visits has been used strategically to monitor and encourage continued participation in activities, including group sessions and online telerehabilitation.[66] These efforts are critical in frail older adults, because they have significantly lower rates of sustained independent adherence.

Consider Frailty to Tailor Interventions After Cardiac Rehabilitation

In addition to aerobic exercises recommended after CR, such as brisk walking for at least 150 minutes per week, frail patients benefit from extra exercises aimed at maintaining functional mobility and strength. In an RCT by Molino-Lova and colleagues,[67] 140 cardiac surgery patients with an SPPB of 9 or greater after completing CR were randomly allocated to usual home exercises versus usual home exercises plus functional strength exercises 30 minutes 3 times per week. One year later, the intervention group had achieved a mean +1.3-point improvement in SPPB, whereas the usual care group had not improved.

Care after CR should be tailored to the physical, psychological, and social needs of the individual to foster their recovery of function and autonomy at home. For those with persistent physical limitations or mobility issues, follow-up with a physical therapist may be beneficial. For those with difficulties performing ADLs in their home environment, consultation with an occupational therapist or home help services may be beneficial. For those with persistent depressive symptoms, follow-up with a mental health professional may be needed on a longitudinal basis. Finally, for those with complex or multidomain impairments, consultation and outpatient follow-up with a geriatrician should be considered.

SUMMARY

By integrating the concept of frailty in CR, practitioners can be better equipped to proactively identify vulnerable patients in need of CR and adapt their assessment and intervention plan. The initial assessment should begin by screening for geriatric impairments and environmental barriers that may impede the participant's progress throughout CR, and subsequently, by administering physical performance tests (6MWT and SPPB) that provide incremental prognostic value and help to individualize the exercise prescription, ideally aiming to improve cardiopulmonary fitness concurrently with sarcopenia and overall frailty. A one-size-fits-all approach is not applicable to the heterogenous demographic of older adults; rather, a tailored geriatric-friendly approach is needed to maximize participation and person-centered benefits.

REFERENCES

1. Cesari M, Calvani R, Marzetti E. Frailty in older persons. Clin Geriatr Med 2017;33(3):293–303.
2. Walker DM, Gale CP, Lip G, et al. Editor's Choice - frailty and the management of patients with acute cardiovascular disease: a position paper from the Acute Cardiovascular Care Association. Eur Heart J Acute Cardiovasc Care 2018;7(2):176–93.
3. Schopfer DW, Forman DE. Cardiac rehabilitation in older adults. Can J Cardiol 2016;32(9):1088–96.
4. Taylor RS, Sagar VA, Davies EJ, et al. Exercise-based rehabilitation for heart failure. Cochrane Database Syst Rev 2014;(4):CD003331.
5. Anderson L, Oldridge N, Thompson DR, et al. Exercise-based cardiac rehabilitation for coronary heart disease: Cochrane systematic review and meta-analysis. J Am Coll Cardiol 2016;67(1):1–12.
6. Ribeiro GS, Melo RD, Deresz LF, et al. Cardiac rehabilitation programme after transcatheter aortic valve implantation versus surgical aortic valve replacement: systematic review and meta-analysis. Eur J Prev Cardiol 2017;24(7):688–97.
7. Suaya JA, Stason WB, Ades PA, et al. Cardiac rehabilitation and survival in older coronary patients. J Am Coll Cardiol 2009;54(1):25–33.
8. Afilalo J, Alexander KP, Mack MJ, et al. Frailty assessment in the cardiovascular care of older adults. J Am Coll Cardiol 2014;63(8):747–62.
9. Ferrucci L, Maggio M, Ceda GP, et al. Acute postoperative frailty. J Am Coll Surg 2006;203(1):134–5.
10. Kortebein P, Ferrando A, Lombeida J, et al. Effect of 10 days of bed rest on skeletal muscle in healthy older adults. JAMA 2007;297(16):1772–4.

11. Kortebein P, Symons TB, Ferrando A, et al. Functional impact of 10 days of bed rest in healthy older adults. J Gerontol A Biol Sci Med Sci 2008;63(10):1076–81.
12. Krumholz HM. Post-hospital syndrome–an acquired, transient condition of generalized risk. N Engl J Med 2013;368(2):100–2.
13. Pack QR, Mansour M, Barboza JS, et al. An early appointment to outpatient cardiac rehabilitation at hospital discharge improves attendance at orientation: a randomized, single-blind, controlled trial. Circulation 2013;127(3):349–55.
14. Martínez-Velilla N, Casas-Herrero A, Zambom-Ferraresi F, et al. Effect of exercise intervention on functional decline in very elderly patients during acute hospitalization: a randomized clinical trial. JAMA Intern Med 2018. https://doi.org/10.1001/jamainternmed.2018.4869.
15. Goldfarb M, Afilalo J, Chan A, et al. Early mobility in frail and non-frail older adults admitted to the cardiovascular intensive care unit. J Crit Care 2018;47:9–14.
16. Doyle MP, Indraratna P, Tardo DT, et al. Safety and efficacy of aerobic exercise commenced early after cardiac surgery: a systematic review and meta-analysis. Eur J Prev Cardiol 2019;26(1):36–45.
17. McCann M, Stamp N, Ngui A, et al. Cardiac prehabilitation. J Cardiothorac Vasc Anesth 2019. https://doi.org/10.1053/j.jvca.2019.01.023.
18. Stammers AN, Kehler DS, Afilalo J, et al. Protocol for the PREHAB study-Pre-operative Rehabilitation for reduction of Hospitalization after coronary Bypass and valvular surgery: a randomised controlled trial. BMJ Open 2015;5(3):e007250.
19. Waite I, Deshpande R, Baghai M, et al. Home-based preoperative rehabilitation (prehab) to improve physical function and reduce hospital length of stay for frail patients undergoing coronary artery bypass graft and valve surgery. J Cardiothorac Surg 2017;12(1):91.
20. Flint K, Kennedy K, Arnold SV, et al. Slow gait speed and cardiac rehabilitation participation in older adults after acute myocardial infarction. J Am Heart Assoc 2018;7(5). https://doi.org/10.1161/JAHA.117.008296.
21. Kimber DE, Kehler DS, Lytwyn J, et al. Pre-operative frailty status is associated with cardiac rehabilitation completion: a retrospective cohort study. J Clin Med 2018;7(12). https://doi.org/10.3390/jcm7120560.
22. Gielen S, Simm A. Frailty and cardiac rehabilitation: a long-neglected connection. Eur J Prev Cardiol 2017;24(14):1488–9.
23. Rogers P, Al-Aidrous S, Banya W, et al. Cardiac rehabilitation to improve health-related quality of life following trans-catheter aortic valve implantation: a randomised controlled feasibility study: RECOVER-TAVI Pilot, ORCA 4, for the Optimal Restoration of Cardiac Activity Group. Pilot Feasibility Stud 2018;4(1):185.
24. El-Khoury F, Cassou B, Charles M-A, et al. The effect of fall prevention exercise programmes on fall induced injuries in community dwelling older adults: systematic review and meta-analysis of randomised controlled trials. BMJ 2013;347(20):f6234.
25. Dedeyne L, Dewinter L, Lovik A, et al. Nutritional and physical exercise programs for older people: program format preferences and (dis)incentives to participate. Clin Interv Aging 2018;13:1259–66.
26. Balady GJ, Ades PA, Bittner VA, et al. Referral, enrollment, and delivery of cardiac rehabilitation/secondary prevention programs at clinical centers and beyond: a presidential advisory from the American Heart Association. Circulation 2011;124(25):2951–60.
27. Taylor RS, Dalal H, Jolly K, et al. Home-based versus centre-based cardiac rehabilitation. Cochrane Database Syst Rev 2015;(8):CD007130.

28. Prescott E, Meindersma EP, van der Velde AE, et al. A EUropean study on effectiveness and sustainability of current Cardiac Rehabilitation programmes in the Elderly: design of the EU-CaRE randomised controlled trial. Eur J Prev Cardiol 2016;23(2 suppl):27–40.
29. Cesari M, Araujo de Carvalho I, Amuthavalli Thiyagarajan J, et al. Evidence for the domains supporting the construct of intrinsic capacity. J Gerontol A Biol Sci Med Sci 2018;73(12):1653–60.
30. van Dam van Isselt EF, van Wijngaarden J, Lok DJA, et al. Geriatric rehabilitation in older patients with cardiovascular disease: a feasibility study. Eur Geriatr Med 2018;9(6):853–61.
31. Eichler S, Salzwedel A, Reibis R, et al. Multicomponent cardiac rehabilitation in patients after transcatheter aortic valve implantation: predictors of functional and psychocognitive recovery. Eur J Prev Cardiol 2017;24(3):257–64.
32. Forman DE, Fleg JL, Kitzman DW, et al. 6-min walk test provides prognostic utility comparable to cardiopulmonary exercise testing in ambulatory outpatients with systolic heart failure. J Am Coll Cardiol 2012;60(25):2653–61.
33. Boxer RS, Wang Z, Walsh SJ, et al. The utility of the 6-minute walk test as a measure of frailty in older adults with heart failure. Am J Geriatr Cardiol 2008; 17(1):7–12.
34. Kamiya K, Hamazaki N, Matsue Y, et al. Gait speed has comparable prognostic capability to six-minute walk distance in older patients with cardiovascular disease. Eur J Prev Cardiol 2018;25(2):212–9.
35. Vigorito C, Abreu A, Ambrosetti M, et al. Frailty and cardiac rehabilitation: a call to action from the EAPC Cardiac Rehabilitation Section. Eur J Prev Cardiol 2017; 24(6):577–90.
36. Guralnik JM, Simonsick EM, Ferrucci L, et al. A short physical performance battery assessing lower extremity function: association with self-reported disability and prediction of mortality and nursing home admission. J Gerontol 1994; 49(2):M85–94.
37. Guralnik JM, Ferrucci L, Simonsick EM, et al. Lower-extremity function in persons over the age of 70 years as a predictor of subsequent disability. N Engl J Med 1995;332(9):556–61.
38. Perera S, Mody SH, Woodman RC, et al. Meaningful change and responsiveness in common physical performance measures in older adults. J Am Geriatr Soc 2006;54(5):743–9.
39. Chiarantini D, Volpato S, Sioulis F, et al. Lower extremity performance measures predict long-term prognosis in older patients hospitalized for heart failure. J Card Fail 2010;16(5):390–5.
40. Afilalo J, Lauck S, Kim DH, et al. Frailty in older adults undergoing aortic valve replacement: the FRAILTY-AVR study. J Am Coll Cardiol 2017;70(6):689–700.
41. Veronese N, Stubbs B, Fontana L, et al. A comparison of objective physical performance tests and future mortality in the elderly people. J Gerontol A Biol Sci Med Sci 2016;glw139. https://doi.org/10.1093/gerona/glw139.
42. Landi F, Calvani R, Cesari M, et al. Sarcopenia as the biological substrate of physical frailty. Clin Geriatr Med 2015;31(3):367–74.
43. Afilalo J. Conceptual models of frailty: the sarcopenia phenotype. Can J Cardiol 2016;32(9):1051–5.
44. Rockwood K. Conceptual models of frailty: accumulation of deficits. Can J Cardiol 2016;32(9):1046–50.
45. Woo J. Sarcopenia. Clin Geriatr Med 2017;33(3):305–14.

46. Liu P, Hao Q, Hai S, et al. Sarcopenia as a predictor of all-cause mortality among community-dwelling older people: a systematic review and meta-analysis. Maturitas 2017;103:16–22.
47. Cruz-Jentoft AJ, Bahat G, Bauer J, et al. Sarcopenia: revised European consensus on definition and diagnosis. Age Ageing 2019;48(1):16–31.
48. Mullie L, Afilalo J. CoreSlicer: a web toolkit for analytic morphomics. BMC Med Imaging 2019;19(1):15.
49. Mamane S, Mullie L, Piazza N, et al. Psoas muscle area and all-cause mortality after transcatheter aortic valve replacement: the Montreal-Munich study. Can J Cardiol 2016;32(2):177–82.
50. Drudi LM, Phung K, Ades M, et al. Psoas muscle area predicts all-cause mortality after endovascular and open aortic aneurysm repair. Eur J Vasc Endovasc Surg 2016. https://doi.org/10.1016/j.ejvs.2016.09.011.
51. Zuckerman J, Ades M, Mullie L, et al. Psoas muscle area and length of stay in older adults undergoing cardiac operations. Ann Thorac Surg 2016. https://doi.org/10.1016/j.athoracsur.2016.09.005.
52. Bibas L, Saleh E, Al-Kharji S, et al. Muscle mass and mortality after cardiac transplantation. Transplantation 2018;102(12):2101–7.
53. Lozano-Montoya I, Correa-Pérez A, Abraha I, et al. Nonpharmacological interventions to treat physical frailty and sarcopenia in older patients: a systematic overview - the SENATOR Project ONTOP Series. Clin Interv Aging 2017;12:721–40.
54. Bibas L, Levi M, Bendayan M, et al. Therapeutic interventions for frail elderly patients: part I. Published randomized trials. Prog Cardiovasc Dis 2014;57(2):134–43.
55. Dedeyne L, Deschodt M, Verschueren S, et al. Effects of multi-domain interventions in (pre)frail elderly on frailty, functional, and cognitive status: a systematic review. Clin Interv Aging 2017;12:873–96.
56. Busch JC, Lillou D, Wittig G, et al. Resistance and balance training improves functional capacity in very old participants attending cardiac rehabilitation after coronary bypass surgery. J Am Geriatr Soc 2012;60(12):2270–6.
57. Bauer J, Biolo G, Cederholm T, et al. Evidence-based recommendations for optimal dietary protein intake in older people: a position paper from the PROT-AGE Study Group. J Am Med Dir Assoc 2013;14(8):542–59.
58. Gill TM, Gahbauer EA, Allore HG, et al. Transitions between frailty states among community-living older persons. Arch Intern Med 2006;166(4):418–23.
59. Rengo JL, Savage PD, Shaw JC, et al. Directly measured physical function in cardiac rehabilitation. J Cardiopulm Rehabil Prev 2017;37(3):175–81.
60. de Vries NM, Staal JB, van Ravensberg CD, et al. Outcome instruments to measure frailty: a systematic review. Ageing Res Rev 2011;10(1):104–14.
61. Tamuleviciute-Prasciene E, Drulyte K, Jurenaite G, et al. Frailty and exercise training: how to provide best care after cardiac surgery or intervention for elder patients with valvular heart disease. Biomed Res Int 2018;2018:9849475.
62. Hardy SE, Perera S, Roumani YF, et al. Improvement in usual gait speed predicts better survival in older adults. J Am Geriatr Soc 2007;55(11):1727–34.
63. Nasreddine ZS, Phillips NA, Bédirian V, et al. The Montreal Cognitive Assessment, MoCA: a brief screening tool for mild cognitive impairment. J Am Geriatr Soc 2005;53(4):695–9.
64. Costa AS, Reich A, Fimm B, et al. Evidence of the sensitivity of the MoCA alternate forms in monitoring cognitive change in early Alzheimer's disease. Dement Geriatr Cogn Disord 2014;37(1–2):95–103.

65. Alagiakrishnan K, Mah D, Gyenes G. Cardiac rehabilitation and its effects on cognition in patients with coronary artery disease and heart failure. Expert Rev Cardiovasc Ther 2018;16(9):645–52.
66. Peretti A, Amenta F, Tayebati SK, et al. Telerehabilitation: review of the state-of-the-art and areas of application. JMIR Rehabil Assist Technol 2017;4(2):e7.
67. Molino-Lova R, Pasquini G, Vannetti F, et al. Effects of a structured physical activity intervention on measures of physical performance in frail elderly patients after cardiac rehabilitation: a pilot study with 1-year follow-up. Intern Emerg Med 2013;8(7):581–9.

Resistance Training for Older Adults in Cardiac Rehabilitation

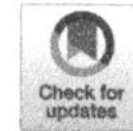

Sherrie Khadanga, MD*, Patrick D. Savage, MS, Philip A. Ades, MD

KEYWORDS

• Resistance training • Older adults • Cardiac rehabilitation • Strength training • Aging • Physical function

KEY POINTS

- Resistance training has been shown to increase muscle strength, endurance, exercise performance and physical function in older adults with coronary heart disease and heart failure.
- Resistance training can help to improve selected cardiovascular risk factors.
- Combining aerobic exercise with resistance training in cardiac patients is more effective at improving muscle strength and cardiorespiratory fitness compared with isolated aerobic or resistance training.

BACKGROUND/INTRODUCTION

The prevalence of atherosclerotic cardiovascular disease and chronic heart failure (HF) increase with age and accounts for more than 50% of cardiovascular related deaths in the United States.[1] Cardiac rehabilitation (CR) plays a key role in improving clinical outcomes, quality of life, exercise capacity, and physical function in older patients with heart disease. Participation in CR is recommended for patients after an acute myocardial infarction, coronary revascularization (percutaneous or surgical), or for patients with chronic stable angina pectoris, systolic HF (ejection fraction of ≤35%), or heart valve surgery. This multidisciplinary program promotes a comprehensive and individualized treatment program of aerobic exercise, resistance training (RT), lifestyle modifications, and counseling, which can be particularly valuable for the aging

Disclosures: This work was supported by the Center of Biomedical Research Excellence award P20GM103644 from the National Institute of General Medical Sciences and the Vermont Center for Behavior and Health.
Department of Medicine, Division of Cardiology, Cardiac Rehabilitation and Prevention, University of Vermont Medical Center, 62 Tilley Drive, South Burlington, VT 05403, USA
* Corresponding author.
E-mail address: Sherrie.Khadanga@uvmhealth.org

Clin Geriatr Med 35 (2019) 459–468
https://doi.org/10.1016/j.cger.2019.07.005

population. The purpose of this review is to focus on the effects of RT on physical function for older participants in CR.

PHYSIOLOGIC RESPONSE IN RESISTANCE TRAINING

RT is a form of anaerobic exercise that uses repeated movements against resistance to stimulate a stronger muscle contraction. It is generally guided by exercise intensity as defined by the single-repetition maximal lift (1-RM), which can be safely determined in older adults by an experienced exercise specialist. The 1-RM is the maximum amount of weight that can be lifted once while maintaining proper form.

Gains in strength result from an overload beyond a minimal threshold of resistance. In the initial phase of RT (weeks), there is an increase in strength owing to neuromuscular adaptation.[2] Over time (months), the muscle fibers respond to the repeated resistance stimulus by increasing in size (muscle hypertrophy), leading to improvements in function and efficiency. The acute cardiovascular response during RT is an augmented pressure load on the heart that can transiently increase heart rate and blood pressure (BP).[3] The BP effect from RT depends on the load intensity and the magnitude of resistance.

Breathing techniques to avoid straining and rest between sets can help to attenuate the BP response to RT. Breath holding (Valsalva maneuver) during exertion should be avoided to mitigate increases in intrathoracic pressure and an exaggerated BP response. By exhaling during the exertion phase of RT, destabilizing hemodynamic responses are minimized.[3]

RESISTANCE TRAINING IN FRAIL OLDER ADULTS

Sarcopenia, the loss of muscle mass and strength owing to aging or chronic disease such as HF and cancer often leads to frailty and physical impairment. Frailty is a clinical syndrome owing to age-associated decreases in function and physiologic reserve, leading to increased vulnerability to acute stressors.[4] Frailty consists of 5 domains: physical exhaustion, mobility, muscular strength, low energy expenditure, and nutrition. The physical frailty phenotype is widely used as a screening tool to assess frailty in the elderly.[5] Frail patients with cardiovascular disease, which includes coronary heart disease, stroke, and HF, have twice the morbidity and mortality compared with non-frail individuals.[6] Furthermore, frailty in patients with cardiovascular disease is associated with higher disability and hospitalization rates. RT can help to combat frailty by improving several components of physical function, including muscular strength, walking endurance, and balance.[3]

Fiatarone and colleagues[7] studied the effects of RT in a cohort of frail adults aged 72 to 98 years who participated in high intensity progressive RT of the hip and knee extensors. Muscle strength and size improved with RT, allowing for better mobility and increased level of physical activity. Similarly, a randomized controlled trial in 40 nonagenarians aged 90 to 97 years assessed the effects of an 8-week RT program consisting of light to moderate intensity RT characterized as 30% to 70% of 1-RM 3 times a week and found an increase in muscle strength and a decrease in fall risk.[8]

Another study examined the efficacy of RT at different intensities in older, frail adults. Individuals participating in RT, starting at 20% and increasing to 80% of 1-RM over a 12-week period, had greater increase in muscle strength compared with those who trained exclusively at 20% of 1-RM.[9] No training related adverse events occurred in either groups. Thus, RT in frail, older adults is well-tolerated and can improve gait speed, strength, and balance, thereby reducing the number of falls and fractures.[7–9]

FUNCTIONAL BENEFITS OF RESISTANCE TRAINING IN CARDIAC REHABILITATION PATIENTS

The functional benefits of RT on measures of physical performance were carefully evaluated in 42 disabled female cardiac patients age 65 or older. Subjects were randomized to either high-intensity RT (ie, 80% of 1-RM) or light yoga (control).[10,11] RT improved the performance on a wide range of physical activities such as simulated grocery carrying or lifting heavier luggage onto a bus more rapidly. There was a close relationship between increases in muscle strength and increases in the total physical function score (**Fig. 1**).[10] Additionally, there were measured improvements in endurance activities such as the stair climb and 6-minute walk and tasks involving flexibility and coordination such as pouring milk or vacuuming. Thus, RT safely improves performance on a wide variety of daily activities in older women with coronary heart disease.

Patients with HF have decreased exercise tolerance for many reasons, including diminished cardiac function, autonomic dysfunction, and skeletal muscle abnormalities.[3,12] For those with HF, exercise intolerance is strongly associated with quality of life, morbidity, and mortality.[12] Historically, there has been apprehension regarding RT in patients with systolic HF owing to a theoretic concern of adverse remodeling of the left ventricle owing to increased afterload with exertion. This, however, has not been the case. Two studies randomized patients with systolic HF to RT versus usual care and noted that left ventricular volumes remained unchanged without deterioration of ejection fraction in the RT group.[13,14]

The relationship of RT and muscle function in older women with HF was examined in a randomized, controlled trial.[15] Participants had significantly lower muscle strength, but similar aerobic capacity, compared with age-matched peers without HF. High-intensity RT resulted in improvements in muscle strength, endurance, and exercise performance owing to peripheral muscle adaptations seen on biopsy. These benefits occurred despite a lack of change in skeletal muscle mass or cardiac function. Another study measured performance in activities of daily living and muscle strength before and after an 18-week RT program in patients 71 to 75 years of age with HF.[16] At baseline, measured performance of daily activities was 30% lower in HF patients compared with healthy age-matched controls owing to decreased aerobic capacity and diminished muscle strength. RT resulted in significant improvements in activities of daily living, such as carrying groceries, loading and unloading a washing machine

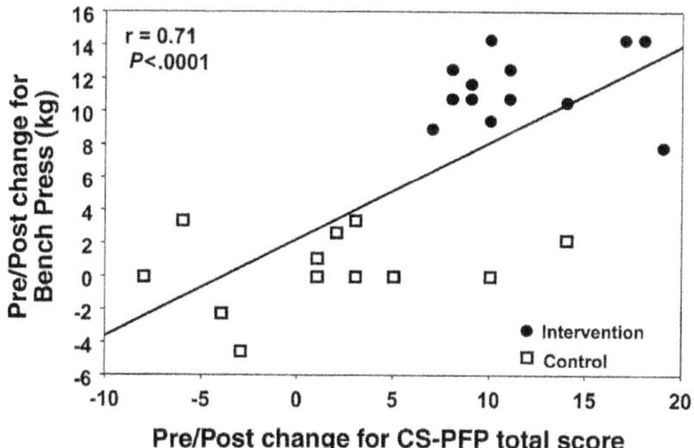

Fig. 1. Association between percent changes in total Continuous-Scale Physical Functional Performance test (CS-PFP) physical performance score and percent changes in maximal strength on the bench press. Pre, before exercise; Post, after exercise. (*From* Brochu M, Savage P, Lee M, et al. Effects of resistance training on physical function in older disabled women with coronary heart disease. J Appl Physiol 2002;92:676.)

and dryer, and picking up items off the floor, without change in aerobic capacity. Muscle weakness, therefore, is a key determinant of physical disability in individuals with HF and RT can improve physical functioning.[3,15,17] Although much research has centered on abnormalities of skeletal muscle in patients with HF and relative benefits of exercise training, recent efforts highlight similar skeletal muscle changes associated with diastolic HF, and similar benefits of exercise training.[18]

METABOLIC BENEFITS OF RESISTANCE TRAINING IN OLDER CARDIAC REHABILITATION PATIENTS

The loss of muscle mass owing to aging diminishes total body glucose use and lowers caloric expenditure thus contributing to insulin resistance, diabetes mellitus type 2 (T2DM), hypertension, dyslipidemia, and obesity. Strength is inversely associated with the prevalence of metabolic syndrome independent of aerobic activity.[2]

Insulin Resistance

Insulin resistance and T2DM are significant risk factors for the development and progression of atherosclerotic cardiovascular disease. In 1 study, the combined prevalence of insulin resistance and T2DM for individuals enrolled in CR was remarkably high at 67%.[19]

RT is associated with increase insulin sensitivity and glucose uptake in patients with abnormal glucose tolerance, improving glycosylated hemoglobin levels, and should, therefore, be considered in patients with insulin resistance and/or T2DM.[20,21] A large prospective cohort study followed 32,000 men aged 40 to 75 over 18 years to examine the role of RT in primary prevention of T2DM.[22] Engaging in RT alone, for at least 150 minutes per week, had a 34% risk reduction in developing T2DMs; but for participants in combined RT and aerobic exercise, a 59% risk reduction was observed. Therefore, RT is an important intervention for the prevention and management of insulin resistance and T2DM.

Blood Pressure

The effect of RT on BP has been examined in 2 meta-analyses.[3] An analysis of 11 studies found that following RT, both resting systolic BP (SBP) and diastolic BP (DBP) decreased by 3.0 to 3.5 mm Hg.[23] Similarly, another meta-analysis of RT reported resting reductions of 3 mm Hg and 6 mm Hg in DBP and SBP, respectively.[24] A caveat to both of these analyses, however, is that only one-third of the study patients were deemed to be hypertensive at baseline (ie, initial resting SBP of >140 mm Hg or DBP >90 mm Hg). Although the decreases seem to be minimal at the individual level, an SBP reduction of 3 mm Hg has been associated with a decrease in stroke and cardiac morbidity and overall mortality at the population level.[3]

For patients with hypertension, there is more benefit when RT is combined with aerobic exercise. In another study, 104 individuals between ages 55 to 75 with untreated mild hypertension (SBP of 130–159 mm Hg or DBP of 85–99 mm Hg) were randomized to combined aerobic and RT versus usual care.[25] A reduction of 5 mm Hg and 3 mm Hg in SBP and DBP, respectively, was observed in the intervention group. Although the evidence for RT alone as a form of exercise to reduce BP is limited, the American Heart Association has recommended moderate intensity RT as an adjunct to aerobic exercise in treating and preventing hypertension.[3]

Effects of Resistance Training on Dyslipidemia

RT seems to have no significant effects on lipid metabolism.[3] One large study, which consisted of approximately 1190 women and 5460 men, found no association between muscle strength and low-density lipoprotein cholesterol or total cholesterol.[26] A randomized, controlled trial examining the effects of high intensity RT (85%–90% of 1-RM) in men aged 60 to 75 years and found no significant improvement in lipid profiles.[27] In another study, 15 postmenopausal women underwent low intensity RT and no significant alterations in low-density lipoprotein cholesterol or total cholesterol were seen.[28] Based on these studies, there is no good evidence that RT affects dyslipidemia.

Resistance Training and Weight Management

More than 80% of participants in CR are overweight.[29] Although aerobic activity is greatly emphasized regarding weight management owing to an increase in caloric expenditure, RT plays a role as well. Several studies have reported an increase in lean body mass and a decrease in adipose tissue for older adults undergoing RT.[3] For example, Hunter and colleagues[30] examined the effects of RT on fat distribution in older men and women aged 61 to 77 years. Interestingly, there seem to be sex-specific differences. Women lost a significant amount of visceral adiposity, whereas men did not. Both men and women, however, had significant increase in muscle mass and similar loss of total body fat. This increase in muscle mass increases the basal metabolic rate, which is responsible for up to two-thirds of total energy expenditure in healthy adults.[3,29] Furthermore, given that visceral fat has been associated with the metabolic syndrome, T2DM, and hypertension, a decrease in visceral adipose tissue is beneficial in older adults in CR.

EFFECT OF RESISTANCE TRAINING ON AEROBIC CAPACITY

Aerobic capacity, defined by peak oxygen consumption (Vo_2), reflects the overall functional capacity of the cardiorespiratory system. It has been postulated that increased muscle strength, resulting from RT, would improve peak aerobic capacity. However, studies examining the link between RT and measures of peak Vo_2 have been equivocal.

In a randomized, controlled trial of 24 healthy older adults who underwent RT, a significant improvement in leg strength and walking endurance was seen, but peak Vo_2 remained unchanged.[31] A recent meta-analysis of 34 studies examined the effects of RT on aerobic fitness and strength in older adults with coronary heart disease and found that although RT improved muscle strength, peak Vo_2 and work capacity remained the same.[32]

Another review, however, examined whether RT enhanced peak Vo_2 in older patients and 6 of the 9 studies reported an improvement in peak Vo_2 after RT regardless of the intensity.[33] Interestingly, a negative correlation was seen between the initial peak Vo_2 and RT-induced change in peak Vo_2, suggesting that the increase in Vo_2 from RT is dependent on the Vo_2 at baseline. Older adults with an initial peak Vo_2 of less than 25 $mL/kg^{-1}/min^{-1}$ were more likely to increase peak Vo_2 with RT. Although the data remain mixed regarding the effect of RT on peak Vo_2, RT clearly improves walking endurance and muscle strength thereby increasing physical function among older adults.

COMBINATION OF AEROBIC EXERCISE AND RESISTANCE TRAINING MORE BENEFICIAL THAN RESISTANCE TRAINING ALONE

Decreases in muscle mass and strength owing to aging affects the performance of daily living and leisure activities, mobility, and aerobic fitness. Although RT alone can help to counteract some of the changes associated with aging, the combination of RT with aerobic exercise has proven to be more beneficial. Several randomized, controlled trials have demonstrated improvement in muscle strength, endurance, and quality of life in cardiac patients with the combination of RT and aerobic exercise.[34,35]

The effects of high-intensity RT on quality of life were studied in 34 older CR participants.[36] Among those randomized to RT with aerobic training, a significant improvement was seen in exercise treadmill time, muscle endurance, and self-reported ability to lift weights, to do push-ups, and to climb stairs.

Furthermore, combined RT and aerobic exercise in cardiac patients was more effective at improving peak Vo_2 and upper/lower body strength compared with isolated RT or aerobic exercise alone.[37] Thus, the combination of aerobic and RT can ameliorate the effects of frailty and improve physical function. Given the overall benefits, all CR programs should be incorporating both RT and endurance exercise.

SAFETY OF RESISTANCE TRAINING

Supervised RT seems to be quite safe, even among the elderly in CR. Nonetheless, a small risk for injury remains and is likely associated with an individual's age, baseline fitness level, intensity of RT, and the quality of supervision.

Absolute and relative contraindications to RT and CR overlap and include decompensated HF, severe and symptomatic aortic stenosis, uncontrolled hypertension (≥180/110 mm Hg), unstable coronary heart disease, Marfan syndrome, enlarging aortic aneurysms, and severe pulmonary hypertension (mean arterial pressure of >55 mm Hg).[3] Patients with recently implanted pacemakers or defibrillators should consult their physician before initiating an RT program because upper body activity can cause lead fractures or dislodgment. For patients who recently underwent valvular or coronary artery bypass surgery with a full sternonotomy, upper body RT should be delayed by 12 weeks from the date of surgery to ensure proper healing of the sternum.[3]

After an acute myocardial infarction, patients can engage in weight lifting activity as early as 4 to 6 weeks after the event. In 1 study, RT combined with aerobic exercise was implemented in patients 6 weeks after an myocardial infarction and an improvement in strength was seen with no adverse events.[38]

Although very intense RT can temporarily increase the BP substantially, such increases are not seen when RT is performed with proper technique and avoidance of Valsalva maneuver in the CR setting. Even for those with controlled hypertension, no adverse events were observed when RT was performed at low to moderate intensity.[39]

Many older patients who enter CR may have comorbidities such as osteoporosis, neuropathy, arthritis, or complications from prior stroke. Although individuals with comorbid conditions are at an increased risk for physical complications, they can still benefit from RT. With appropriate guidance, the RT program can be adapted to accommodate patients with physical limitations.[3]

PRESCRIPTION OF RESISTANCE TRAINING IN OLDER CARDIAC REHABILITATION PATIENTS

The critical components of RT prescription include intensity, frequency, type, and the number of sets and repetitions. The primary types of RT are weight lifting stations, free weights, wall pulleys, resistance bands, and weight cuffs/hand weights[3] (**Table 1**).

Once RT is initiated, proper technique and progression need to be prioritized. Initially, patients should perform single-set of 8 to 10 lifts per station at least twice a

Table 1
Types of RT

	Advantages	Disadvantages
Weight lifting machines	Low risk of injury with proper technique Able to target specific muscle groups Proper form fostered by going through a machine dictated range of motion Requires less counseling	More expensive Space consuming or requires facility membership Range of motion is not individualized and is dictated by the constraints of the machine May not be appropriate for individuals who are on the extremes for body habitus Not versatile (each station is muscle group specific) Machine may allow for dominate limb to compensate for strength deficiencies in the other limb Requires maintenance/repairs
Free weights	Relatively compact Allows for free range of motion Requires engaging axillary stabilizing muscles Versatile (same equipment can be used for multiple exercises) Exercise can be more functional (recreating everyday activities)	May cause injury if weight is mishandled May be difficult to target specific muscle groups without adjunct equipment (ie, bench) Need to master proper form Requires more counseling
Resistance bands	Inexpensive Portable, compact Allows for free range of motion Requires engaging axillary stabilizing muscles Low risk of equipment being mishandled Versatile	May not provide a sufficient resistance for some muscle groups. With repeated use, bands lose resistance Bands need to be replaced when broken Need to master proper form
Resistance balls, sand bags	Inexpensive Portable, relatively compact Allows for free range of motion Requires engaging axillary stabilizing muscles	Difficult to target specific muscle groups May not provide an adequate resistance for some muscle groups
Individual's body weight	No expense Portable Allows for free range of motion Requires engaging axillary stabilizing muscles	May not provide an adequate resistance for some muscle groups Need to master proper form Difficult to target specific muscle groups

week and strength intensity should be 30% to 40% of 1-RM in the upper body and 50% to 60% of 1-RM in the legs and hips.[3,40] Participants should work to a perceived exertion of 11 to 14 (fairly light to somewhat hard) on the Borg scale.[2] Periodically during the workout, heart rate, BP, and perceived exertion should be assessed. If adverse signs or symptoms such as dizziness, angina equivalent, and heart rhythm irregularities occur, RT should be temporarily terminated.

As the individual adapts, parameters can be advanced to further facilitate improvement. Once the upper limit of a prescribed repetition range is achieved, for example, 10 to 12 repetitions, resistance or weight load can be increased up to 80% of 1-RM.

Typically, this translates to increases of 2 to 5 lb for arm exercises and 5 to 10 lb for leg exercises.[3] Over time, the prescription can include multiple set programs to ensure all major muscle groups are being trained. For many older people in CR, RT is often a new form of exercise and should be counseled as to when it is appropriate to make these changes.

SUMMARY

Many patients entering CR are older with diminished muscle mass and reduced strength and functional capacity. RT can play a pivotal role because it enhances muscular strength and exercise capacity, allowing for improvement in physical function and quality of life. The benefits of RT are distinct yet complementary to aerobic exercise. Under appropriate guidance and supervision, RT is safe and can be implemented with minimal adverse events in the CR setting. It is, therefore, a safe and effective way to improve exercise capacity, ameliorate cardiovascular risk factors, and reduce disability in older CR patients.

REFERENCES

1. Available at: https://www.heart.org/-/media/data-import/downloadables/heart-disease-and-stroke-statistics-2018—at-a-glance-ucm_498848.pdf. Accessed February 5, 2019.
2. Williams MA, Stewart KJ. Impact of strength and resistance training on cardiovascular disease risk factors and outcomes in older adults. Clin Geriatr Med 2009; 25(4):703–14.
3. Williams MA, Haskell WL, Ades PA, et al. Resistance exercise in individuals with and without cardiovascular disease: 2007 update: a scientific statement from the American Heart Association Council on Clinical Cardiology and Council on Nutrition, Physical Activity, and Metabolism. Circulation 2007;116:572–84.
4. Singh M, Alexander K, Roger VL, et al. Frailty and its potential relevance to cardiovascular care. Mayo Clin Proc 2008;83(10):1146–53.
5. Fried LP, Tangen CM, Walston J, et al. Frailty in older adults: evidence for a phenotype. J Gerontol A Biol Sci Med Sci 2001;56:M146–56.
6. Afilalo J, Karunananthan S, Eisenberg MJ, et al. Role of frailty in patients with cardiovascular disease. Am J Cardiol 2009;103(11):1616–21.
7. Fiatarone MA, O'Neill EF, Ryan ND, et al. Exercise training and nutritional supplementation for physical frailty in very elderly people. N Engl J Med 1994;330: 1769–75.
8. Serra-Rexach JA, Bustamante-Ara N, Hierro Villarán M, et al. Short-term, light- to moderate-intensity exercise training improves leg muscle strength in the oldest old: a randomized controlled trial. J Am Geriatr Soc 2011;59:594–602.
9. Sullivan DH, Roberson PK, Smith ES, et al. Effects of muscle strength training and megestrol acetate on strength, muscle mass, and function in frail older people. J Am Geriatr Soc 2007;55:20–8.
10. Brochu M, Savage PD, Lee M, et al. Effects of resistance training on physical function in older disabled women with coronary heart disease. J Appl Physiol (1985) 2002;92:672–8.
11. Ades PA, Savage PD, Cress ME, et al. Resistance training on physical performance in disabled older female cardiac patients. Med Sci Sports Exerc 2003; 35:1265–70.

12. Tucker WJ, Haykowsky MH, Seo Y, et al. Impaired exercise tolerance in heart failure: role of skeletal muscle morphology and function. Curr Heart Fail Rep 2018; 15:323–31.
13. Palevo G, Keteyian SJ, Kang M, et al. Resistance exercise training improves heart function and physical fitness in stable patients with heart failure. J Cardiopulm Rehabil Prev 2009;29:294–8.
14. Levinger I, Bronks R, Cody DV, et al. The effect of resistance training on left ventricular function and structure of patients with chronic heart failure. Int J Cardiol 2005;105:159–63.
15. Pu CT, Johnson MT, Forman DE, et al. Randomized trial of progressive resistance training to counteract the myopathy of chronic heart failure. J Appl Physiol (1985) 2001;90:2341–50.
16. Savage PA, Shaw AO, Miller MS, et al. Effect of resistance training on physical disability in chronic heart failure. Med Sci Sports Exerc 2011;43(8):1379–86.
17. Selig SE, Carey MF, Menzies DG, et al. Moderate-intensity resistance exercise training in patients with chronic heart failure improves strength, endurance, heart rate variability, and forearm blood flow. J Card Fail 2004;10(1):21–30.
18. Kitzman DW, Nicklas B, Kraus WE, et al. Skeletal muscle abnormalities and exercise intolerance in older patients with heart failure and preserved ejection fraction. Am J Physiol Heart Circ Physiol 2014;306(9):H1364–70.
19. Khadanga S, Savage PD, Ades PA. Insulin resistance and diabetes mellitus in contemporary cardiac rehabilitation. J Cardiopulm Rehabil Prev 2016;36:331–8.
20. Cauza E, Hanusch-Enserer U, Strasser B, et al. Strength and endurance training lead to different postexercise glucose profiles in diabetic participants using a continuous subcutaneous glucose monitoring system. Eur J Clin Invest 2005; 35:745–75.
21. Sigal RJ, Kenny GP, Boule NG, et al. Effects of aerobic training, resistance training, or both on glycemic control in type 2 diabetes: a randomized trial. Ann Intern Med 2007;147:357–69.
22. Grontved A, Rimm E, Willet W. A prospective study of weight training and risk of type 2 diabetes mellitus in men. Arch Intern Med 2012;172(17):1306–12.
23. Kelley GA, Kelley KS. Progressive resistance exercise and resting blood pressure: a meta-analysis of randomized controlled trials. Hypertension 2000;35: 838–43.
24. Cornelissen VA, Fagard RH. Effect of resistance training on resting blood pressure: a meta-analysis of randomized controlled trials. J Hypertens 2005;23: 251–9.
25. Stewart KJ, Bacher AC, Turner KL, et al. Effect of exercise on blood pressure in older persons: a randomized controlled trial. Arch Intern Med 2005;165:756–62.
26. Stewart KJ, Bacher AC, Turner K, et al. Exercise and risk factors associated with metabolic syndrome in older adults. Am J Prev Med 2005;28:9–18.
27. Hagerman FC, Walsh SJ, Staron RS, et al. Effects of high-intensity resistance training on untrained older men. I. Strength, cardiovascular, and metabolic responses. J Gerontol A Biol Sci Med Sci 2000;55:B336–46.
28. Elliott KJ, Sale C, Cable NT. Effects of resistance training and detraining on muscle strength and blood lipid profiles in postmenopausal women. Br J Sports Med 2002;36:340–4.
29. Ades PA, Savage PD, Harvey-Berino J. The treatment of obesity in cardiac rehabilitation. J Cardiopulm Rehabil Prev 2010;30(5):289–98.

30. Hunter GR, Bryan DR, Wetzstein CJ, et al. Resistance training and intra-abdominal adipose tissue in older men and women. Med Sci Sports Exerc 2002;34:1023–8.
31. Ades PA, Ballor DL, Ashikaga T, et al. Weight training improves walking endurance in healthy elderly persons. Ann Intern Med 1996;124:568–72.
32. Hollings M, Mavros Y, Freeston J, et al. The effect of progressive resistance training on aerobic fitness and strength in adults with coronary heart disease: a systematic review and meta-analysis of randomized controlled trials. Eur J Prev Cardiol 2017;24(12):1242–59.
33. Ozaki H, Loenneke JP, Thiebaud RS, et al. Resistance training induced increase in VO_2max in young and older subjects. Eur Rev Aging Phys Act 2013;10:107.
34. Beniamini Y, Rubenstein JJ, Faigenbaum AD, et al. High-intensity strength training of patients enrolled in an outpatient cardiac rehabilitation program. J Cardiopulm Rehabil 1999;19:8–17.
35. McCartney N, McKelvie RS, Haslam DR, et al. Usefulness of weightlifting training in improving strength and maximal power output in coronary artery disease. Am J Cardiol 1991;67:939–45.
36. Beniamini Y, Rubenstein JJ, Zaichkowsky LD, et al. Effects of high intensity strength training on quality of life parameters in cardiac rehabilitation patients. Am J Cardiol 1997;80(7):841–6.
37. Stewart KJ, Williams MA. Safety and efficacy of weight training soon after acute myocardial infarction. J Cardiopulm Rehabil 1998;18(1):37–44.
38. Gordon NF, Kohl HW, Pollock ML, et al. Cardiovascular safety of maximal strength testing in healthy adults. Am J Cardiol 1995;76:851–3.
39. Haslam DR, McCartney SN, McKelvie RS, et al. Direct measurements of arterial blood pressure during formal weightlifting in cardiac patients. J Cardiopulm Rehabil 1988;8:213–25.
40. American College of Sports Medicine. ACSM's guidelines for exercise testing and prescription. Philadelphia: Lippincott Williams & Wilkins; 2018.

High-Intensity Interval Training in Cardiac Rehabilitation

Yaoshan Dun, MD, PhD[a,b], Joshua R. Smith, PhD[b], Suixin Liu, MD, PhD[a,*], Thomas P. Olson, PhD[b,*]

KEYWORDS

- Interval training • Cardiac rehabilitation • Peak oxygen uptake • Cardiovascular disease • Exercise prescription • Old age • Frailty

KEY POINTS

- High-intensity interval training has been shown to result in greater improvements in peak oxygen uptake (Vo_2) when compared with moderate-intensity continuous training for patients at high risk of developing and those with overt cardiovascular disease (CVD).
- The presence of CVD and frailty increases with advanced age. High-intensity interval training has shown positive effects in improving cardiovascular outcomes and frailty in older adults.
- High-intensity interval training can be prescribed using a combination of objective and subjective measures of exercise intensity with similar results for older patients with CVD in cardiac rehabilitation settings.
- Multisystem integrative physiologic adaptations in respiratory, cardiovascular, and skeletal muscle systems induced by high-intensity interval training contribute to improvements in peak Vo_2.

INTRODUCTION

Comprehensive exercise-based cardiac rehabilitation (CR) is a secondary prevention tool used worldwide to improve prognosis in patients with various forms of cardiovascular disease (CVD). A key component of a comprehensive CR program is exercise training, which has been shown to reduce the incidence of falls[1] and mortality as well as improve quality of life, frailty, and cardiovascular fitness (defined as peak

Disclosure Statement: This work was supported by the National Institutes of Health (HL126638) and Human Development and Reform Commission Foundation of China (Grant no. [2012] 1521).

[a] Division of Cardiac Rehabilitation, Department of Physical Medicine and Rehabilitation, Xiangya Hospital Central South University, 87 Xiangya Road, Changsha, Hunan, P.R. China; [b] Division of Preventive Cardiology, Department of Cardiovascular Medicine, Mayo Clinic, 200 First Street Southwest, Rochester, MN 55905, USA
* Corresponding authors.
E-mail addresses: liusuixin@csu.edu.cn (S.L.); olson.thomas2@mayo.edu (T.P.O.)

Clin Geriatr Med 35 (2019) 469–487
https://doi.org/10.1016/j.cger.2019.07.011

oxygen uptake [V_{O_2}]), which is an independent predictor of hospitalizations and mortality in patients with CVD.[2] Moderate-intensity continuous training (MICT) has traditionally been a foundation of aerobic-based exercise prescription resulting in short- and long-term clinical benefits for patients with CVD.[3]

High-intensity interval training (HIIT) has recently emerged as an alternative or adjunct strategy to MICT and has been shown to result in similar or greater improvements in peak V_{O_2} compared with MICT.[4] Specifically, HIIT has been found to be as effective, if not superior, to MICT with respect to improving clinical outcomes for older patients with CVD, including quality of life (QoL),[5] heart rate (HR) response to exercise,[6] and myocardial function.[7] Importantly, HIIT also seems to be as safe as MICT for older patients with CR.[8,9] HIIT involves repeated bouts of relatively higher-intensity exercise interspersed with periods of lower-intensity recovery.[10] Unfortunately, to date, there is no clear consensus on the optimal HIIT prescriptive variables that elicit the greatest benefits for patients at high risk of or with overt CVD.

The most common uncertainties surrounding the prescription and implementation of HIIT for older patients with CVD include the specific exercise intensity for the high and low intervals, durations and ratio of high and low intervals, the method to prescribe exercise intensity (eg, percentage of peak HR, rating of perceived exertion, etc.), and patient safety. This review discusses the principles of HIIT prescription and provides suggestions for the prescribing of HIIT for patients with CVD in the CR setting. Further, the authors discuss specific HIIT considerations in relation to frailty, falls, and other risks associated with older age in patients with CVD; the physiologic mechanisms by which HIIT contributes to improvements in peak V_{O_2}; and finally, the impact and safety of HIIT in older patients with coronary artery disease(CAD) and heart failure (HF) in the CR setting.

GENERAL PRINCIPLES AND SPECIFIC CONSIDERATIONS FOR PRESCRIBING HIGH-INTENSITY INTERVAL TRAINING FOR OLDER ADULTS WITH CARDIOVASCULAR DISEASE

Common Methods for Prescribing the Intensity of High-Intensity Interval Training

The American College of Sports Medicine provides guidance on objective and subjective methods for prescribing exercise intensity, which results in improvements in peak V_{O_2},[11] some of which have been used to prescribe HIIT for older patients with CR with CVD.[6,12–14] The most common objective metrics include the HR measured at peak exercise (peak HR), peak V_{O_2}, and metabolic equivalents (METs). Subjective measures that are commonly used include the Borg rating of perceived exertion (RPE, Borg: 6–20) and the perceived dyspnea on exertion (DoE: 0–10) scales. For patients with CVD, the methodology used to measure these objective and subjective measurements have been discussed previously.[11] In this section, the authors discuss the advantages and disadvantages of these objective and subjective methods for prescribing exercise intensity during HIIT in older patients with CR. In addition, they propose a guide for prescribing intensity for HIIT in older patients with CR.

Peak V_{O_2} is the gold-standard measure of exercise capacity and/or physical fitness. In addition, peak HR is a widely used metric to prescribe exercise intensity due to its relative ease of acquisition. The percentage of peak V_{O_2} and peak HR methods for determining optimal exercise intensity during HIIT are the most widely researched and have the most robust evidence supporting their efficacy[12,15,16]; however, known limitations exist for using percentage of peak V_{O_2} and peak HR. First, patients entering into CR who undergo baseline exercise stress testing may not reach a true maximum HR or V_{O_2} due to early termination of the exercise stress test for a variety of reasons including heightened symptomology, early onset of peripheral fatigue, and/or anxiety.[17,18] In addition, some patients with CR may have conditions for which maximal exercise stress testing may be contraindicated and thus only perform submaximal exercise testing because of specific clinical conditions such as advanced HF, known obstructive left main coronary artery stenosis, and moderate to severe aortic stenosis.[17,18] Second, a large proportion of patients in CR are prescribed rate modulating pharmacotherapy (eg, beta-blocker medication), which blunts the HR response at rest and during exercise and may lead to lower peak HR and Vo_2 values during the exercise stress test.[19] Third, not all CR centers are equipped with cardiopulmonary exercise testing equipment, which would preclude the direct measurement of peak Vo_2. Finally, peak HR prediction equations (eg, 220-age) can underestimate or overestimate measured peak HR[20–22] leading to an inappropriate prescription of exercise intensity for exercise training purposes.

Although there are several considerations when using percentage of peak Vo_2 and peak HR for prescribing exercise intensity, they are the most widely used methods to prescribe exercise intensity for HIIT in older patients with CR.[12,15,16] Specifically, 2 recent multicenter randomized controlled trials, the Study of Aerobic Interval Exercise Training in CAD patients (SAINTEX-CAD, mean age: 58 $\pm$ 9 years)[5] and the Study of Myocardial Recovery after Exercise Training in Heart Failure (SMARTEX-HF, age range: 58–68 years),[15] used percentage of peak HR (ie, 90%–95% peak HR) to prescribe exercise intensity for HIIT. These studies found that although HIIT resulted in improved peak Vo_2 (~23%), not all patients were able to maintain the prescribed exercise intensity[5,15] (ie, 51% of the patients in the HIIT group exercised at a lower intensity than prescribed[15]). As a result, supplementary strategies may be advantageous to optimize exercise intensity prescription during HIIT in the CR setting particularly in older adults who may present with additional comorbidities and/or musculoskeletal concerns.

The RPE (6–20) and DoE scales (0–10) are the 2 most common subjective methods used to prescribe exercise intensity[23–25] and recent studies highlight the practical importance of incorporating subjective measures of intensity for older adults in the CR setting.[5,15] Previous studies have shown that RPE is significantly related to HR, ventilation, and Vo_2 in patients with HF,[23,25] CAD, and atrial fibrillation[24] and is not influenced by beta-blocker mediation.[25] The European Association for Cardiovascular Prevention and Rehabilitation, American Association of Cardiovascular and Pulmonary Rehabilitation (AACVPR), and Canadian Association of Cardiac Rehabilitation have published a joint position statement[10] recommending the use of RPE and DoE scales as the primary prescription tool for exercise intensity or as an adjunct to objective measures in CR. Iellamo and colleagues[23] demonstrated that RPE is an easy-to-use and validated method for prescription of intensity in HIIT. In contrast, Aamot and colleagues[26] recently demonstrated that when RPE was solely used in CR the exercise intensity was less than the target intensity during the HIIT bouts, suggesting that the combination of both an objective and a subjective metric may be needed to prescribe exercise intensity for HIIT in older adults with CVD. In an attempt to provide clinicians and researchers with a framework for implementation of HIIT in CR, where most of the participants are older patients with CVD, the authors recommend using a combination of objective and subjective measures to prescribe exercise intensity of HIIT. Specifically, the breadth of literature supports a protocol that prescribes high-intensity intervals at an exercise intensity between 85% and 95% peak HR and RPE between 15 and 17 (Borg) and low-intensity intervals at 50% to 75% peak HR and RPE between 12 and 14 (Borg) with differing high- and low-intensity interval durations that depend on the patient's level of deconditioning, symptomology, disease severity, and comorbidity burden. While using objective and subjective measures to prescribe exercise intensity, there may be instances when discrepancies can occur between peak HR and RPE (eg, peak HR is <85%, but RPE is >15). In this case, the authors recommend using RPE as the primary method because of limitations associated with peak HR and to optimize patient adherence to HIIT in the CR setting.

Older patients with CVD present with predictable complexity that makes specific considerations necessary when HIIT is prescribed in the CR setting. Specifically, older patients may exhibit frailty, multimorbidity, impaired balance and cognition, as well as other liabilities with age.[1] As a result, the approach to HIIT may need to be modified to best accommodate these factors and to facilitate HIIT adherence in this population. The primary strategies to alter the HIIT protocol are by modifying the exercise modality (especially for patients with musculoskeletal conditions and higher risk of falling) and using subjective measures to prescribe exercise intensity (ie, RPE) to a greater extent than objective measures.

Short-, Medium-, and Long-Interval High-Intensity Interval Trainings for Older Patients with Cardiovascular Disease

The duration and ratio of high-intensity and low-intensity intervals are key parameters that differentiate HIIT from MICT and contribute to the HIIT-enhanced physiologic response and health benefits.[27,28] There are 3 classic categories for HIIT used for competitive sports that differ in both duration and exercise intensity: long, medium, and short. Each category of HIIT protocols elicit specific physiologic responses and can be sports specific[29,30] (**Table 1**). Interval training for patients with CVD in CR settings is often termed HIIT or aerobic interval training and defined as "near-maximal" efforts generally performed at an intensity less than peak V_{O_2} or peak power output that elicits greater than or equal to 80% peak HR (often in the range of 85%–95%). For many deconditioned individuals, this may be similar to that encountered during activities of daily living.[31] There are also 3 types of HIIT protocols widely used in patients with CVD with varying durations of the high- and low-intensity intervals, whereas the exercise intensity is typically constant at 85% to 95% peak V_{O_2} or peak HR (see **Table 1**).

Long-interval HIIT is the most widely used protocol for older patients with CVD, and this may include 4 sets of high-intensity intervals, each lasting 4 minutes interspersed with 3 sets of low-intensity intervals, each lasting 3 minutes.[4–6,12,13,32–34] Medium-interval HIITs, such as 8 $\times$ 2 minute high-intensity intervals interspersed with 7 $\times$ 2 minute low-intensity intervals, have also been used, albeit to a lesser extent, in older patients with CVD.[35] For older patients with HF with reduced ejection fraction (HFrEF, NYHA II-III), medium- and short-interval protocols have been used[14,15,36] such as 10 $\times$ 1 minute high-intensity intervals interspersed with 9 $\times$ 2 minute low-intensity intervals. All 3 protocols are safe and contribute to significant improvements in peak V_{O_2} and QoL.[5,6,8,9,15] At this time, there are no studies that have compared long-, medium-, and short-interval HIIT in patients with CVD to determine the most appropriate duration. However, a recent meta-analysis found that long-interval HIIT may elicit greater improvements in peak V_{O_2} compared with short-interval HIIT.[37] However, as previous studies have found, some older patients with CVD newly enrolled in CR may not be able to maintain the long intervals at high intensity. Thus, over the course of CR, health care providers or clinical exercise physiologists may recommend patients with CR to begin with short-, then progress to medium, and finally progress to long intervals as they accumulate the benefits of exercise training and increase their exercise tolerance.

Table 1
Short-, medium-, and long-interval high-intensity interval trainings for athletes and older patients with cardiovascular disease

	Interval Duration Category	Duration (High/Low Intervals)	Intensity	Ratio of Interval Duration	Key Goals or Benefits
Athletes[29,30]	Long	3–15/3–15 min	85%–90% peak HR or peak Vo_2	1:1	Improving functions of aerobic metabolism system
	Medium	1–3/1–3 min	95%–100% peak HR or peak Vo_2	1:1	Improving functions of anaerobic and aerobic metabolism systems
	Short	10–60/10–60 s	100%–120% peak HR or peak Vo_2	1:1	Improving function of ATP-CP system
Older Patients with CVD	Long	3–4/3–4 min	85%–95% peak HR or peak Vo_2	1:1	VO_2peak, V_E/VCO_2, VAT, QoL[4–6,12,13,32–34]
	Medium	1–2/1–4 min	85%–95% peak HR or peak Vo_2	1:1–4	VO_2peak, Vo_2/Pulse, QoL[15,35,66]
	Short	15–60/15–120 s	85%–95% peak HR or peak Vo_2	1:1–8	VO_2peak, Vo_2/Pulse[14,27,28,68]

Abbreviations: ATP-CP, adenosine triphosphate-creatine phosphate; VAT, ventilatory anaerobic threshold; VCO_2 volume of carbon dioxide produced; V_E, ventilation; VO_2, volume of oxygen consumed.

As detailed in **Fig. 1**, based on the evidence described, the authors propose the use of short-interval protocols for patients with CVD with low exercise capacity (<5 METs) or in the beginning stage of CR (0–4 weeks) and the use of medium- or long-interval protocols for patients with CVD with intermediate or high exercise capacity (≥5 METs) as well as for those in the improvement (4–12 weeks) and maintenance stages (>12 weeks) of CR (see **Fig. 1**).

PHYSIOLOGIC MECHANISMS BY WHICH HIGH-INTENSITY INTERVAL TRAINING CONTRIBUTES TO IMPROVED PEAK VO_2

Despite compelling evidence that HIIT is a useful strategy to improve peak VO_2 in individuals with and without CVD,[12,37] the specific mechanisms underpinning the increased peak VO_2 in these patients have not been well documented. Peak VO_2 is

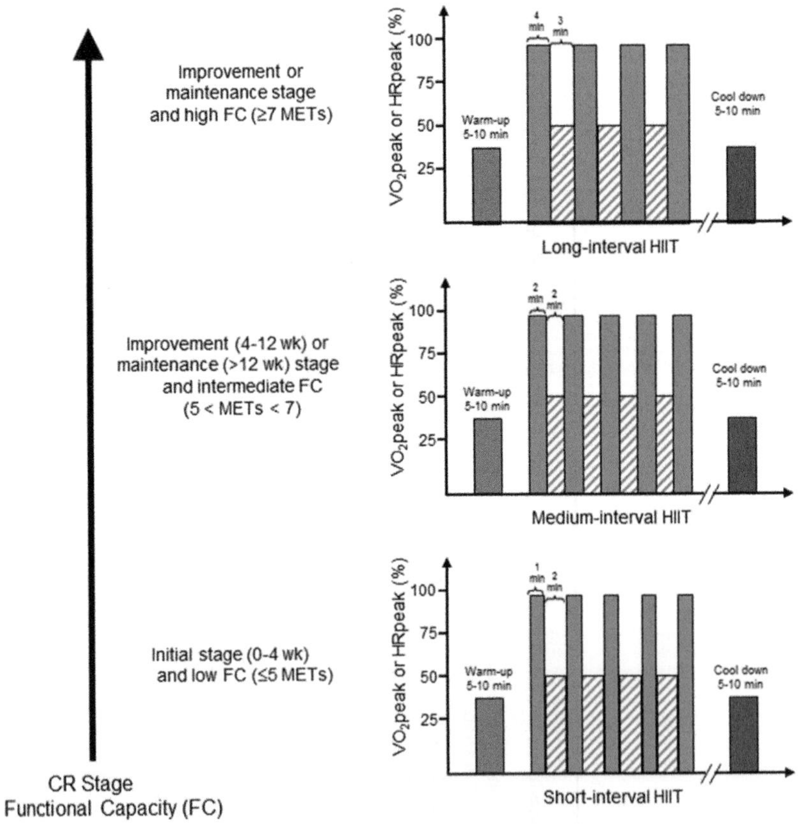

Fig. 1. Principles of HIIT prescription and progression. Examples of long-, medium-, and short-interval HIITs. The short-interval HIIT may be appropriate for patients with CVD with low functional capacity (<5 METs) or in the initiation stage of CR (0–4 weeks), and the medium- or long-interval HIIT protocols may be recommended for patients with CVD with intermediate or high functional capacity (≥5 METs) and in the improvement (4–12 weeks) and/or maintenance stages (>12 week) of CR. The exercise intensity is constant for each of these HIIT protocols with the high- and low-intensity intervals eliciting 85% to 95% peak HR at RPE of 15% to 17% and 50% to 75% peak HR at RPE of 12% to 14%, respectively. FC, functional capacity.

primarily determined by the systems that transport and use oxygen, including the respiratory (oxygen uptake from the atmosphere), heart (oxygen transport), peripheral vasculature (oxygen transport, tissue perfusion, tissue diffusion), and skeletal muscle (oxygen extraction and utilization) as highlighted in **Fig. 2**.[18] In this section, the authors review the physiologic adaptations in response to HIIT in terms of these systems.

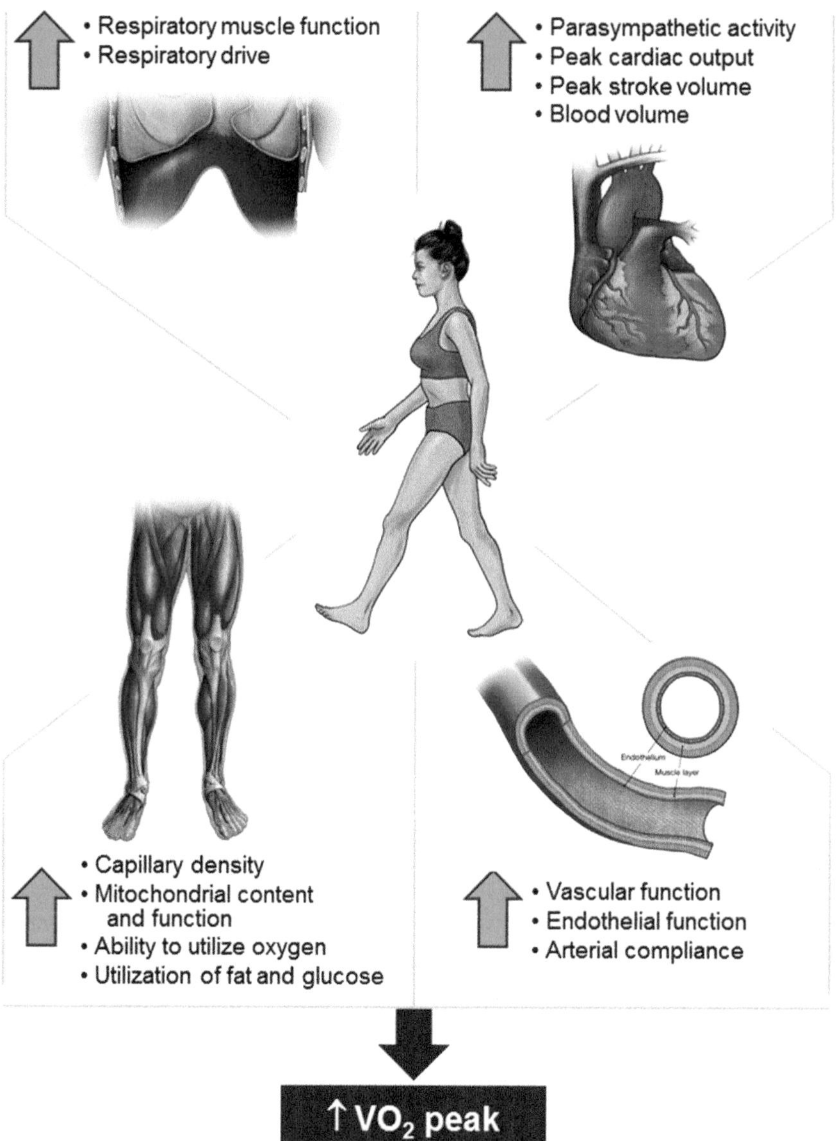

Fig. 2. Key physiologic mechanisms of HIIT for improvement of peak V_{O_2}. This summary figure illustrates the key physiologic systems that contribute to the increased VO_2peak with HIIT. As discussed in the text, HIIT enhances the functions of the respiratory, cardiovascular, and skeletal muscle systems contributing to the improvement in VO_2peak. ()

The Impact of High-Intensity Interval Training on the Respiratory System

Respiratory muscle dysfunction is a common manifestation in patients with CVD, especially older patients with HF, and contributes to exercise intolerance.[38–40] Tasoulis and colleagues[41] demonstrated that 12 weeks of HIIT significantly improved respiratory muscle function in older patients with HF. Moreover, Dunham and Harms[42] demonstrated that 4 weeks of both HIIT and MICT elicited significant increases in respiratory muscle function (HIIT ~43%, MICT ~25%), with a greater increase with HIIT. Furthermore, Tasoulis[41] and Christensen[43] have shown that HIIT improves pulmonary Vo_2 kinetics, ventilatory drive ($P_{0.1}$/PImax), and ventilatory patterns (resting inspiratory flow [V_T/T_I] and V_T/T_I at identical exercise testing workloads) in patients with HF[41] and healthy adults.[43] Thus, HIIT has the potential to improve the pulmonary system's ability to take in oxygen for distribution to working skeletal muscle during exercise. This has important implications for overall exercise capacity/tolerance in older patients undergoing CR.

The Impact of High-Intensity Interval Training on the Cardiovascular System

Peak stroke volume (SV), HR, and cardiac output (CO), as well as blood volume are cardinal parameters that influence peak Vo_2 according to the Fick equation.[44] Astorino and colleagues[45] recently showed that 10 sessions of short-interval HIIT increased peak CO. This finding is supported by previous studies demonstrating that 6 weeks of long-interval HIIT increased resting SV and CO, peak exercise CO, plasma volume, and hemoglobin mass with greater improvement than[46,47] or similar to[48,49] MICT. In addition, resting HR variability (HRV) is a predictor of peak Vo_2 and an independent predictor of all-cause mortality.[50,51] An increase (improvement) in HRV has been identified as one of the early cardiac adaptations in response to exercise training likely due to improvement of intrinsic HR (SA node) and vagal activity (parasympathetic activity).[52,53] Alansare and colleagues[54] demonstrated that 8 sessions of short-interval HIIT are superior to MICT at improving HRV in sedentary adults. These studies suggest that HIIT may have a greater effect on improving cardiovascular and autonomic nervous system function than MICT in sedentary adults; however, additional research is warranted to extend these findings to older patients with CVD in the CR setting. Collectively, HIIT seems to be more effective or at least equivalent to MICT with respect to increasing peak SV, HR, and CO and improving cardiovascular and autonomic nervous system function, which together contributes to improved peak Vo_2.

Flow-mediated dilation (FMD), an indicator of endothelial function, is closely associated with peak Vo_2 where individuals with lower FMD exhibit lower peak Vo_2.[55] Van and colleagues reported that both MICT and HIIT improved peak Vo_2 and FMD in patients with CVD undergoing CR, with a close relationship between the improvement in peak Vo_2 and FMD. A meta-analysis by Ramos[56] reported that 12 weeks of MICT and long-interval HIIT increased brachial artery FMD by 2.15% and 4.31%, respectively, with a greater improvement demonstrated in the HIIT group. Moreover, Mora-Rodriguez and colleagues[57] recently demonstrated that 6 months of long-interval HIIT reduced arterial stiffness in patients with metabolic syndrome. Thus, although the available research suggests that HIIT has the capacity to improve vascular function, more studies are necessary to fully elucidate the impact of HIIT on vascular function in older patients undergoing CR.

The Impact of High-Intensity Interval Training on the Skeletal Muscle System

Skeletal muscle total fiber amount and type proportions, capillary density, mitochondrial content, and function all play a role in regulating the efficiencies of oxygen extraction and utilization of energy substrates, such as fat and glucose, and as a result significantly contribute to exercise tolerance.[58] Early studies investigating the effect of HIIT on skeletal muscle fiber type changes date back 30 years to a landmark study by Simoneau[59] who showed that HIIT significantly increased total muscle fiber quantity and the proportion of type I fibers and decreased the proportion of type IIb fibers, whereas the proportion of type IIa remained unchanged in the vastus lateralis muscle of healthy adults. A recent study by Tan[60] further showed that 18 sessions of short-interval HIIT over 6 weeks increased the total amount of type I and II muscle fibers, capillary density, and the protein expression of cytochrome oxidase IV (a marker of skeletal muscle oxidative capacity) in overweight women. Besides skeletal muscle structure alterations induced by HIIT, several studies also[61–63] demonstrate that HIIT improves skeletal muscle deoxygenation, which indicates oxygen extraction, as well as the content and activity of glucose and fat oxidative metabolism markers in patients with obesity[61,62] and HF.[63] In summary, HIIT is a powerful strategy to improve skeletal muscle total fiber amount and type proportions, capillary density, as well as mitochondrial content and function. However, very few studies have been conducted in this area specific to older patients with CVD, and thus additional research is critical to extend these findings to the older patients in the CR setting.

APPLICATION OF HIGH-INTENSITY INTERVAL TRAINING FOR OLDER PATIENTS WITH CARDIOVASCULAR DISEASE

High-Intensity Interval Training for Older Patients with Cardiovascular Disease

Guiraud and colleagues[64] and Ribeiro and colleagues[65] reviewed the application of HIIT in CR globally and patients with CAD, respectively in 2012 and 2017. To further evaluate the effects of HIIT exclusively in older patients with CAD using recent data, the authors reviewed randomized controlled trials from the last 5 years that compared the effects of HIIT and MICT in older patients with CAD (**Table 2**). All reviewed studies demonstrated that both MICT and HIIT led to improvements in peak Vo_2,[4–6,12,13,32,35] oxygen pulse,[35] ventilatory efficiency (ie, V_E/VCO_2 slope),[35] oxygen uptake efficiency slope,[13,35] QoL,[5] HR recovery,[6] and submaximal HR during cardiopulmonary exercise stress testing.[4]

Of these 7 studies, 4 studies reported a superior effect of HIIT over MICT in improving peak Vo_2[4,6,32] and oxygen pulse.[35] For example, Keteyian and colleagues[4] found that long-interval HIIT and MICT resulted in significant decreases in resting HR, systolic blood pressure, and increases in peak Vo_2 in older patients with CAD, with greater improvements observed in the HIIT group. These results are consistent with the result of Kim and colleagues[6] who demonstrated that the 6 weeks of HIIT resulted in greater increases in peak Vo_2 and HR recovery after exercise in patients with CR with CVD compared with MICT.

Three studies[5,13,32] demonstrated that HIIT and MICT elicited numerous physiologic benefits for patients with CAD to a similar degree. For example, a multicenter randomized controlled trial, SAINTEX-CAD,[5] included 200 older patients with CAD and examined the impact of 12 weeks of either HIIT (4 $\times$ 4 minute at 90%–95% peak HR, with 3-minute active recovery) or MICT (32 minutes at 70%–75% peak HR) on peak Vo_2, peripheral endothelial function, cardiovascular risk factors, and QoL. The improvements in peak Vo_2, endothelial function, QoL, and resting diastolic blood pressure were similar for HIIT and MICT groups.

Collectively, HIIT seems to be more effective or at least equally beneficial compared with MICT in terms of improving peak Vo_2 for older patients with CAD. However, future

Table 2
Study characteristics of randomized control trials comparing high-intensity interval training and moderate-intensity continuous training for older patients with coronary artery disease and heart failure

Author (y)	No. of Randomized Patients (HIIT/MICT)	Age (y) and Sex (Male %) (HIIT/MICT)	Average Exercise Capacity (HIIT/MICT)	Intervention (Frequency/Duration)	HIIT (Intensity/Duration/Mode)	MICT (Intensity/Duration/Mode)	Cardiovascular AEs (HIIT/MICT)	Delta of Main Effects (HIIT vs MICT)
Coronary Artery Disease								
Van De Heyning et al,[12] 2018	100/100	60/57 91/89	NS	F: 3 × wk D: 12 wk	I: 4 × 4 min 85%–95% peak HR Rec: 3 × 3 min 50%–70% HR peak D: 25 min Mode: bicycle	I: 70%–75% peak HR D: 32 min M: bicycle	NS	Peak V_{O_2}: 23% vs 21%.
Prado et al,[13] 2016	17/18	57/61 82/77	Medium/medium	F: 3 × wk D: 12 wk	I: 7 × 3 min VAT Rec: 7 × 3 min RCP D: 42 min Mode: treadmill	I: VAT D: 50 min M: treadmill	NS	Peak V_{O_2}: 25% vs 22%. AT: 14% vs 20%
Conraads et al,[5] 2015	100/100	57/59 91/89	Medium/medium	F: 3 × wk D: 12 wk	I: 4 × 4 min 90%–95% peak HR Rec: 3 × 3 min 50%–70% HR peak D: 38 min Mode: bicycle	I: 70%–75% peak HR D: 30 min M: bicycle	No AEs during training sessions MICT: 1 AMI, after the last session (PCI was performed; 2 significant ST-depression during the exercise test at 6 wk (2 PCI performed)	V_{O_2} peak: 23% vs 20%. No effect on BP

Cardozo et al,[35] 2015	23/24	56/62 63/66	Medium/medium	F: 3 × wk D: 16 wk	I: 2 min × 90% peak HR Rec: 2 min at 60% peak HR D: 30 min Mode: treadmill	I: 70%–75% HR peak D: 30 min M: treadmill	0/0	Peak V_{O_2}: 18% vs 0.5%. No effect on BP
Kim et al,[6] 2015	14/14	57/60 86/71	High/high	F: 3 × wk D: 6 wk	I: 4 × 4 min 85%–95% HRR Rec: 3 × 3 min 50%–70% HRR D: 25 min Mode: treadmill	I: 70%–85% HRR D: 25 min M: treadmill	0/0	Peak V_{O_2}: 22% vs 9%
Madssen et al,[32] 2014	15/21	56/60 93/71	High/high	F: 3 × wk D: 12 wk	I: 4 × 4 min 85%–95% peak HR Rec: 3 × 3 min 70% peak HR D: 28 min Mode: treadmill	I: 60% peak HR D: 46 min M: treadmill	HIIT: cerebral hemorrhage	PEAK V_{O_2}: 11% vs 7%
Keteyian et al,[4] 2014	21/18	60/58 73/92	Low/low	F: 3 × wk D: 10 wk	I: 4 × 4 min 80%–90% HRR Rec: 3 × 3 min 60%–70% HRR D: 25 min Mode: treadmill	I: 60%–80% HRR D: 30 min M: treadmill	1 keen pain (HIIT) 1 leg pain (MICT) No events that required hospitalization during or within 3 h after exercise	Peak V_{O_2}: 16% vs 8%. AT: 21% vs 5% No effect on BP

(*continued on next page*)

Table 2 *(continued)*

Author (y)	No. of Randomized Patients (HIIT/MICT)	Age (y) and Sex (Male %) (HIIT/MICT)	Average Exercise Capacity (HIIT/MICT)	Intervention (Frequency/Duration)	HIIT (Intensity/Duration/Mode)	MICT (Intensity/Duration/Mode)	Cardiovascular AEs (HIIT/MICT)	Delta of Main Effects (HIIT vs MICT)
Heart failure								
Ellingsen et al,[15] 2017	77/65	65/65 82/81 EF: 29/29 NYHA: II-III	Low/low	F: 3 × wk D: 12 wk	I: 4 × 4 min 90%–95% peak HR Rec: 3 × 3 min 60%–70% peak HR D: 25 min Mode: bicycle	I: 60%–70% peak HR D: 32 min M: bicycle	HIIT: 2 ventricular arrhythmia, 4 worsening HF, 3 other cardiovascular events MICT: 1 fatal cardiovascular event, 1 ventricular arrhythmia, 3 worsening HF, 1 other cardiovascular event	Peak Vo_2: 8% vs 5%. LVEF: 2% vs −2%
Ulbrich et al,[66] 2016	12/10	53/54 100/100 NYHA: II-III	Medium/medium	F: 3 × wk D: 12 wk	I: 6 × 3 min ~ 90% peak HR Rec: 5 × 3 min 50% peak HR D: 33 min Mode: treadmill	I: 70%–75% peak HR D: 40 min M: treadmill	NS	Peak Vo_2: 11% vs 8%.
Benda et al,[14] 2015	10/10	63/64 90/100 EF: 37%/38% NYHA: II-III	Medium/medium	F: 3 × wk D: 12 wk	I: 10 × 1 min 90% PPO peak (RPE 15–17) Rec: 9 × 2.5 min 30% PPO D: 35 min Mode: bicycle	I: 60%–70% HR PPO (RPE 12–14) D: 30 min M: bicycle	NS	Peak Vo_2: 7% vs 1%.

Angadi et al,[33] 2015	9/6	69/71 89/50 HFpEF	Medium/medium	F: 3 × wk D: 4 wk	I: 4 × 4 min 85%–90% peak HR Rec: 3 × 3 min 30%–50% peak HR D: 25 min Mode: treadmill	I: 70% peak HR D: 40 min M: treadmill	No AEs during exercise	Peak Vo_2: 9% vs 0%.
Dall et al,[36] 2015	16/16	51/51 75/75 Heart transplant	Medium/medium	F: 3 × wk D: 12 wk	I: 4, 2, 4, 2 plus 4 × 1 min >80% Vo_2 peak Rec: 7 × 2 min 70% peak Vo_2 D: 30 min Mode: bicycle	I: 60% peak HR D: 45 min M: bicycle	NS	Peak Vo_2: 21% vs 11%
Koufaki et al,[34] 2014	16/17	60/60 88/76 EF: 42/35 NYHA: II-III	Low/low	F: 3 × wk D: 12 wk	I: 4 × 4 min 90%–95% peak HR Rec: 3 × 3 min 50%–70% peak HR D: 38 min Mode: bicycle	I: 60%–70% peak HR D: 47 min M: bicycle	NS	Peak Vo_2: 13% vs 13%.

Abbreviations: AE, adverse event; BP, blood pressure; EF, ejection fraction; NS: data not shown; NYHA, New York Heart Association classification; PPO: peak power output; RCP: respiratory compensation point; RPE, rating of perceived exertion (Borg 6-20 scale); VAT, ventilatory anaerobic threshold; Vo_2, volume of oxygen consumed.

Exercise capacities were classified as low, medium, and high levels according to the stratification for cardiac events during exercise participation exercise risk classification guidelines of ACCVPR, low level, METs $\leq$5; medium level, 5< METs < 7; high level, METs $\geq$7; 1 MET = 3.5 mL/kg/min oxygen uptake.

studies are needed to determine the long-term effect of HIIT on mortality, morbidity, rehospitalization, and recurrent MI in older patients with CAD.

High-Intensity Interval Training for Older Patients with Heart Failure

The authors reviewed randomized controlled trials for the last 5 years that compared the effects of HIIT and MICT in older patients with HF (see **Table 2**). Among all reviewed studies, 4 studies recruited patients with HF with HFrEF,[14,15,34,66] one study recruited patients with HF with preserved ejection fraction (HFpEF),[33] and one study recruited heart transplant patients.[36]

With respect to patients with HFrEF, a multicenter randomized controlled trial, SMARTEX-HF,[15] included 210 older patients with HFrEF and examined the impact of 12 weeks of either HIIT (4 × 4 minute at 90%–95% peak HR, with 3-minute active recovery) or MICT (32 minutes at 60%–70% peak HR) on left ventricular end-diastolic diameter (LVEDD) and peak V_{O_2}. The investigators report a significant decrease in LVEDD and increase in peak V_{O_2} in both HIIT and MICT groups compared with the control group from pre- to posttraining, with no differences between the HIIT and MICT groups.

In patients with HFpEF, Angadi and colleagues[33] compared the effects of 4 weeks of HIIT (4 × 4 min at 85%–90% peak HR, with 3-minute active recovery) versus MICT (30 min at 70% peak HR) on peak V_{O_2}, left ventricular diastolic dysfunction, and endothelial function in older patients with HFpEF. HIIT improved peak V_{O_2} and left ventricular diastolic dysfunction, whereas no changes were observed following MICT.

In heart transplant patients, Dall and colleagues[36] used a randomized controlled crossover trial to study the impact of 12 weeks of HIIT and MICT on peak V_{O_2}, endothelial function, arterial stiffness, QoL, anxiety, depression, and biomarkers, such as glucose, insulin, IL-6, and adiponectin. There were significant improvements in peak V_{O_2}, SF-36 physical function score and depression score in HIIT compared with MICT. In contrast, arterial stiffness, biomarkers, and endothelial function did not change following HIIT or MICT.

In summary, HIIT can elicit numerous physiologic benefits in older patients with HF, such as peak V_{O_2}, QoL, left ventricular diastolic function, and endothelial function. However, future large prospective studies are needed to determine if HIIT is superior to MICT with respect to different types of patients with HF (ie, HFrEF, HFpEF, and patients following heart transplant).

SAFETY CONSIDERATIONS OF USING HIGH-INTENSITY INTERVAL TRAINING FOR OLDER PATIENTS WITH CARDIOVASCULAR DISEASE IN CARDIAC REHABILITATION SETTINGS

The safety of HIIT for clinical populations is an important topic, especially for older patients with CVD in whom the potential for adverse events is heighted.[67] It must be noted that HIIT protocols have been modified for clinical populations to include less strenuous exercise intensities (ie, usually 85%–95% of HRpeak) compared with those used for athletes. Rognmo and colleagues[9] examined the risk of cardiovascular events during HIIT and MICT among 4846 patients with CR with CVD (mean age of 58 years). These investigators report only 1 fatal cardiac arrest during MICT and 2 nonfatal cardiac arrests during HIIT. Further, the rate of complications to number of patient-exercise hours was 1 per 129,456 hours of MICT and 1 per 23,182 hours of HIIT. The SMARTEX-HF study[15] demonstrated no differences between the HIIT and MICT groups in terms of total number of serious adverse events during the 12-week intervention and follow-up period (ie, from weeks 13–52) in older patients with HFrEF.

Thus, current studies suggest that the risk of a cardiovascular event is low for both HIIT and MICT in older patients with CVD in the CR setting.

As always, it is important to recognize standard CR procedures whenever developing an exercise prescription using either HIIT or MICT. These procedures, as described in the joint position statement of the European Association for Cardiovascular Prevention and Rehabilitation, AACVPR, and Canadian Association of Cardiac Rehabilitation,[10] include performing a preexercise evaluation, recognizing the relative and absolute indications for avoiding and terminating exercise, as well as taking into account special considerations for older patients with CVD who may present with various comorbidities attributable to aging (frailty, sarcopenia, balance disorders, cognitive decline, etc.).

SUMMARY AND PERSPECTIVES

As part of a comprehensive CR program, HIIT results in similar or even superior physiologic exercise training adaptations compared with MICT. These physiologic adaptations contribute to greater improvements in risk factors and exercise capacity/tolerance for these patients. It should be recognized that numerous studies have demonstrated that HIIT is a safe exercise training strategy. Because solely using an objective or subjective method for determining the appropriate intensity of exercise is prone to misrepresent actual exercise intensity, it may be more appropriate to use a combination of objective and subjective methods when prescribing HIIT in clinical populations. Exercise training using high-intensity (85%–95% peak HR or peak Vo_2 and RPE 15–17) and low-intensity intervals (50%–75% peak HR or peak Vo_2 and RPE 12–14) is proposed for older patients undergoing CR. With respect to the duration of HIIT, the authors propose short-interval HIIT for patients with low exercise capacity or in the initial stage of CR (0–4 week) and medium- or long-interval HIIT for patients with intermediate or high exercise capacity ($\geq$5 METs) and in the improvement (4–12 week) and maintenance stages (>12 week) of CR.

REFERENCES

1. Schopfer DW, Forman DE. Cardiac rehabilitation in older adults. Can J Cardiol 2016;32(9):1088–96.
2. Myers J, Prakash M, Froelicher V, et al. Exercise capacity and mortality among men referred for exercise testing. N Engl J Med 2002;346(11):793–801.
3. Piepoli MF, Hoes AW, Agewall S, et al. 2016 European guidelines on cardiovascular disease prevention in clinical practice: the Sixth joint Task Force of the European Society of Cardiology and other Societies on cardiovascular disease prevention in clinical Practice (constituted by representatives of 10 societies and by invited experts)Developed with the special contribution of the European Association for Cardiovascular Prevention & Rehabilitation (EACPR). Eur Heart J 2016;37(29):2315–81.
4. Keteyian SJ, Hibner BA, Bronsteen K, et al. Greater improvement in cardiorespiratory fitness using higher-intensity interval training in the standard cardiac rehabilitation setting. J Cardiopulm Rehabil Prev 2014;34(2):98–105.
5. Conraads VM, Pattyn N, De Maeyer C, et al. Aerobic interval training and continuous training equally improve aerobic exercise capacity in patients with coronary artery disease: the SAINTEX-CAD study. Int J Cardiol 2015;179(1):203–10.
6. Kim C, Choi HE, Lim MH. Effect of high interval training in acute myocardial Infarction patients with Drug-Eluting stent. Am J Phys Med Rehabil 2015;94(10 Suppl 1):879–86.

7. Molmen-Hansen HE, Stolen T, Tjonna AE, et al. Aerobic interval training reduces blood pressure and improves myocardial function in hypertensive patients. Eur J Prev Cardiol 2012;19(2):151–60.
8. Hannan AL, Hing W, Simas V, et al. High-intensity interval training versus moderate-intensity continuous training within cardiac rehabilitation: a systematic review and meta-analysis. Open Access J Sports Med 2018;9(1):1–17.
9. Rognmo O, Moholdt T, Bakken H, et al. Cardiovascular risk of high- versus moderate-intensity aerobic exercise in coronary heart disease patients. Circulation 2012;126(12):1436–40.
10. Mezzani A, Hamm LF, Jones AM, et al. Aerobic exercise intensity assessment and prescription in cardiac rehabilitation: a joint position statement of the European Association for Cardiovascular Prevention and Rehabilitation, the American Association of Cardiovascular and Pulmonary Rehabilitation and the Canadian Association of Cardiac Rehabilitation. Eur J Prev Cardiol 2013;20(3):442–67.
11. Garber CE, Blissmer B, Deschenes MR, et al. American College of Sports Medicine position stand. Quantity and quality of exercise for developing and maintaining cardiorespiratory, musculoskeletal, and neuromotor fitness in apparently healthy adults: guidance for prescribing exercise. Med Sci Sports Exerc 2011;43(7):1334–59.
12. Van De Heyning CM, De Maeyer C, Pattyn N, et al. Impact of aerobic interval training and continuous training on left ventricular geometry and function: a SAINTEX-CAD substudy. Int J Cardiol 2018;257:193–8.
13. Prado DM, Rocco EA, Silva AG, et al. Effects of continuous vs interval exercise training on oxygen uptake efficiency slope in patients with coronary artery disease. Braz J Med Biol Res 2016;49(2):e4890.
14. Benda NM, Seeger JP, Stevens GG, et al. Effects of high-intensity interval training versus continuous training on physical fitness, cardiovascular function and quality of life in heart failure patients. PLoS One 2015;10(10):e0141256.
15. Ellingsen O, Halle M, Conraads V, et al. High-intensity interval training in patients with heart failure with reduced ejection fraction. Circulation 2017;135(9):839–49.
16. Taylor JL, Holland DJ, Spathis JG, et al. Guidelines for the delivery and monitoring of high intensity interval training in clinical populations. Prog Cardiovasc Dis 2019;9(1):1–17.
17. Guazzi M, Adams V, Conraads V, et al. EACPR/AHA scientific statement. Clinical recommendations for cardiopulmonary exercise testing data assessment in specific patient populations. Circulation 2012;126(18):2261–74.
18. Fletcher GF, Ades PA, Kligfield P, et al. Exercise standards for testing and training: a scientific statement from the American Heart Association. Circulation 2013;128(8):873–934.
19. Diaz-Buschmann I, Jaureguizar KV, Calero MJ, et al. Programming exercise intensity in patients on beta-blocker treatment: the importance of choosing an appropriate method. Eur J Prev Cardiol 2014;21(12):1474–80.
20. Zhu N, Suarez-Lopez JR, Sidney S, et al. Longitudinal examination of age-predicted symptom-limited exercise maximum HR. Med Sci Sports Exerc 2010;42(8):1519–27.
21. Gulati M, Shaw LJ, Thisted RA, et al. Heart rate response to exercise stress testing in asymptomatic women: the st. James women take heart project. Circulation 2010;122(2):130–7.
22. Gellish RL, Goslin BR, Olson RE, et al. Longitudinal modeling of the relationship between age and maximal heart rate. Med Sci Sports Exerc 2007;39(5):822–9.

23. Iellamo F, Manzi V, Caminiti G, et al. Validation of rate of perceived exertion-based exercise training in patients with heart failure: insights from autonomic nervous system adaptations. Int J Cardiol 2014;176(2):394–8.
24. Tang LH, Zwisler AD, Taylor RS, et al. Self-rating level of perceived exertion for guiding exercise intensity during a 12-week cardiac rehabilitation programme and the influence of heart rate reducing medication. J Sci Med Sport 2016; 19(8):611–5.
25. Levinger I, Bronks R, Cody DV, et al. Perceived exertion as an exercise intensity indicator in chronic heart failure patients on Beta-blockers. J Sports Sci Med 2004;3(YISI 1):23–7.
26. Aamot IL, Forbord SH, Karlsen T, et al. Does rating of perceived exertion result in target exercise intensity during interval training in cardiac rehabilitation? A study of the Borg scale versus a heart rate monitor. J Sci Med Sport 2014;17(5):541–5.
27. Townsend LK, Islam H, Dunn E, et al. Modified sprint interval training protocols. Part II. Psychological responses. Appl Physiol Nutr Metab 2017;42(4):347–53.
28. Islam H, Townsend LK, Hazell TJ. Modified sprint interval training protocols. Part I. Physiological responses. Appl Physiol Nutr Metab 2017;42(4):339–46.
29. Billat VL, Flechet B, Petit B, et al. Interval training at VO2max: effects on aerobic performance and overtraining markers. Med Sci Sports Exerc 1999;31(1): 156–63.
30. MacDougall D, Sale D. Continuous vs. interval training: a review for the athlete and the coach. Can J Appl Sport Sci 1981;6(2):93–7.
31. Haykowsky MJ, Daniel KM, Bhella PS, et al. Heart failure: exercise-based cardiac rehabilitation: who, when, and how intense? Can J Cardiol 2016;32(10 Suppl 2): S382–7.
32. Madssen E, Moholdt T, Videm V, et al. Coronary atheroma regression and plaque characteristics assessed by grayscale and radiofrequency intravascular ultrasound after aerobic exercise. Am J Cardiol 2014;114(10):1504–11.
33. Angadi SS, Mookadam F, Lee CD, et al. High-intensity interval training vs. moderate-intensity continuous exercise training in heart failure with preserved ejection fraction: a pilot study. J Appl Physiol (1985) 2015;119(6):753–8.
34. Koufaki P, Mercer TH, George KP, et al. Low-volume high-intensity interval training vs continuous aerobic cycling in patients with chronic heart failure: a pragmatic randomised clinical trial of feasibility and effectiveness. J Rehabil Med 2014; 46(4):348–56.
35. Cardozo GG, Oliveira RB, Farinatti PT. Effects of high intensity interval versus moderate continuous training on markers of ventilatory and cardiac efficiency in coronary heart disease patients. ScientificWorldJournal 2015;2015(2): e192479.
36. Dall CH, Gustafsson F, Christensen SB, et al. Effect of moderate- versus high-intensity exercise on vascular function, biomarkers and quality of life in heart transplant recipients: a randomized, crossover trial. J Heart Lung Transplant 2015;34(8):1033–41.
37. Bacon AP, Carter RE, Ogle EA, et al. VO2max trainability and high intensity interval training in humans: a meta-analysis. PLoS One 2013;8(9):e73182.
38. Meyer FJ, Borst MM, Zugck C, et al. Respiratory muscle dysfunction in congestive heart failure: clinical correlation and prognostic significance. Circulation 2001;103(17):2153–8.
39. Olson TP, Joyner MJ, Dietz NM, et al. Effects of respiratory muscle work on blood flow distribution during exercise in heart failure. J Physiol 2010;588(13): 2487–501.

40. Smith JR, Hageman KS, Harms CA, et al. Effect of chronic heart failure in older rats on respiratory muscle and hindlimb blood flow during submaximal exercise. Respir Physiol Neurobiol 2017;243(9):20–6.
41. Tasoulis A, Papazachou O, Dimopoulos S, et al. Effects of interval exercise training on respiratory drive in patients with chronic heart failure. Respir Med 2010;104(10):1557–65.
42. Dunham C, Harms CA. Effects of high-intensity interval training on pulmonary function. Eur J Appl Physiol 2012;112(8):3061–8.
43. Christensen PM, Jacobs RA, Bonne T, et al. A short period of high-intensity interval training improves skeletal muscle mitochondrial function and pulmonary oxygen uptake kinetics. J Appl Physiol (1985) 2016;120(11):1319–27.
44. Boyle J 3rd. Graphic analysis of the Fick equation to evaluate oxygen transport. Respiration 1984;45(4):353–9.
45. Astorino TA, Edmunds RM, Clark A, et al. Increased cardiac output and maximal oxygen uptake in response to ten sessions of high intensity interval training. J Sports Med Phys Fitness 2018;58(1):164–71.
46. Matsuo T, Saotome K, Seino S, et al. Effects of a low-volume Aerobic-type interval exercise on VO2max and cardiac mass. Med Sci Sports Exerc 2014;46(1):42–50.
47. Baekkerud FH, Solberg F, Leinan IM, et al. Comparison of three popular exercise modalities on V O2max in overweight and obese. Med Sci Sports Exerc 2016; 48(3):491–8.
48. Warburton DE, Haykowsky MJ, Quinney HA, et al. Blood volume expansion and cardiorespiratory function: effects of training modality. Med Sci Sports Exerc 2004;36(6):991–1000.
49. Esfandiari S, Sasson Z, Goodman JM. Short-term high-intensity interval and continuous moderate-intensity training improve maximal aerobic power and diastolic filling during exercise. Eur J Appl Physiol 2014;114(2):331–43.
50. Jensen MT, Suadicani P, Hein HO, et al. Elevated resting heart rate, physical fitness and all-cause mortality: a 16-year follow-up in the Copenhagen Male Study. Heart 2013;99(12):882–7.
51. Nauman J, Aspenes ST, Nilsen TI, et al. A prospective population study of resting heart rate and peak oxygen uptake (the HUNT Study, Norway). PLoS One 2012; 7(9):e45021.
52. Rave G, Fortrat JO. Heart rate variability in the standing position reflects training adaptation in professional soccer players. Eur J Appl Physiol 2016;116(8): 1575–82.
53. da Silva VP, de Oliveira NA, Silveira H, et al. Heart rate variability indexes as a marker of chronic adaptation in athletes: a systematic review. Ann Noninvasive Electrocardiol 2015;20(2):108–18.
54. Alansare A, Alford K, Lee S, et al. The effects of high-intensity interval training vs. Moderate-intensity continuous training on heart rate variability in physically inactive adults. Int J Environ Res Public Health 2018;15(7):e1508.
55. Buscemi S, Canino B, Batsis JA, et al. Relationships between maximal oxygen uptake and endothelial function in healthy male adults: a preliminary study. Acta Diabetol 2013;50(2):135–41.
56. Ramos JS, Dalleck LC, Tjonna AE, et al. The impact of high-intensity interval training versus moderate-intensity continuous training on vascular function: a systematic review and meta-analysis. Sports Med 2015;45(5):679–92.
57. Mora-Rodriguez R, Ramirez-Jimenez M, Fernandez-Elias VE, et al. Effects of aerobic interval training on arterial stiffness and microvascular function in patients with metabolic syndrome. J Clin Hypertens 2018;20(1):11–8.

58. Baum O, Torchetti E, Malik C, et al. Capillary ultrastructure and mitochondrial volume density in skeletal muscle in relation to reduced exercise capacity of patients with intermittent claudication. Am J Physiol Regul Integr Comp Physiol 2016; 310(10):R943–51.
59. Simoneau JA, Lortie G, Boulay MR, et al. Human skeletal muscle fiber type alteration with high-intensity intermittent training. Eur J Appl Physiol Occup Physiol 1985;54(3):250–3.
60. Tan R, Nederveen JP, Gillen JB, et al. Skeletal muscle fiber-type-specific changes in markers of capillary and mitochondrial content after low-volume interval training in overweight women. Physiol Rep 2018;6(5):e13597.
61. Guadalupe-Grau A, Fernandez-Elias VE, Ortega JF, et al. Effects of 6-month aerobic interval training on skeletal muscle metabolism in middle-aged metabolic syndrome patients. Scand J Med Sci Sports 2018;28(2):585–95.
62. De Matos MA, Vieira DV, Pinhal KC, et al. High-intensity interval training improves markers of oxidative metabolism in skeletal muscle of individuals with obesity and insulin resistance. Front Physiol 2018;9(10):e1451.
63. Spee RF, Niemeijer VM, Wijn PF, et al. Effects of high-intensity interval training on central haemodynamics and skeletal muscle oxygenation during exercise in patients with chronic heart failure. Eur J Prev Cardiol 2016;23(18):1943–52.
64. Guiraud T, Nigam A, Gremeaux V, et al. High-intensity interval training in cardiac rehabilitation. Sports Med 2012;42(7):587–605.
65. Ribeiro PAB, Boidin M, Juneau M, et al. High-intensity interval training in patients with coronary heart disease: prescription models and perspectives. Ann Phys Rehabil Med 2017;60(1):50–7.
66. Ulbrich AZ, Angarten VG, Schmitt Netto A, et al. Comparative effects of high intensity interval training versus moderate intensity continuous training on quality of life in patients with heart failure: study protocol for a randomized controlled trial. Clin Trials Regul Sci Cardiol 2016;13:21–8.
67. Thompson PD, Franklin BA, Balady GJ, et al. Exercise and acute cardiovascular events placing the risks into perspective: a scientific statement from the American Heart Association Council on Nutrition, Physical Activity, and Metabolism and the Council on Clinical Cardiology. Circulation 2007;115(17):2358–68.
68. Astorino TA, Vella CA. Predictors of change in affect in response to high intensity interval exercise (HIIE) and sprint interval exercise (SIE). Physiol Behav 2018;196: 211–7.

Can Older Adults Benefit from Smart Devices, Wearables, and Other Digital Health Options to Enhance Cardiac Rehabilitation?

Julie Redfern, PhD, BAppSc (Physiotherapy Hons 1), BSc[a,b,*]

KEYWORDS

• Cardiovascular disease • Cardiac rehabilitation • Digital health interventions

KEY POINTS

- Improving reach, access, and effectiveness of postdischarge care through cardiac rehabilitation and secondary prevention strategies is currently an international priority.
- Proliferation in availability of mobile technology has resulted in widespread development and availability of digital health interventions that have the potential to reduce cardiovascular risk.
- Some text-messaging programs and apps have been shown to improve health outcomes, whereas research investigating the wearable devices are still emerging and lack robust data.
- User-centered design processes for development and training programs can help older adults engage with digital health technology; however, more robust research is needed.

CARDIOVASCULAR DISEASE AND EVIDENCE-PRACTICE GAPS

Cardiovascular disease (CVD), including coronary heart disease (CHD) and stroke, is the leading cause of death and disease burden globally.[1] CVD resulted in greater than 1.1 million hospitalizations in 2015 to 2016 and incurs the highest level of health care sector expenditure in Australia (11%–12% of total health expenditure).[2] CHD accounts for the greatest single disease morbidity (>500,000 bed-days annually) and nearly one-fifth of all deaths with a total cost of $1.14 billion annually.[2]

Disclosure: Dr. Redfern s supported by a NHMRC Career Development Fellowship (APP1143538).
[a] University of Sydney, Westmead Applied Research Centre, Faculty of Medicine and Health; [b] The George Institute for Global Health, UNSW Medicine, Sydney, Australia
[*] The University at Westmead Hospital, PO Box 154, Westmead, New South Wales 2154, Australia.
E-mail address: julie.redfern@sydney.edu.au

Clin Geriatr Med 35 (2019) 489–497
https://doi.org/10.1016/j.cger.2019.07.004
0749-0690/19/

Over 65,000 Australians experience an acute coronary event (heart attack or unstable angina) each year[3] and, importantly, around a third of these occur in people who have previous CHD and are therefore largely preventable.[4,5] With an aging population, more people surviving initial events, and an epidemic of lifestyle-related health problems, the health burden is escalating globally.[6] Thus, improving postdischarge care through cardiac rehabilitation and secondary prevention strategies (healthy living, adherence to medicines) is a current national and international priority.[7,8]

CARDIAC REHABILITATION AND ITS EVOLUTION

Cardiac rehabilitation, which originated in the 1970s and is generally a 6- to 10-week program after discharge, has been found to improve morbidity, mortality, and improve quality of life.[9] Yet, despite international[10–12] guidelines recommending cardiac rehabilitation and secondary prevention, adherence, access, and sustainability remain suboptimal.[13,14] Indeed, research consistently shows unacceptably poor rates for referral (30% of those eligible), attendance (9% of eligible), and completion (<5% of eligible).[15] Reasons are well documented and include transport, work/social commitments, and lack of perceived need.[16] Further, certain groups are less likely to attend including women, and those from culturally/linguistically diverse or low socioeconomic backgrounds.[15] From a systems perspective, the practicalities and costs of providing traditional programs to all who are eligible across diverse geographic areas with cultural and linguistic diversity is a major barrier.[7]

Understanding the historical context underscores the need to reform postdischarge management in light of societal changes (eg, cultural, linguistic and geographic diversity, and proliferation of technology) and medical and surgical advancements (**Fig. 1**).[17–19] Modern day "rehabilitation" was born at a time[20] when *bed rest and physical inactivity were recommended* for people with heart disease. Despite being established more than 50 years ago, this traditional model is still followed by 70% to 80% of programs (Australian and international) in today's completely different social and medical environments.[15,21] Delivering management and systems reform to address current evidence-practice gaps is a major challenge for current health care and requires a unified, efficient and multidisciplinary approach. Innovative and scalable solutions are needed.

THE POTENTIAL OF DIGITAL HEALTH INTERVENTIONS

In the past decade, there has been rapid proliferation in the number of people (now around 4.7 billion) around the world who own and use a mobile phone.[22] Further, the number of mobile broadband subscriptions has increased more than 15

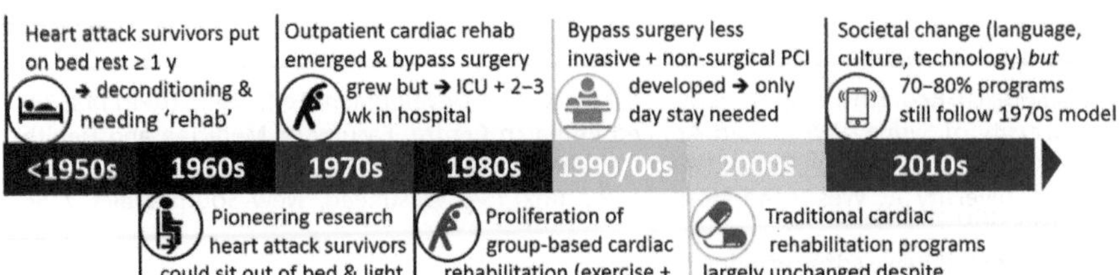

Fig. 1. Historical context underscores the current need for reform. PCI, percutaneous coronary intervention.

times in the last 10 years, which has enabled millions of people to have access to the Internet through their mobile devices.[23] This advancement in affordable mobile technology offers an opportunity to maximize the effectiveness and reach of health care. mHealth is defined as the use of mobile wireless technologies to support the achievement of health objectives, especially for public health purposes.[24]

In the past 20 years, technology has expanded from personal digital assistants to basic mobile phones, and then more recently to smartphones that are Internet-enabled and are now synchronized with other devices such as wearable devices and smartwatches. In society today, mobile and digital technology is of potential value in health care because of the widespread availability, broad acceptance, and diverse and simple functionality.[25] As a result there has been growing research and development of strategies that target secondary prevention of cardiovascular disease that are directly relevant to the cardiac rehabilitation context.

DIGITAL HEALTH INTERVENTIONS AND SECONDARY PREVENTION OF CARDIOVASCULAR DISEASE

In 2009, a systematic review and meta-analysis of telehealth (phone, Internet, and videoconference communication between patient and health care provider) interventions identified a total of 11 trials.[26] Results found that telehealth interventions were associated with nonsignificant lower all-cause mortality than controls (relative risk [RR] = 0.70, 95% confidence interval [CI], 0.45 to 1.1; $P = .12$). The telehealth interventions also resulted in significantly lower weighted mean difference (WMD) at medium long-term follow-up than controls for total cholesterol (WMD = 0.37 mmol/L, 95% CI, 0.19–0.56, $P<.001$), systolic blood pressure (WMD = 4.69 mm Hg, 95% CI, 2.91–6.47, $P<.001$), and fewer smokers (RR = 0.84, 95% CI, 0.65–0.98, $P = .04$).[26] The same team repeated the review in 2019 and identified 30 trials and found that telehealth interventions were associated with significantly lower rehospitalization or cardiac events (RR = 0.56, 95% CI, 0.39–0.81, $P<.0001$) compared with nonintervention groups.[27] Similar to the 2009 findings, there was again a significantly lower WMD at medium- to long-term follow-up than comparison groups for total cholesterol (WMD = −0.26 mmol/L, 95% CI,= −0.4 to −0.11, $P<.001$), low-density lipoprotein (LDL) (WMD = −0.28, 95% CI = −0.50 to −0.05, $P = .02$), and smoking status (RR = 0.77, 95% CI, 0.59–0.99, $P = .04$).[27]

Interestingly, the 2009 review identified only 1 trial in which the intervention was delivered primarily via the Internet.[26] In contrast, the 2019 review found 4 studies using the Internet as the intervention, 2 used text messaging alone, and 7 studies that tested an intervention with various combinations of the Internet, mobile phone, text message, and smartphone apps.[27] In both reviews, the interventions were delivered by a combination of nurses, allied health professionals, and other health care providers. In the 2019 review, the authors report that contact time was not rarely quantified and varied considerably with durations ranging from 6 weeks to 48 months and contact times ranging from 9 minutes to 9 hours. Telehealth intervention time varied from 6 weeks to 48 months. These wide variations in delivery, contact and modes of delivery make it difficult to synthesize evidence, implementation requirements, and costs. However, the authors concluded that telehealth interventions, with a range of delivery modes, could be offered to patients who cannot attend cardiac rehabilitation, or as an adjunct to cardiac rehabilitation for effective secondary prevention.[27]

TEXT MESSAGES

Text messages are simple, instant, and popular, they offer a widely available medium for delivery of health-related communication and can be sent remotely to large numbers of people in an unobtrusive manner. Many international randomized controlled trials (RCTs) have now demonstrated effectiveness of text message programs addressing management of chronic disease and CVD risk including smoking cessation,[28] weight loss,[29] physical activity,[30] BP lowering,[31] and diabetes care.[32] The Australian TEXTME RCT (n = 710) showed that the text message intervention group (4 messages/wk for 6 months sent on random days and times to minimize habituation) achieved lower LDL cholesterol (−0.13 mmol/L), systolic blood pressure (SBP) (−7.6 mm Hg), body mass index (BMI) (−1.3 kg/m^2), and smoking rates.[33] In subgroup analyses, patients ≥58 years achieved similar benefits to their younger counterparts for SBP and BMI, although not as a significant reduction in LDL cholesterol.[33]

TEXTME was particularly novel in that it demonstrated the ability of a texting program to achieve simultaneous improvement across multiple cardiovascular risk factors. In over 5 years of qualitative and analytical research, the team have also shown that patients find the texting programs useful (91%), easy to understand (97%), and motivating (77%).[34] Patients have also repeatedly stated that the program "*is excellent*" and "*should be available to everyone*."[34] Further, cost-effectiveness evaluation (assuming implementation to 50,000 patients) found to deliver the 6-month text message program in Australia it would cost $US24/patient (eg, including message, human resources, and information technology costs) and the program was found to be cost-effective and cost-saving for the health system.[35]

WHAT ABOUT APPS?

In the past decade there has been a proliferation of Web sites and mobile applications (apps) that claim to support secondary prevention of heart disease. These apps are computer software programs that operate on smartphones, tablets, and other mobile devices such as smartwatches.[36] Apps are generally readily available and relatively easy to use via touchscreens on the mobile devices. A 2015 review summarizes the literature related to apps and their potential in the prevention of CVD.[37] The review highlights how many apps are developed without evidence and become marketing and business strategy without an evidence base for effective behavior change; and also the lag time from development and app release to publication of trial results. By the time researchers have determined any clinical benefit of a new app, technology has evolved and, consequently, the app being studied might well be superseded by new developments and technologies.[37] However, a recent study has shown that use of freely available apps by people with CHD improves medication adherence.[38]

In 2013, the authors of a review identified 710 cardiology-related apps available for users of smartphones, most of which were heart monitors and medical calculators, with very few specifically targeting cardiac rehabilitation or prevention.[39] A more recent paper provides a systematic review of apps themselves, in which a systematic process was used to assess the quality, effectiveness, and features of apps (available in Australia) targeting medication adherence for management of CHD.[40] This review identified 272 medication reminder apps, of which 109 apps were available for free and 124 had been updated within the previous 2 years. The review found that the median number of features per app was 3.0 (interquartile range 4.0) and the most common features were flexible scheduling, medication tracking history, snooze option, and visual aids.[40] Further, using the MARS instrument, the authors found that less than half the apps were classified as high quality (combined score based on interest, interactivity, customizability, intuitiveness, ease of navigation, visual appeal, and information quality).[40]

The 2015 review by Neubeck and colleagues[37] outlined the important features for apps if behavior change in the context of cardiac rehabilitation is to be achieved. These included simplicity: that information is clear and unambiguous with a minimal number of steps to navigate from 1 feature in the app. Also, that information presented must be from a source that is considered credible by consumers: that information is perceived to be from a source of expertise and authority, is verified, and is endorsed by third parties and health professionals. Successful apps should also consider positive and supportive behavior change concepts in areas such as goal-setting, visual feedback, social support, and planning features. Other features, such as real-time data tracking supports engagement and regular use, as well as the app being personalizable based on individual circumstances. A further and important component of health-related apps is privacy, because consumers value the privacy of their health information and prefer the presence of a robust privacy policy.

WEARABLE DIGITAL HEALTH INTERVENTION

Perhaps the concept of wearable devices started with the simple battery-operated pedometer, with which people could track daily step counts in a simple and cost-effective way. There is reasonable scientific evidence that use of pedometers enhances physical activity and hence reduces cardiovascular risk and increases physical activity levels in people participating in cardiac rehabilitation.[41] In more recent years, and as technology has expanded, the market for wearable devices has also proliferated. Some smartphones have integrated systems (including accelerometers) for monitoring risk factors, such as physical activity and sensors to measure heart rate. However, there is little evidence regarding the accuracy of the information produced and hence the technology still remains limited in terms of wearable devices and their role in diagnosis, treatment, and prevention, and caution is important. There are currently many studies, large and small, underway in this area but there is little scientific evidence of effectiveness to date. One RCT (n = 800) found that 12-month use of an activity tracker had no significant impact on health outcomes.[42] Overall, the potential of wearable devices in relation to reach is appealing and will be an area of interest in the coming years.

CONCEPTUAL BENEFITS AND FEASIBILITY FOR OLDER ADULTS

One potential concern with digital heal interventions for secondary prevention of CVD is that many patients are of an older age and that mobile technology may be less widely adopted by this demographic.[43] However, 2016 data suggest that, among over 65 year olds in the United States, 42% own a smartphone and 80% a mobile phone of any sort.[44] Although this is somewhat lower than younger age groups it still represents a doubling in ownership compared with 3 years previously and rapidly increasing adoption rates among seniors.[44] The rate of smartphone ownership does decline with age and is only 31% of those over 75 years.[37] Importantly, age itself is not a barrier to digital health usage and some apps have been successfully used in the older population to improve physical activity[45] and cognitive function.[46] However, the challenges of complicated data-usage plans and apps that have not been developed with simple features or for those with declining vision can reduce the likelihood of apps being downloaded and used by older adults.[47] Some smartphones have even been suggested as being too small for older users to hold and present challenges are associated with small buttons.[37,48] Further, as authors such as Neubeck and

Leung highlight, older people may be less comfortable with a trial-and-error approach without step-by-step printed instructions than those from younger generations.[37,49]

DIGITAL HEALTH INTERVENTIONS DESIGN AND DEVELOPMENT CONSIDERATIONS FOR OLDER ADULTS

Overall, older adults generally have more difficulty than younger ones in learning new skills, particularly in learning to use new technology.[50] Leung and colleagues[49] summarize these difficulties as a number of user characteristics, such as declines in spatial working memory, lower information-processing speed, reduced technology experience, and a higher negative reaction to errors. To overcome these challenges it is essential to involve older people in the design of any digital health interventions that they will be potentially using. Further, user-centered design processes should be used, in which end users are involved at all stages and have active input to all areas of development, including the usability, functionality, and visual design.[51] These processes support greater usability and are likely to enhance eventual engagement with the technology. Another, potential strategy to support older adults using technology is to make practical training programs available with relevant hard-copy manuals, in which step-by-step instructions and screenshots can be followed,[49] and also providing positive feedback, and reassurance that they will not break the device and lose data by accident.[49] Further, technologies such as text messaging offer a more simple introductory approach in which older people do not need to interact heavily with the device, and for which evidence has shown that health benefits are similar across age groups.

SUMMARY

CVD is the leading cause of death and disease burden globally, yet it is largely preventable. With an aging population, more people surviving initial events, and an epidemic of lifestyle-related health problems, the health burden is escalating globally. Improving reach, access, and effectiveness of postdischarge care through cardiac rehabilitation, and secondary prevention strategies is currently an international priority. The current proliferation in availability of mobile technology has resulted in the widespread development and availability of digital health interventions that have the potential to reduce cardiovascular risk. Some studies have demonstrated the effectiveness of text messaging and apps in improving health outcomes. Other areas of research investigating the use of wearable devices are still emerging, but currently lack robust data. Importantly, mobile and smartphone ownership is rapidly increasing among older populations, and digital health is not limited by age. Hence, these interventions are potentially suitable for all age groups depending on personal preference and need. User-centered design processes for development and training programs can help older adults engage with digital health technology; however, more robust research to needed.

REFERENCES

1. Roth GA, Huffman MD, Moran AE, et al. Global and regional patterns in cardiovascular mortality from 1990 to 2013. Circulation 2015;132:1667–78.
2. Australian Institute of Health and Welfare. Cardiovascular disease snapshot. Canberra (Australia): AIHW; 2018. Cat. no. CVD 83.
3. Australian Institute of Health and Welfare. Australia's health 2016. Australia's health series no. 15. Canberra (Australia): AIHW; 2016. Cat. no. AUS 199.

4. Briffa TG, Hobbs MST, Tonkin A, et al. Population trends of recurrent coronary heart disease event rates remain high. Circ Cardiovasc Qual Outcomes 2011; 4:107–13.
5. Chew D, French J, Briffa T, et al. Acute coronary syndrome care across Australia and New Zealand: the SNAPSHOT ACS study. Med J Aust 2013;199:185–91.
6. Roxon N. Department of Health and Ageing. Taking preventative action: a response to Australia: the healthiest country by 2020 - the report of the national preventative health taskforce/[Australian Government]; [introduction from the Minister, Nicola Roxon]. Capital Hill, ACT: Commonwealth of Australia; 2010. Available at: https://trove.nla.gov.au/work/37303999?q&versionId=50352168. Accessed July 26, 2019.
7. Redfern J, Chow CK, on behalf of Secondary Prevention Alliance. Secondary prevention of coronary heart disease in Australia: a blueprint for reform. Med J Aust 2013;198:70–1.
8. Perel P, Avezum A, Huffman M, et al. Reducing premature cardiovascular morbidity and mortality in people with vascular disease. WHF Roadmap for secondary prevention. Glob Heart 2015;10:99–110.
9. Taylor RS, Brown A, Ebrahim S, et al. Exercise-based rehabilitation for patients with coronary heart disease: systematic review of RCTs. Am J Med 2004;116: 682–92.
10. Chew DP, Scott IA, Cullen L, et al. National Heart Foundation of Australia and Cardiac Society of Australia and New Zealand: Australian clinical guidelines for the management of acute coronary syndromes 2016. Med J Aust 2016;205:128–33.
11. Task Force on the management of ST-segment elevation acute myocardial infarction of the European Society of Cardiology (ESC), Steg PG, James SK, Atar D, et al. ESC guidelines for the management of acute myocardial infarction in patients presenting with ST-segment elevation. Eur Heart J 2012;33:2569–619.
12. Anderson JL, Adams CD, Antman EM, et al, 2011 Writing Group Members, ACCF/AHA Task Force Members. 2011 ACCF/AHA focused update incorporated into the ACC/AHA 2007 guidelines for the management of patients with unstable angina/non-ST-elevation myocardial infarction: a report of the American College of Cardiology Foundation/American Heart Association Task Force on practice guidelines. Circulation 2011;123:e426–579.
13. Scott IA, Lindsay KA, Harden HE. Utilisation of cardiac rehabilitation in Queensland. Med J Aust 2003;179:341–5.
14. Redfern J, Hyun K, Chew DP, et al. Prescription of secondary prevention medications, lifestyle advice and referral to rehabilitation among ACS inpatients. Heart 2014;100:1281–8.
15. Astley CM, Chew DP, Keech W, et al. The impact of cardiac rehabilitation and secondary prevention programs on 12-month outcomes: linked data analysis. Heart Lung Circ 2019. https://doi.org/10.1016/j.hlc.2019.03.015.
16. Grace SL, Gravely-Witte S, Brual J, et al. Contribution of patient and physician factors to cardiac rehabilitation enrollment: a prospective multilevel study. Eur J Cardiovasc Prev Rehabil 2008;15:548–56.
17. Redfern J. The evolution of physical activity and recommendations for patients with coronary heart disease. Heart Lung Circ 2016;25:759–64.
18. Brauwald E. Evolution of management of AMI: a 20th century saga. Lancet 1998; 352:1771–4.
19. Herrick JB. Clinical features of obstruction of the coronary arteries. JAMA 1912; 59:2015–20.

20. Levine SA, Lown B. Armchair treatment of coronary thrombosis. JAMA 1952;148: 1365–9.
21. Briffa T, Kinsman L, Maiorana AJ, et al. An integrated and coordinated approach to preventing recurrent coronary heart disease events in Australia: a policy statement. Med J Aust 2009;190:683–6.
22. Statistica (2018). Number of mobile phone users worldwide from 2013 to 2019 (in billions).
23. International Telecommunication Union (ITU). Measuring the information society report. Geneva (Switzerland): ITU; 2017. Available at: https://www.itu.int/en/ITU-D/Statistics/Documents/publications/misr2017/MISR2017_Volume1.pdf. Accessed June 15, 2019.
24. World Health Organization (WHO). mHealth: new horizons for health through mobile technologies: second global survey on eHealth. Switzerland: WHO; 2011. Available at: http://www.who.int/goe/publications/goe_mhealth_web.pdf. Accessed June 15, 2019.
25. World Health Organization (WHO). mHealth - use of appropriate digital technologies for public health. Switzerland: WHO; 2018. Available at: https://apps.who.int/gb/ebwha/pdf_files/WHA71/A71_20-en.pdf. Accessed June 2, 2019.
26. Neubeck L, Redfern J, Briffa T, et al. Telehealth interventions for the secondary prevention of heart disease: a systematic review. Eur J Cardiovasc Prev Rehabil 2009;16(3):281–9.
27. Jin K, Khonsari S, Gallagher R, et al. Telehealth interventions for the secondary prevention of coronary heart disease: a systematic review and meta-analysis. Eur J Cardiovasc Nurs 2019;18(4):260–71.
28. Whittaker R, McRobbie H, Bullen C, et al. Mobile phone-based interventions for smoking cessation. Cochrane Database Syst Rev 2016;(4):CD006611.
29. Patrick K, Raab F, Adams MA, et al. A text message-based intervention for weight loss: randomized controlled trial. J Med Internet Res 2009;11:e1.
30. Hurling R, Catt M, Boni MD, et al. Using internet and mobile phone technology to deliver an automated physical activity program: RCT. J Med Internet Res 2007; 9:e7.
31. Bobrow K, Farmer AJ, Springer D, et al. Mobile phone text messages to support treatment adherence in adults with high blood pressure (StAR): a single-blind, randomized trial. Circulation 2016;133(6):592–600.
32. Buis LR, Hirzel L, Turske SA, et al. Use of a text message program to raise type 2 diabetes risk awareness and promote health behavior change (part I): assessment of participant reach and adoption. J Med Internet Res 2013;15(12):e281.
33. Chow CK, Redfern J, Hills GS, et al. Effect of lifestyle-focused text messaging on risk factor modification in patients with CHD: a randomized clinical trial. JAMA 2015;314:1255–63.
34. Redfern J, Santo K, Coorey G, et al. Factors influencing engagement, perceived usefulness and behavioral mechanisms associated with a text message support program. PLoS One 2016;11(10):e0163929.
35. Burn E, Nghiem S, Jan S, et al. Cost-effectiveness of a text-message program for cardiovascular disease secondary prevention. Heart 2017;103(12):893–4.
36. Janssen C. Mobile application (mobile app) 2014. Available at: https://www.techopedia.com/definition/2953/mobile-application-mobile-app. Accessed June 19, 2019.
37. Neubeck L, Lowres N, Benjamin EJ, et al. The mobile revolution – can smartphone apps help prevent cardiovascular disease? Nat Rev Cardiol 2015;12: 350–60.

38. Santo K, Chow C, Singleton A, et al. MEDication reminder APPs to improve medication adherence in Coronary Heart Disease (MedApp-CHD) study: results of a randomised controlled trial. Heart 2018. https://doi.org/10.1136/heartjnl-2018-313479.
39. Martínez-Pérez B, de la Torre-Díez I, López-Coronado M, et al. Mobile apps in cardiology: review. JMIR Mhealth Uhealth 2013;1:e15.
40. Santo K, Richtering SS, Chalmers J, et al. Smartphone apps to improve medication adherence: a systematic stepwise process to identify high-quality apps. JMIR Mhealth Uhealth 2016;4(4):e132.
41. Sangster J, Furber S, Phongsavan P, et al. Effects of a pedometer-based telephone coaching intervention on physical activity among people with cardiac disease in urban, rural and semi-rural settings: a replication study. Heart Lung Circ 2017;26(4):354–61.
42. Finkelstein EA, Haaland BA, Bilger M, et al. Effectiveness of activity trackers with and without incentives to increase physical activity (TRIPPA): a randomised controlled trial. Lance Diabetes Endocrinol 2016;4(12):983–95.
43. Leung R, McGrenere J, Graf P. Age-related differences in the initial usability of mobile device icons. Behav Inform Tech 2011;30:629–42.
44. Anderson M, Perrin A. Technology use among seniors. Pew research center internet and technology 2016. Available at: https://www.pewinternet.org/2017/05/17/technology-use-among-seniors/. Accessed June 19, 2019.
45. Brox E, Luque LF, Evertsen GJ, et al. Exergames for elderly: social exergames to persuade seniors to increase physical activity [abstract]. Presented at 5th International ICST Conference on Pervasive Computing Technologies for Healthcare. Dublin, Ireland, May 23–26, 2011. p. 546–9.
46. Omatu S, Rodríguez S, Villarrubia G, et al, editors. Distributed computing, artificial intelligence, bioinformatics, soft computing, and ambient assisted living. Springer; 2009. p. 756–63.
47. Deloitte. The smartphone generation gap: over-55?. 2014. there's no app for that [online], Available at: https://www2.deloitte.com/ug/en/pages/technology-media-and-telecommunications/articles/2014predictions-the-smart phone-generation-gap.html. Accessed July 26, 2019.
48. Plaza I, Martín L, Martin S, et al. Mobile applications in an aging society: status and trends. J Syst Softw 2011;84:1977–88.
49. Leung R, Tang C, Haddad S, et al. How older adults learn to use mobile devices: survey and field investigations. ACM Trans Access Comput 2012;4:11.
50. Fisk AD, Rogers WA, Charness N, et al. Designing for older adults: principles and creative human factors approaches. 2nd edition. Boca Raton (FL): CRC Press; 2009. Available at: http://sutlib2.sut.ac.th/sut_contents/H128786.pdf. Accessed July 26, 2019.
51. Fogg BJ. Persuasive technology: using computers to change what we think and do. Burlington (MA): Morgan Kaufmann Publishers; 2003.

Utility of Home-Based Cardiac Rehabilitation for Older Adults

Theresa M. Beckie, PhD

KEYWORDS

- Home-based cardiac rehabilitation • Older adults • Patient-centered
- Exercise training

KEY POINTS

- Home-based cardiac rehabilitation programs have been shown to be safe, cost effective, acceptable, and as efficacious as center-based cardiac rehabilitation programs.
- Home-based cardiac rehabilitation programs for older adults should include assessment and management of frailty, disability, cognition, comorbidity, mobility, and cardiovascular disease risk.
- Home-based cardiac rehabilitation can extend the breadth and depth of education, counseling, and monitoring modalities because these services can be accessed 24 hours a day, 7 days a week.

EPIDEMIOLOGY OF CARDIOVASCULAR DISEASE IN OLDER ADULTS

Coronary heart disease is the leading cause of morbidity and mortality, chronic disability, loss of independence and impaired quality of life in older adults.[1,2] Cardiovascular disease (CVD) deaths have increased steadily since 1990 driven by aging and population growth, whereas improvements in prevention health care strategies have reduced mortality in recent years.[3] Adults aged 65 years or older comprised 13% of the US population (49.2 million) in 2016, with numbers projected to reach 72.1 million (19% of the population) by 2030.[4] Further, the number of adults 85 years and older is projected to increase to 14.6 million by 2040. Because of these growing demographic trends, secondary prevention of CVD, maintaining functional status, ameliorating the age-related physiologic changes of the cardiovascular system, and preserving the physical independence and quality of life of older adults present major challenges with substantial health care implications.

Disclosure Statement: The author has nothing to disclose.
College of Nursing, University of South Florida, MDC Box 22, 12901 Bruce B. Downs Boulevard, Tampa, FL 33612, USA
E-mail address: tbeckie@health.usf.edu

Clin Geriatr Med 35 (2019) 499–516
https://doi.org/10.1016/j.cger.2019.07.003

CARDIAC REHABILITATION: THE GOLD STANDARD OF CARE FOR OLDER ADULTS WITH CARDIOVASCULAR DISEASE

More than 2.4 million patients are eligible for center-based cardiac rehabilitation (CBCR) annually in the United States.[1] The benefits of CBCR for secondary prevention of CVD are compelling and well-established. In the United States, CBCR typically consists of up to 36 outpatient electrocardiogram-monitored sessions over 12 weeks. The American Heart Association, the American College of Cardiology, and the European Society of Cardiology provide a class I recommendation for CBCR after an acute coronary syndrome or after coronary revascularization.[5–9] Eligibility for CBCR now includes heart failure, valvular heart disease, and peripheral arterial disease.[10] A comprehensive, multidisciplinary CBCR program comprising medical evaluation, prescriptive exercise, education, psychosocial and tobacco cessation counseling, and diet and weight management can substantially improve CVD risk factors and quality of life and decrease hospital admissions and recurrent ischemic events.[11–14] These CBCR programs also provides noncardiovascular benefits (eg, social support, improved cognition, mood).[15–22] Geriatric syndromes common to older adults including multiple morbidities, deconditioning, age-related muscle atrophy, polypharmacy, frailty, poor sleep quality, and declining cognition can be improved with CBCR.[15] Afilalo and colleagues[23] noted the bidirectional relationship between physical frailty and CVD, and provided comprehensive recommendations for implementing frailty assessment and management in the CVD care of older adults.[24]

Evidence substantiates the role of CBCR exercise participation for improving CVD risk factors, and reducing recurrent CVD adverse events and mortality in older adults.[15,25] Among US Medicare beneficiaries hospitalized with acute coronary syndrome or coronary revascularization, patients participating in at least 25 CBCR sessions showed a significant 19% decreased mortality in the subsequent 5 years compared with those attending 24 or fewer sessions.[25] Moreover, compared with participants aged 65 to 74 years, mortality reductions increased progressively with older age ($P<.001$ for 75–84 years and $P<.013$ for $\geq$85 years). The advantage of CBCR for older adults is the direct multidisciplinary supervision; the standardized delivery model; the individualized exercise training; nutrition, tobacco cessation, and psychological counseling; and the coordinated management of lipids, diabetes, blood pressure, and weight according to criteria established by the American Association of Cardiovascular and Pulmonary Rehabilitation.[26] Schopfer and Forman[15] provide a thorough review of the numerous benefits of CBCR for older adults. Unfortunately, CBCR programs are financially and logistically prohibitive for many older adults, resulting in profound underuse.

MAINTENANCE OF CENTER-BASED CARDIAC REHABILITATION ACHIEVEMENTS

Even when adults complete CBCR programs, the maintenance of improvements is often not achieved.[27,28] Previous reports show decreased exercise adherence and increased weight and lipid levels as early as 6 months after CBCR.[29,30] Studies have reported that patients in long-term home-based cardiac rehabilitation (HBCR) programs show better sustainability of physical activity (PA) compared with CBCR programs that end.[31–33] An alternative approach is to integrate comprehensive education, counseling, and PA into daily life routines in the context of work, social contacts, and other daily activities based on personalized goals and interests.[34] Rejeski and colleagues[35] demonstrated that interventions that promote behavioral skills and develop resources to sustain home-based PA yield stronger long-term effects than traditional structured exercise programs. Health habits are thought to be context dependent and might explain why PA in CBCR programs may not translate well to a sedentary home environment.[36] Healthy behaviors become habits when they are executed repeatedly, in the same context, and over an extended length of time.[37] Interventions delivered during everyday life may be more effective for helping older adults improve their health behaviors in the moment compared with more traditional interventions that occur outside daily lived contexts.

BARRIERS TO CENTER-BASED CARDIAC REHABILITATION PARTICIPATION BY OLDER ADULTS

Participation of older patients in CBCR programs remains suboptimal internationally.[11,19,38,39] Barriers related to program availability, referrals, attendance, and completion are multifactorial and widely researched.[5,40,41] An enduring barrier to CBCR participation by older adults is the lackluster or absent encouragement by physicians.[42–44] Indeed, too few referrals jeopardize the financial viability of many CBCR programs.[45] Yet, even with referral to CBCR, an enrollment gap exists with only 50% of referred patients actually enrolling and participating in CBCR.[46–48] Patient-specific barriers to CBCR participation include older age, comorbid conditions that limit PA, low motivation or lack of awareness, geographic inaccessibility, limited transportation, financial cost, and competing domestic or vocational responsibilities.[19,45,49–54] Understanding patient values and goals regarding quality of life and longevity is essential.[55]

To address barriers to attendance and extend the reach of secondary prevention services, there is an urgent need for alternative cardiac rehabilitation models. These models may include structured education and exercise interventions supplemented with mobile technology used in the home.[56] Among Australian patients, 43% strongly preferred cardiac rehabilitation delivered in the home. Convenience, independence, work commitments, travel issues, flexibility, and a dislike of social groups influenced the patients' decision.[57] This research concurs with a prior study reporting that 45% of patients preferred a home-based setting.[58]

HOME-BASED CARDIAC REHABILITATION FOR OLDER ADULTS

HBCR consists of the core components of CBCR programs but instead is delivered through regular contact with health care professionals via telephone calls or mobile technology.[31] Further, HBCR can extend the breadth and depth of education, counseling, and monitoring modalities for patients because these services can be accessed 24 hours a day, 7 days a week compared with the more restricted contact with CBCR personnel. A challenge for the scalability of HBCR programs in the United States is the lack of reimbursement by the Centers for Medicare & Medicaid Services and third-party payers.

Table 1 presents a summary of 4 randomized controlled trials evaluating the effectiveness of CBCR compared with HBCR that included adults with a mean age of at least 65 years (range, 35–85 years). Only 1 study evaluated the primary outcomes by age.[59] All 4 studies were conducted in countries outside the United States and most included low-risk male participants who were capable of completing a symptom-limited graded exercise test, a 6-minute walk test, or an incremental shuttle walk test. The format and delivery of HBCR varied in content and quality, and the frequency and method of contact with health care professionals, was heterogeneous. All interventions included exercise training of varying length with most protocols involving walking with support via telephone calls or home visits by a physical therapist, exercise physiologist, or nurse. Additional components included nutrition counseling, psychological support, and risk factor management.

Table 1
Summary of HBCR studies

Study Design	Patient Population	Interventions	Outcomes
Cowie 2012[98,99] *UK* RCT	N = 60 HF class II/III Age 65.8 *Range: 35–85* 85% men	*Exercise-only programs* *HBCR n = 20* (DVD, booklet, phone calls 2× a month). Exercise: WU and CD. Aerobic: 2 × 15-min circuits (10 exercises, eg, knee lifts, side steps); and low-paced recovery; 90 s each. ↑ time in aerobic exercise. Education: symptoms; HR monitor. 12–14 on Borg *CBCR n = 20* (2 supervised sessions/wk for 1 h each – 2 × 15-min circuits); WU and CD. Same instructions as HBCR. Control n = 20.	Primary outcome: 8 wk FU Incremental Shuttle Walk Test: HBCR vs CBCR NS group differences. Secondary outcome: HRQOL: NS group differences Adherence (16 sessions) HBCR 77% and CBCR 86% (NS group differences) 5/20 (25%) CBCR and 5/20 (25%) dropped out. Adverse events: NR
Marchionni 2003[59] *Italy* RCT; factorial	N = 270; MI 3 age groups: 45–65, 66–75, and >75 y *Range: 46–86 y* 67.8% male	*Comprehensive Program: CBCR n = 90*: 40 exercise sessions (24 sessions; 3/wk) cycle ergometer (WU, 20-min workload, CD; 16 (2/wk) 60-min sessions stretching and flexibility; ECG monitored. Intensity 70% to 85% of HR. Risk factor counseling 2/wk and monthly support group. *HBCR n = 90*: 4–8 supervised sessions in CBCR. Risk factor counseling each session and invite to join monthly support group. Exercise similar to CBCR, wristwatch HR monitor, cycle ergometer, logbook. Home visits 2/mo for 2 mo. *Control group n = 90*: Single education session of risk factors, no exercise.	Primary outcome: 8 wk, 6 and 12 mo later Total work capacity: NS group differences at 14 mo Secondary outcomes: HRQOL: NS group difference; in *older adults*, HRQOL ↑ significantly with either active treatment. Adverse events: NS group difference in new events Drop-out: HBCR (16/90); CBCR (11/90); control (11/90) Adherence exercise sessions: HBCR: 37.3 (3.4); CBCR: 34.4 (4.4); *P*<.0001; favors HBCR

Oerkild 2011[100] *Denmark* RCT	N = 75 MI, PCI, CABG HBCR: n = 36 Men 52.8%; age: 74 (6) *Range: 69–80 y* CBCR: N = 39 Men 67% Age: 74.7 (5.9) *Range: 69–81*	*Comprehensive program* *HBCR n = 36*: PT home visit every 6 wk; telephone between 2 visits. Exercise: 30 min/d, 6 d/wk; intensity 11–13 on Borg. Self-paced brisk walking and bike. Lifestyle counseling. *CBCR n = 39*: PT tailored 6-wk intensive group program; exercise 60 min 2×/week at home. 6 lectures: dietary, cooking, and smoking cessation. Cardiologist counseled both groups. Both interventions 12 wk but encouraged to exercise 30 min 6 d/wk.	Primary outcomes: 3, 6, 12 mo FU Peak V_{O_2} and 6MWT. NS group differences 3 mo and significant ↓ in both groups at 12 mo. Secondary outcomes: NS group differences Self-reported activity, BP, lipid profile, smoking status, BMI, WHR, HRQOL, Anxiety, depression; Charlson Comorbidity Index. AE: NS differences up to 12 m. Mortality: 7; drop-out: 4
Piotrowicz 2010[101–103] *Poland* RCT	N = 152; HF NYHA functional classes II and III; 95% men in CBCR and 85% in HBCR. Age: CBCR: 61 (8.8) *Range: 52–69* HBCR: 65 (10.9) *Range: 55–76*	*Comprehensive programs: 8 wk*. First week both groups: meet with psychologist. *HBCR n = 77*: telemetry monitored via mobile device. WU; aerobic exercise: walking; 40%–70% of HR reserve; 11 on Borg. Start point based on baseline peak V_{O_2}; ↑ to 20–30 min/session/d; CD. Support via telephone; 2 meetings in person. *CBCR: n = 75*: WU; aerobic exercise: interval training on cycle ergometer at 40%–70% of HR reserve; 11 on Borg. 10–15 min/session/d; (intermittent exercise 1-2-3 min, then 1–2 min of recovery). ↑ to 30 min/d (intermittent exercise 4 min, then 2 min recovery); CD. Psychologist available during session. Education.	Outcomes 8 wk: Functional capacity: treadmill test with V_{O_2} peak (NS group difference) Adherence: 59/75 (79%) completed CBCR; 77/77 (100%) HBCR; *P*<.001 CBCR: 19/75 (25%) HBCR: 2/77 (3%) failed to provide 8-wk data Drop outs (only in CBCR- N = 20%, owing to financial constraints and transportation difficulties) HRQOL: NS group difference. AE: 0

Abbreviations: ↑, increased; ↓, decreased; 6MWT, 6-utemin walk test; AE, adverse event; BMI, body mass index; BP, blood pressure; CABG, coronary artery bypass graft; CD, cool down; ECG, electrocardiogram; FU, follow-up; HF, heart failure; HR, heart rate; HRQOL, health related quality of life; MI, myocardial infarction; NR, not reported; NS, not significant; NYHA, New York Heart Association; PCI, percutaneous coronary intervention; PT, physical therapist; RCT, randomized controlled trial; WHR, waist-hip ratio; WU, warm up.

These HBCR programs have been shown to be safe, cost effective, and acceptable, and as efficacious as CBCR.[60–62] Buckingham and colleagues[61] found no significant differences in the short-term (<12 months) or long-term patient outcomes, including exercise capacity, modifiable CVD risk factors, quality of life, and cardiac events (mortality, coronary revascularization, and hospital readmissions) among patients participating in HBCR or CBCR programs. Compared with CBCR, a modestly greater proportion of participants completed HBCR programs. This finding is consistent with a report of slightly better maintenance of exercise capacity with HBCR.[62] The self-monitoring and self-management inherent in HBCR compared with CBCR may make the transition from active intervention to lifelong disease self-management more seamless; this finding needs further investigation with older adults 70 years of age and older. The generalizability of findings from the studies comparing CBCR and HBCR is very limited for older frail or cognitively challenged adults, non-white ethnic minorities, rural, uninsured, and low socioeconomic individuals, as well as women.

HOME-BASED CARDIAC REHABILITATION: SPECIAL CONSIDERATIONS FOR OLDER ADULTS

Collectively, the studies of HBCR show little evidence of addressing the needs of disabled, frail, socially isolated or high-risk older adults with CVD. Before implementing an HBCR program for older adults, assessments of frailty, disability, comorbidity and, CVD risk are essential to providing patient-centered care (**Table 2**).[24] Frailty and decreased muscle mass present a challenge for maintaining independence, mobility, and quality of life.[63,64] It is important to evaluate functional capacity in older adults in HBCR for both improved health and quality of life.[65] Ideally, HBCR programs for older adults should include guidance from experts in geriatrics, cognition, nutrition, and physical function. It is important to assess older adults' cognitive and functional status because these factors determine their ability to communicate, their level of independence, and their ability to adhere to prescribed regimens.

Regular PA is key to preventing and managing chronic diseases and for preserving physical function and mobility to delay the onset of major disability.[66] Physically active older adults are less likely to fall, less likely to be seriously injured if they do fall, and more likely to maintain independence and functional ability compared with those who are inactive. The American Heart Association Scientific Statement on Secondary Prevention of Atherosclerotic Cardiovascular Disease in Older Adults noted that exercise training is associated with preventing falls, maintaining ambulation, and improving muscular strength, function, and quality of life.[2] This and other secondary prevention strategies strive to slow the progression of age-associated cardiovascular dysfunction.[67]

Healthy lifestyle strategies with stress management, optimal nutrition, PA, and weight management have the strongest established evidence for efficacy in secondary prevention of adverse cardiovascular aging and frailty.[68] Frail older adults with cognitive deficits can also benefit from exercise training.[69,70] In the 3C Study, a heart-healthy diet and lifestyle modifications were associated with reduced all-cause mortality in individuals greater than 70 years of age.[71] There was also a significant association between increased PA and decreased mortality over time. **Table 3** presents the most current PA guidelines for older adults.

Empirical data support the integration of patient preferences into behavioral and exercise programs to optimize the receptivity for, and adherence to, a given program[72] and to maximize regular and sustained PA.[73] A systematic review of studies of PA

Table 2
Special considerations HBCR for older adults

Risk Category	Recommendations and Implications
Frailty (slow walking speed, weakness, inactivity, exhaustion, shrinking) Activities of daily living	Careful screening and assessment for safety, frailty, risk for falls Consider using the Short Physical Performance Battery[104] and the Katz Index of Independence in activities of daily living.[105] PA improves walking, balance, activities of daily living for individuals with functional impairments, and counteracts frailty. Individualize exercise training starting slow and gradually increasing. Resistance training for strength.
Cardiovascular risk	Assess for multimorbidity. Using appropriate screening, risk stratification, and monitoring procedures in higher risk individuals, HBCR can be feasible and safe, including patients with stable heart failure.[70,99,101] Assess the utility of alternative methods to traditional exercise testing to assess functional status such as walk tests, gait speed, strength indices to guide coronary heart disease management.[96] Perform a thorough medical history and physical examination to determine cardiac contraindications to exercise. Activities should be defined relative to the older adult's fitness within the context of perceived physical exertion using a 0–10 point scale with 0 considered an effort equivalent to sitting, a moderate-intensity activity defined as 5 or 6, and a vigorous-intensity activity as a 7 or 8.
Cognition	Individuals with deficits in cognition and executive function can benefit from exercise including improved neuropsychological performance (executive function, processing speed, memory).[69,106] Careful assessment and screening for health literacy and the process of symptom recognition.
Individual preference and patient-centered outcomes	HBCR programs that integrate individual preferences, values and goals in the decision-making process are needed.[96] Implement evidence-based behavior change interventions such as goal setting, social support, self-efficacy for improving clinical outcomes.
Attitudes toward exercise, purpose in life, independence	Patients' attitudes toward exercise, personal wishes, and desired outcomes should be incorporated in the design and delivery.
Psychological symptoms	Evaluate the relationship between depressive symptoms and cognitive dysfunction in older patients. Fewer depressive symptoms with or without major depression; exercise reduces state anxiety.

preferences for adults 65 years of age and older found that most prefer to walk and engage in PA continuously for about 30 minutes during the morning hours.[74] Of relevance to the cardiac rehabilitation population, the review showed that the ease of access to the location for performing PA (eg, alone, at home, with companions) was more important than the type of location. The authors highlighted the usefulness of matching the contact or format of PA to the older adult's social context preferences.

Many sedentary older adults also hold erroneous, negative, and self-defeating views about their ability to exercise. They may assume that they are too old to

Table 3
PA guidelines for older adults

Exercise Type	Recommendation	Examples
Aerobic activities	Older adults with chronic conditions should understand whether and how their conditions affect the ability to do regular PA safely. Older adults should determine their level of effort for PA relative to their level of fitness. Older adults should do at least 150 min/wk of moderate-intensity or 75 min/wk of vigorous-intensity aerobic activity, preferably, spread throughout the week. When older adults cannot do 150 min of moderate-intensity activity a week, they should be as physically active as their abilities and conditions allow. Older adults should move more and sit less during the day as some PA is better than none. Adults who sit less and do any amount of moderate-to-vigorous PA gain health benefits.	Walking or hiking, dancing, swimming, water aerobics, jogging, aerobics exercise classes, bicycle riding (stationary or outdoors), some yard work such as raking and pushing a lawn mower, tennis, walking as part of golf
Muscle-strengthening exercises	Older adults should do muscle-strengthening activities of moderate or greater intensity that involve all major muscle groups on ≥2 d per week for additional health benefits. No specific amount of time is recommended for muscle strengthening, but these exercises should be performed to the point at which it would be difficult to do another repetition. When resistance training is used to enhance muscle strength, one set of 8–12 repetitions of each exercise is effective, although 2 or 3 sets may be more effective.	Exercises using exercise bands, weight machines or hand-held weights, body-weight exercises (eg, push-ups, pull-ups, squats), digging, lifting and carrying when gardening, carrying groceries, some yoga postures, some forms of tai chi
Flexibility exercises	Flexibility activities enhance the ability of a joint to move through the full range of motion. Stretching before and after PA should be part of warm-up and cool-down.[107]	Neck stretches, shoulder shrugs, should protraction, arm circles, anterior chest stretch

(*continued on next page*)

Table 3
(continued)

Exercise Type	Recommendation	Examples
Balance exercises	Balance activities can improve the ability to resist forces within or outside the body that cause falls. Fall prevention programs that include balance training and other exercises to improve activities of daily living can also significantly reduce the risk of injury such as bone fractures if a fall does occur.	Walking heel-to-toe, walking backwards, sideways, stand on 1 foot while doing an upper body muscle-strengthening activity such as bicep curls, practice standing from a sitting position, use a wobble board
Safety	Understand the risks, yet be confident that PA can be safe for almost everyone. Choose types of PA that are appropriate for their current fitness level and health goals, because some activities are safer than others. Increase PA gradually over time to meet key guidelines or health goals. Inactive people should start with lower intensity activities and gradually increase and making sensible choices about when, where and how to be active. Be under the care of a health care provider if they have chronic conditions or symptoms. Consult a health care professional or PA specialist about the types and amounts of activity appropriate for them.	Appropriate weather, adequate hydration, proper exercise equipment, appropriate footwear and clothing, safety equipment as appropriate.

Data from U.S. Department of Health and Human Services. 2018 Physical activity guidelines for Americans. 2nd edition. Available at: https://health.gov/paguidelines/second-edition/pdf/Physical_Activity_Guidelines_2nd_edition.pdf.

exercise, that exercise will not be beneficial, or that exertion will be harmful or painful.[34] Novel HBCR exercise strategies may be useful for older adults and a relatively simpler emphasis on increasing PA may be more successful than formal exercise training.[65] These patient-centered considerations to address barriers to increasing PA and correcting misconceptions about exercise and behavior change are critical.

The consequences of inattention to noncardiovascular impediments to PA training was evident in the Heart Failure: A Controlled Trial Investigating Outcomes of Exercise Training (HF-ACTION) trial.[75] Limited consideration for patient multimorbidity, frailty, depression, and cognitive impairment led to poor adherence to the exercise intervention. Psychological comorbidities also can influence cardiovascular health. The Stabilization of Atherosclerotic Plaque by Initiation of Darapladib Therapy (STABILITY) trial found that women older than 65 years of age with CVD were more likely than their male counterparts to experience psychosocial stress and depression with a correspondingly stronger association between psychosocial stress, depression, and adverse events.[76]

INNOVATIVE OPPORTUNITIES IN HOME-BASED CARDIAC REHABILITATION FOR OLDER ADULTS

The ubiquity of smartphones and wearable sensors provides opportunities to leverage advances in mobile computing for improved monitoring and CVD health outcomes in HBCR. Of older adults who own cellphones, 50% have some type of smartphone compared with just 23% in 2013 (http://www.pewinternet.org/2017/05/17/technology-use-among-seniors/). Smartphone ownership among older adults varies by age: 65 to 69 years (59%), 70 to 74 years (49%), and 75 to 79 years (31%), and 80 years or older (17%). Smartphone ownership is also associated with income and education. Fully 81% of older Americans with an annual income of $75,000 or more report owning smartphones, compared with 27% of those earning less than $30,000 a year. HBCR programs using smartphone technology and wearable sensors can overcome inaccessibility barriers by allowing health care professionals to deliver real-time individualized support.[77] Access to a health professional through a web portal dashboard has the potential to be a low cost strategy for fostering adherence to sustained healthy behavior changes. Consideration of health and technology literacy as well as sensory and manual dexterity deficits among older adults that may interfere with optimal HBCR delivery is essential. Although age is an important consideration in the development and implementation of technology-enhanced HBCR, the effect is likely to be rapidly diluted in the future with the rapidly changing technology landscape.

The use of mobile health (mHealth) technologies to promote lifestyle improvements in patients with chronic diseases is increasing. Mobile health interventions have been demonstrated as effective for improving CVD outcomes, body weight, and body mass index, and to increase adherence to medical therapy.[78,79] Mobile health can deliver interventions to CVD patients that are personalized, sustainable, engaging, and adaptive to their personal context, and improve access to health care services. HBCR using mHealth is shown to be feasible with high rates of participant engagement, acceptance, use, and adherence.[77,80] For example, Varnfield and colleagues[81] reported that technology-assisted HBCR with middle-aged patients who had a myocardial infarction has greater uptake, adherence, and completion compared with CBCR. Moreover, both groups demonstrated improved physiologic and psychosocial health outcomes.

Text messaging and the Internet can be useful for increasing PA levels.[81–84] A meta-analysis found that interventions using pedometers or accelerometers in older adults were acceptable and improved PA in the short term.[85] Two studies implemented brief text messaging intervention reminders for improving the number of sessions attended[86] and for improving CVD risk factors.[87] Using a combination of multiple technology modalities (smartphone, text messaging, and mentoring by phone) may prove superior to using a single modality.[80] A systematic review of exercise-based HCBR reported comparable effectiveness for improving aerobic capacity and superior effectiveness for improving PA level, exercise adherence, diastolic blood pressure, and cholesterol than CBCR.[88]

Mobile health intervention designs informed by behavior change theory are more effective than those without a theoretic foundation.[89,90] Behavioral theories can inform interventions by identifying constructs that are hypothesized to be causally related to the desired behavior, and therefore appropriate, for the intervention.[91] A potential strength of mHealth technologies for delivering behavioral interventions is the high fidelity of delivery, and objectively measuring what parts of the interventions are engaged with by users.[92] Technology and mHealth applications can deliver timely, effective, efficient, and equitable behavior change interventions to foster deeper patient engagement and patient-centered cardiac care.[93]

Long-term data from large, theory-based studies are required to fully understand the effective components for sustaining an active lifestyle in older adults. Although more study is warranted for use in older adults, systematic reviews suggest that mHealth interventions may be beneficial for secondary prevention of CVD.[78] Developing home-based activities tailored to older adults' preferences and goals may increase participation of older adults in cardiac rehabilitation programs.[94] Translating a CBCR program to an mHealth platform can potentially decrease barriers to access, decrease the cost, alleviate patient transportation burden, and increase adherence to health behaviors.[95]

FUTURE RESEARCH

With as few as 10% of eligible adults attending CBCR programs, this model is not meeting the growing need of this patient population and alternative methods of delivery must be developed. The use of mHealth technology and wearable sensors has potential to address this gap through a patient-centered HBCR model. Research that refines and personalizes HBCR programs to optimize functional capacity, decrease disability and fall risk, preserve independence, decrease hospital and long-term care admissions, and decrease health care costs in older adults with CVD are warranted.[96] Special considerations for assessment and management of older adults with multimorbidity, noncardiovascular functional and cognitive limitations, and frailty also require additional scientific inquiry. This goal is best accomplished by considering patient preferences, values, and goals of care in the decision-making process. Limited research has focused on frail, older adults with multimorbidity or women in cardiac rehabilitation programs.[97] Conducting randomized clinical trials of HBCR programs that include older adults, and in particular, older women is needed. Additionally, little is known about the efficacy of HBCR in diverse races and ethnicities, those with low socioeconomic status, and those living in rural areas. Well-designed randomized clinical trials of HBCR models using mHealth technologies with older adults are required to provide efficacy and effectiveness data. These data will increase the likelihood that personalized, patient-centered HBCR models integrated seamlessly into older adult's home routines are feasible and reimbursable.

REFERENCES

1. Benjamin EJ, Blaha MJ, Chiuve SE, et al. Heart disease and stroke statistics-2017 update: a report from the American Heart Association. Circulation 2017;135(10):e146–603.

2. Fleg JL, Forman DE, Berra K, et al. Secondary prevention of atherosclerotic cardiovascular disease in older adults: a scientific statement from the American Heart Association. Circulation 2013;128(22):2422–46.

3. GBD 2017 Causes of Death Collaborators. Global, regional, and national age-sex-specific mortality for 282 causes of death in 195 countries and territories, 1980-2017: a systematic analysis for the Global Burden of Disease Study 2017. Lancet 2018;392(10159):1736–88.

4. Roberts AW, Ogunwole SU, Blakeslee H, et al. The population 65 years and older in the United States: 2016. In: U.S. Census Bureau, editor. American Community survey reports. Washington, DC: U.S. Census Bureau; 2018. p. 1–25.
5. Balady GJ, Ades PA, Bittner VA, et al. Referral, enrollment, and delivery of cardiac rehabilitation/secondary prevention programs at clinical centers and beyond: a presidential advisory from the American Heart Association. Circulation 2011;124(25):2951–60.
6. Smith SC Jr, Benjamin EJ, Bonow RO, et al. AHA/ACCF secondary prevention and risk reduction therapy for patients with coronary and other atherosclerotic vascular disease: 2011 update: a guideline from the American Heart Association and American College of Cardiology Foundation endorsed by the World Heart Federation and the Preventive Cardiovascular Nurses Association. J Am Coll Cardiol 2011;58(23):2432–46.
7. Hillis LD, Smith PK, Anderson JL, et al. 2011 ACCF/AHA guideline for coronary artery bypass graft surgery: executive summary: a report of the American College of Cardiology Foundation/American Heart Association Task Force on practice guidelines. Circulation 2011;124(23):2610–42.
8. Levine GN, Bates ER, Blankenship JC, et al. 2011 ACCF/AHA/SCAI guideline for percutaneous coronary intervention: executive summary: a report of the American College of Cardiology Foundation/American Heart Association Task Force on practice guidelines and the Society for Cardiovascular Angiography and Interventions. Circulation 2011;124(23):2574–609.
9. Piepoli MF, Hoes AW, Agewall S, et al. 2016 European guidelines on cardiovascular disease prevention in clinical practice: the Sixth Joint Task Force of the European Society of Cardiology and other Societies on Cardiovascular Disease Prevention in Clinical Practice: developed with the special contribution of the European Association for Cardiovascular Prevention & Rehabilitation (EACPR). Eur J Prev Cardiol 2016;23(11):NP1–96.
10. Thomas RJ, Balady G, Banka G, et al. 2018 ACC/AHA clinical performance and quality measures for cardiac rehabilitation: a report of the American College of Cardiology/American Heart Association Task Force on performance measures. J Am Coll Cardiol 2018;71(16):1814–37.
11. Williams MA, Fleg JL, Ades PA, et al. Secondary prevention of coronary heart disease in the elderly (with emphasis on patients > or =75 years of age): an American Heart Association scientific statement from the Council on Clinical Cardiology Subcommittee on Exercise, Cardiac Rehabilitation, and Prevention. Circulation 2002;105(14):1735–43.
12. Anderson L, Oldridge N, Thompson DR, et al. Exercise-based cardiac rehabilitation for coronary heart disease: cochrane systematic review and meta-analysis. J Am Coll Cardiol 2016;67(1):1–12.
13. Lavie CJ, Milani RV. Benefits of cardiac rehabilitation and exercise training programs in elderly coronary patients. Am J Geriatr Cardiol 2001;10(6):323–7.
14. Balady GJ, Williams MA, Ades PA, et al. Core components of cardiac rehabilitation/secondary prevention programs: 2007 update: a scientific statement from the American Heart Association Exercise, Cardiac Rehabilitation, and Prevention Committee, the Council on Clinical Cardiology; the Councils on Cardiovascular Nursing, Epidemiology and Prevention, and Nutrition, Physical Activity, and Metabolism; and the American Association of Cardiovascular and Pulmonary Rehabilitation. Circulation 2007;115(20):2675–82.
15. Schopfer DW, Forman DE. Cardiac rehabilitation in older adults. Can J Cardiol 2016;32(9):1088–96.

16. Lavie CJ, Milani RV. Effects of cardiac rehabilitation programs on exercise capacity, coronary risk factors, behavioral characteristics, and quality of life in a large elderly cohort. Am J Cardiol 1995;76(3):177–9.
17. Lavie CJ, Milani RV, Littman AB. Benefits of cardiac rehabilitation and exercise training in secondary coronary prevention in the elderly. J Am Coll Cardiol 1993; 22(3):678–83.
18. Lavie CJ, Milani RV. Disparate effects of improving aerobic exercise capacity and quality of life after cardiac rehabilitation in young and elderly coronary patients. J Cardiopulm Rehabil 2000;20(4):235–40.
19. Menezes AR, Lavie CJ, Forman DE, et al. Cardiac rehabilitation in the elderly. Prog Cardiovasc Dis 2014;57(2):152–9.
20. Stanek KM, Gunstad J, Spitznagel MB, et al. Improvements in cognitive function following cardiac rehabilitation for older adults with cardiovascular disease. Int J Neurosci 2011;121(2):86–93.
21. Lavie CV, Milani RV. Impact of aging on hostility in coronary patients and effects of cardiac rehabilitation and exercise training in elderly persons. Am J Geriatr Cardiol 2004;13(3):125–30.
22. Rutledge T, Redwine LS, Linke SE, et al. A meta-analysis of mental health treatments and cardiac rehabilitation for improving clinical outcomes and depression among patients with coronary heart disease. Psychosom Med 2013;75(4): 335–49.
23. Afilalo J, Karunananthan S, Eisenberg MJ, et al. Role of frailty in patients with cardiovascular disease. Am J Cardiol 2009;103(11):1616–21.
24. Afilalo J, Alexander KP, Mack MJ, et al. Frailty assessment in the cardiovascular care of older adults. J Am Coll Cardiol 2014;63(8):747–62.
25. Suaya JA, Stason WB, Ades PA, et al. Cardiac rehabilitation and survival in older coronary patients. J Am Coll Cardiol 2009;54(1):25–33.
26. American Association of Cardiovascular and Pulmonary Rehabilitation. Guidelines for cardiac rehabilitation and secondary prevention programs. Champaign (IL): Human Kinetics; 2013.
27. Kotseva K, Wood D, De Backer G, et al. Use and effects of cardiac rehabilitation in patients with coronary heart disease: results from the EUROASPIRE III survey. Eur J Prev Cardiol 2013;20(5):817–26.
28. Chase JA. Systematic review of physical activity intervention studies after cardiac rehabilitation. J Cardiovasc Nurs 2011;26(5):351–8.
29. Janssen V, De Gucht V, van Exel H, et al. Beyond resolutions? A randomized controlled trial of a self-regulation lifestyle programme for post-cardiac rehabilitation patients. Eur J Prev Cardiol 2013;20(3):431–41.
30. Lear SA, Spinelli JJ, Linden W, et al. The Extensive Lifestyle Management Intervention (ELMI) after cardiac rehabilitation: a 4-year randomized controlled trial. Am Heart J 2006;152(2):333–9.
31. Dalal HM, Zawada A, Jolly K, et al. Home based versus centre based cardiac rehabilitation: Cochrane systematic review and meta-analysis. BMJ 2010;340: b5631.
32. Ramadi A, Haennel RG, Stone JA, et al. The sustainability of exercise capacity changes in home versus center-based cardiac rehabilitation. J Cardiopulm Rehabil Prev 2015;35(1):21–8.
33. Smith KM, McKelvie RS, Thorpe KE, et al. Six-year follow-up of a randomised controlled trial examining hospital versus home-based exercise training after coronary artery bypass graft surgery. Heart 2011;97(14):1169–74.

34. Lachman ME, Lipsitz L, Lubben J, et al. When adults don't exercise: behavioral strategies to increase physical activity in sedentary middle-aged and older adults. Innov Aging 2018;2(1):igy007.
35. Rejeski WJ, Brawley LR, Ambrosius WT, et al. Older adults with chronic disease: benefits of group-mediated counseling in the promotion of physically active lifestyles. Health Psychol 2003;22(4):414–23.
36. Bailly L, Mosse P, Diagana S, et al. "As du Coeur" study: a randomized controlled trial on quality of life impact and cost effectiveness of a physical activity program in patients with cardiovascular disease. BMC Cardiovasc Disord 2018;18(1):225.
37. Lally P, Gardner B. Promoting habit formation. Health Psychol Rev 2013;7(sup1): S137–58.
38. Jelinek MV, Thompson DR, Ski C, et al. 40 years of cardiac rehabilitation and secondary prevention in post-cardiac ischaemic patients. Are we still in the wilderness? Int J Cardiol 2015;179:153–9.
39. Menezes AR, Lavie CJ, Milani RV, et al. Cardiac rehabilitation and exercise therapy in the elderly: should we invest in the aged? J Geriatr Cardiol 2012;9(1): 68–75.
40. Grace SL, Turk-Adawi K, Santiago de Araujo Pio C, et al. Ensuring cardiac rehabilitation access for the majority of those in need: a call to action for Canada. Can J Cardiol 2016;32(10 Suppl 2):S358–64.
41. Santiago de Araujo Pio C, Chaves GS, Davies P, et al. Interventions to promote patient utilisation of cardiac rehabilitation. Cochrane Database Syst Rev 2019;(2):CD007131.
42. Ades PA, Waldmann ML, McCann WJ, et al. Predictors of cardiac rehabilitation participation in older coronary patients. Arch Intern Med 1992;152(5):1033–5.
43. Grace SL, Gravely-Witte S, Brual J, et al. Contribution of patient and physician factors to cardiac rehabilitation enrollment: a prospective multilevel study. Eur J Cardiovasc Prev Rehabil 2008;15(5):548–56.
44. Brown TM, Hernandez AF, Bittner V, et al. Predictors of cardiac rehabilitation referral in coronary artery disease patients: findings from the American Heart Association's get with the guidelines program. J Am Coll Cardiol 2009;54(6): 515–21.
45. Arena R, Williams M, Forman DE, et al. Increasing referral and participation rates to outpatient cardiac rehabilitation: the valuable role of healthcare professionals in the inpatient and home health settings: a science advisory from the American Heart Association. Circulation 2012;125(10):1321–9.
46. Mazzini MJ, Stevens GR, Whalen D, et al. Effect of an American Heart Association get with the guidelines program-based clinical pathway on referral and enrollment into cardiac rehabilitation after acute myocardial infarction. Am J Cardiol 2008;101(8):1084–7.
47. Weingarten MN, Salz KA, Thomas RJ, et al. Rates of enrollment for men and women referred to outpatient cardiac rehabilitation. J Cardiopulm Rehabil Prev 2011;31(4):217–22.
48. Grace SL, Russell KL, Reid RD, et al. Effect of cardiac rehabilitation referral strategies on utilization rates: a prospective, controlled study. Arch Intern Med 2011; 171(3):235–41.
49. Sandesara PB, Dhindsa D, Khambhati J, et al. Reconfiguring cardiac rehabilitation to achieve panvascular prevention: new care models for a new world. Can J Cardiol 2018;34(10S2):S231–9.

50. Grace SL, Shanmugasegaram S, Gravely-Witte S, et al. Barriers to cardiac rehabilitation: DOES AGE MAKE A DIFFERENCE? J Cardiopulm Rehabil Prev 2009; 29(3):183–7.
51. Sandesara PB, Lambert CT, Gordon NF, et al. Cardiac rehabilitation and risk reduction: time to "rebrand and reinvigorate". J Am Coll Cardiol 2015;65(4): 389–95.
52. Listerman J, Bittner V, Sanderson BK, et al. Cardiac rehabilitation outcomes: impact of comorbidities and age. J Cardiopulm Rehabil Prev 2011;31(6):342–8.
53. Cossette S, Maheu-Cadotte MA, Mailhot T, et al. Sex- and gender-related factors associated with cardiac rehabilitation enrollment: a secondary analysis among systematically referred patients. J Cardiopulm Rehabil Prev 2019;39(4):259–65.
54. Resurreccion DM, Motrico E, Rubio-Valera M, et al. Reasons for dropout from cardiac rehabilitation programs in women: a qualitative study. PLoS One 2018;13(7):e0200636.
55. Forman DE, Rich MW, Alexander KP, et al. Cardiac care for older adults. Time for a new paradigm. J Am Coll Cardiol 2011;57(18):1801–10.
56. Anderson L, Sharp GA, Norton RJ, et al. Home-based versus centre-based cardiac rehabilitation. Cochrane Database Syst Rev 2017;(6):CD007130.
57. Boyde M, Rankin J, Whitty JA, et al. Patient preferences for the delivery of cardiac rehabilitation. Patient Educ Couns 2018;101(12):2162–9.
58. Tang LH, Kikkenborg Berg S, Christensen J, et al. Patients' preference for exercise setting and its influence on the health benefits gained from exercise-based cardiac rehabilitation. Int J Cardiol 2017;232:33–9.
59. Marchionni N, Fattirolli F, Fumagalli S, et al. Improved exercise tolerance and quality of life with cardiac rehabilitation of older patients after myocardial infarction: results of a randomized, controlled trial. Circulation 2003;107(17):2201–6.
60. Clark RA, Conway A, Poulsen V, et al. Alternative models of cardiac rehabilitation: a systematic review. Eur J Prev Cardiol 2015;22(1):35–74.
61. Buckingham SA, Taylor RS, Jolly K, et al. Home-based versus centre-based cardiac rehabilitation: abridged Cochrane systematic review and meta-analysis. Open Heart 2016;3(2):e000463.
62. Claes J, Buys R, Budts W, et al. Longer-term effects of home-based exercise interventions on exercise capacity and physical activity in coronary artery disease patients: a systematic review and meta-analysis. Eur J Prev Cardiol 2017;24(3): 244–56.
63. Paneni F, Diaz Canestro C, Libby P, et al. The aging cardiovascular system: understanding it at the cellular and clinical levels. J Am Coll Cardiol 2017;69(15): 1952–67.
64. Wang J, Maxwell CA, Yu F. Biological processes and biomarkers related to frailty in older adults: a state-of-the-science literature review. Biol Res Nurs 2019;21(1): 80–106.
65. Forman DE, Arena R, Boxer R, et al. Prioritizing functional capacity as a principal end point for therapies oriented to older adults with cardiovascular disease: a scientific statement for healthcare professionals from the American Heart Association. Circulation 2017;135(16):e894–918.
66. Galloza J, Castillo B, Micheo W. Benefits of exercise in the older population. Phys Med Rehabil Clin N Am 2017;28(4):659–69.
67. Seals DR, Brunt VE, Rossman MJ. Keynote lecture: strategies for optimal cardiovascular aging. Am J Physiol Heart Circ Physiol 2018;315(2):H183–8.
68. LaRocca TJ, Martens CR, Seals DR. Nutrition and other lifestyle influences on arterial aging. Ageing Res Rev 2017;39:106–19.

69. Zheng G, Xia R, Zhou W, et al. Aerobic exercise ameliorates cognitive function in older adults with mild cognitive impairment: a systematic review and meta-analysis of randomised controlled trials. Br J Sports Med 2016;50(23):1443–50.
70. Karapolat H, Demir E, Bozkaya YT, et al. Comparison of hospital-based versus home-based exercise training in patients with heart failure: effects on functional capacity, quality of life, psychological symptoms, and hemodynamic parameters. Clin Res Cardiol 2009;98(10):635–42.
71. Gaye B, Canonico M, Perier MC, et al. Ideal cardiovascular health, mortality, and vascular events in elderly subjects: the three-city study. J Am Coll Cardiol 2017; 69(25):3015–26.
72. Morgan PJ, Young MD, Smith JJ, et al. Targeted health behavior interventions promoting physical activity: a conceptual model. Exerc Sport Sci Rev 2016; 44(2):71–80.
73. Ryan RM, Deci EL. Self-determination theory and the facilitation of intrinsic motivation, social development, and well-being. Am Psychol 2000;55(1):68–78.
74. Amireault S, Baier JM, Spencer JR. Physical activity preferences among older adults: a systematic review. J Aging Phys Act 2019;27(2):128–39.
75. O'Connor CM, Whellan DJ, Lee KL, et al. Efficacy and safety of exercise training in patients with chronic heart failure: HF-ACTION randomized controlled trial. JAMA 2009;301(14):1439–50.
76. Guimaraes PO, Granger CB, Stebbins A, et al. Sex differences in clinical characteristics, psychosocial factors, and outcomes among patients with stable coronary heart disease: insights from the STABILITY (Stabilization of Atherosclerotic Plaque by Initiation of Darapladib Therapy) Trial. J Am Heart Assoc 2017;6(9) [pii:e006695].
77. Rawstorn JC, Gant N, Rolleston A, et al. End users want alternative intervention delivery models: usability and acceptability of the REMOTE-CR exercise-based cardiac telerehabilitation program. Arch Phys Med Rehabil 2018;99(11):2373–7.
78. Gandhi S, Chen S, Hong L, et al. Effect of mobile health interventions on the secondary prevention of cardiovascular disease: systematic review and meta-analysis. Can J Cardiol 2017;33(2):219–31.
79. Widmer RJ, Collins NM, Collins CS, et al. Digital health interventions for the prevention of cardiovascular disease: a systematic review and meta-analysis. Mayo Clin Proc 2015;90(4):469–80.
80. Hamilton SJ, Mills B, Birch EM, et al. Smartphones in the secondary prevention of cardiovascular disease: a systematic review. BMC Cardiovasc Disord 2018; 18(1):25.
81. Varnfield M, Karunanithi M, Lee CK, et al. Smartphone-based home care model improved use of cardiac rehabilitation in postmyocardial infarction patients: results from a randomised controlled trial. Heart 2014;100(22):1770–9.
82. Forman DE, LaFond K, Panch T, et al. Utility and efficacy of a smartphone application to enhance the learning and behavior goals of traditional cardiac rehabilitation: a feasibility study. J Cardiopulm Rehabil Prev 2014;34(5):327–34.
83. Maddison R, Pfaeffli L, Whittaker R, et al. A mobile phone intervention increases physical activity in people with cardiovascular disease: results from the HEART randomized controlled trial. Eur J Prev Cardiol 2015;22(6):701–9.
84. Dale LP, Whittaker R, Jiang Y, et al. Improving coronary heart disease self-management using mobile technologies (Text4Heart): a randomised controlled trial protocol. Trials 2014;15:71.

85. Jonkman NH, van Schooten KS, Maier AB, et al. eHealth interventions to promote objectively measured physical activity in community-dwelling older people. Maturitas 2018;113:32–9.
86. Lounsbury P, Elokda AS, Gylten D, et al. Text-messaging program improves outcomes in outpatient cardiovascular rehabilitation. Int J Cardiol Heart Vasc 2015; 7:170–5.
87. Chow CK, Redfern J, Hillis GS, et al. Effect of lifestyle-focused text messaging on risk factor modification in patients with coronary heart disease: a randomized clinical trial. JAMA 2015;314(12):1255–63.
88. Rawstorn JC, Gant N, Direito A, et al. Telehealth exercise-based cardiac rehabilitation: a systematic review and meta-analysis. Heart 2016;102(15):1183–92.
89. Webb TL, Joseph J, Yardley L, et al. Using the internet to promote health behavior change: a systematic review and meta-analysis of the impact of theoretical basis, use of behavior change techniques, and mode of delivery on efficacy. J Med Internet Res 2010;12(1):e4.
90. Moller AC, Merchant G, Conroy DE, et al. Applying and advancing behavior change theories and techniques in the context of a digital health revolution: proposals for more effectively realizing untapped potential. J Behav Med 2017; 40(1):85–98.
91. Michie S, Prestwich A. Are interventions theory-based? Development of a theory coding scheme. Health Psychol 2010;29(1):1–8.
92. Michie S, Yardley L, West R, et al. Developing and evaluating digital interventions to promote behavior change in health and health care: recommendations resulting from an international workshop. J Med Internet Res 2017;19(6):e232.
93. Schwamm LH, Chumbler N, Brown E, et al. Recommendations for the implementation of Telehealth in cardiovascular and stroke care: a policy statement from the American Heart Association. Circulation 2017;135(7):e24–44.
94. Madhavan MV, Gersh BJ, Alexander KP, et al. Coronary artery disease in patients >/=80 years of age. J Am Coll Cardiol 2018;71(18):2015–40.
95. Lear SA. The delivery of cardiac rehabilitation using communications technologies: the "virtual" cardiac rehabilitation program. Can J Cardiol 2018;34(10S2): S278–83.
96. Rich MW, Chyun DA, Skolnick AH, et al. Knowledge gaps in cardiovascular care of the older adult population: a scientific statement from the American Heart Association, American College of Cardiology, and American Geriatrics Society. Circulation 2016;133(21):2103–22.
97. Vigorito C, Abreu A, Ambrosetti M, et al. Frailty and cardiac rehabilitation: a call to action from the EAPC Cardiac Rehabilitation Section. Eur J Prev Cardiol 2017; 24(6):577–90.
98. Cowie A, Thow MK, Granat MH, et al. A comparison of home and hospital-based exercise training in heart failure: immediate and long-term effects upon physical activity level. Eur J Cardiovasc Prev Rehabil 2011;18(2):158–66.
99. Cowie A, Thow MK, Granat MH, et al. Effects of home versus hospital-based exercise training in chronic heart failure. Int J Cardiol 2012;158(2):296–8.
100. Oerkild B, Frederiksen M, Hansen JF, et al. Home-based cardiac rehabilitation is as effective as centre-based cardiac rehabilitation among elderly with coronary heart disease: results from a randomised clinical trial. Age Ageing 2011;40(1): 78–85.
101. Piotrowicz E, Baranowski R, Bilinska M, et al. A new model of home-based telemonitored cardiac rehabilitation in patients with heart failure: effectiveness, quality of life, and adherence. Eur J Heart Fail 2010;12(2):164–71.

102. Piotrowicz E, Stepnowska M, Leszczynska-Iwanicka K, et al. Quality of life in heart failure patients undergoing home-based telerehabilitation versus outpatient rehabilitation–a randomized controlled study. Eur J Cardiovasc Nurs 2015;14(3):256–63.
103. Piotrowicz E, Zielinski T, Bodalski R, et al. Home-based telemonitored Nordic walking training is well accepted, safe, effective and has high adherence among heart failure patients, including those with cardiovascular implantable electronic devices: a randomised controlled study. Eur J Prev Cardiol 2015;22(11):1368–77.
104. Guralnik JM, Ferrucci L, Simonsick EM, et al. Lower-extremity function in persons over the age of 70 years as a predictor of subsequent disability. N Engl J Med 1995;332(9):556–61.
105. Katz S. Assessing self-maintenance: activities of daily living, mobility, and instrumental activities of daily living. J Am Geriatr Soc 1983;31(12):721–7.
106. Groot C, Hooghiemstra AM, Raijmakers PG, et al. The effect of physical activity on cognitive function in patients with dementia: a meta-analysis of randomized control trials. Ageing Res Rev 2016;25:13–23.
107. American College of Sports Medicine. ACSM's resource manual for guidelines for exercise testing and prescription. Baltimore (MD): Williams & Wilkins; 1998.

Cardiac Rehabilitation in Older Adults with Heart Failure: Fitting a Square Peg in a Round Hole

Kelsey M. Flint, MD, MSCS[a,*], Amy M. Pastva, PT, PhD[b], Gordon R. Reeves, MD, MPT[c,d,*]

KEYWORDS

- Cardiac rehabilitation • Older adults • Heart failure • Frailty • Sarcopenia
- Cognitive impairment • Multimorbidity

KEY POINTS

- Cardiac rehabilitation (CR) is a structured exercise and lifestyle program that improves mortality and quality of life in patients with heart failure (HF) with reduced ejection fraction.
- The HF-ACTION trial advanced the scientific understanding of aerobic exercise in patients with HF with reduced ejection fraction in a significant way and led to important policy changes that made CR accessible to a large segment of the HF population, many clinically important questions remain unanswered.
- Such limitations in the current CR landscape guide our discussion of the geriatric-specific complexities in CR for older adults with HF, and the clinical and research implications of those complexities.

Disclosure: The authors have nothing to disclose.
Funding: Dr G.R. Reeves receives funding from National Institutes of Health (NIH) grant R01AG045551. Dr A. Pastva receives funding from NIH R01 AG045551, PCORI PCS-1403-14532 and NIH P30 AG028716. Dr K.M. Flint has no funding sources to report.
[a] Division of Cardiology, Rocky Mountain Regional VA Medical Center, 1700 North Wheeling Street, Cardiology F2 (111B), Aurora, CO 80045, USA; [b] Departments of Medicine, Orthopedic Surgery, and Population Health Sciences, Duke University School of Medicine, Duke Claude D. Pepper Older American Independence Center, 2200 West Main Street, Suite B-230, Wing B, #216, Durham, NC 27705, USA; [c] Department of Medicine, Division of Cardiology, Thomas Jefferson University, Philadelphia, PA 19107, USA; [d] Advanced Heart Failure for the Greater Charlotte Market, Novant Health Heart and Vascular Institute, 1718 E 4th Street, Suite 501, Charlotte, NC 28204, USA
* Corresponding authors.
E-mail addresses: Kelsey.Flint@ucdenver.edu (K.M.F.); gordon.r.reeves@gmail.com (G.R.R.)

Clin Geriatr Med 35 (2019) 517–526
https://doi.org/10.1016/j.cger.2019.07.008
0749-0690/19/Published by Elsevier Inc.

INTRODUCTION

Cardiac rehabilitation (CR) is a structured exercise and lifestyle intervention program initially designed for patients with ischemic heart disease. CR program structure typically requires patients to attend group exercise and education courses at a medical center 3 times per week for 12 weeks. CR is successful in reducing cardiovascular mortality and rehospitalizations among patients with ischemic heart disease.[1] The past decade has seen significant progress in the study of CR for patients with heart failure (HF), spearheaded by the National Institutes of Health (NIH)-sponsored HF-ACTION trial.[2] HF-ACTION is the largest randomized clinical trial of CR to date, randomizing 2331 patients with symptomatic HF with reduced ejection fraction (≤35%; HFrEF) to CR or attention control. Notably, these patients were clinically stable outpatients who had not been hospitalized for at least 6 weeks and were on stable guideline-directed medical therapy. CR sessions occurred 3 times per week at the study center and consisted of traditional moderate-intensity aerobic exercise. Patients were also encouraged to exercise at home and were provided with home exercise equipment and frequent reminder phone calls to reinforce adherence.[2]

To some, the results of HF-ACTION were underwhelming, as the reduction in all-cause mortality and hospitalizations was seen only after prespecified adjustment for highly prognostic baseline characteristics.[2] However, HF-ACTION also showed clinically significant improvement in quality of life measures in the exercise intervention arm,[3,4] a finding supported in smaller studies.[5] Furthermore, HF-ACTION proved unequivocally that moderate-intensity aerobic exercise is *safe* in patients with medically treated and stable HFrEF, an issue that was unresolved before the study. Ultimately, the results of HF-ACTION were instrumental to the decision by the Centers for Medicare and Medicaid Services (CMS) to approve payment for CR for beneficiaries matching the HF-ACTION inclusion criteria. Specifically, this includes those with symptomatic HF with ejection fraction ≤35% who have not been hospitalized for at least 6 weeks and who did not have a planned major cardiovascular hospitalization or procedure in the past 6 months (https://www.cms.gov/medicare-coverage-database/details/nca-decision-memo.aspx?NCAId=270). Most clinical CR programs now use these inclusion criteria when identifying which patients with HF should be enrolled.

Although HF-ACTION advanced the scientific understanding of aerobic exercise in patients with HFrEF in a significant way and led to important policy changes that made CR accessible to a large segment of the HF population, many clinically important questions remain unanswered. First, HF-ACTION did not include patients with HF with preserved ejection fraction (≥45%; HFpEF). HFpEF is now recognized to account for approximately 50% of the total HF population in the United States, and is the most common type of HF among the rapidly growing population of older adults.[6–8] Although smaller studies have demonstrated improvement in exercise capacity, quality of life, and possibly hospital admissions in patients with HFpEF who participate in structured endurance exercise training programs,[9–11] such patients are typically excluded from CR by CMS and most other third-party payers because of lack of evidence.

Second, HF-ACTION enrolled chronic stable patients with HFrEF from the outpatient setting and excluded patients who had been hospitalized in the past 6 weeks. Consequently, recently hospitalized patients with HF patients are explicitly excluded from CR participation under CMS policy; however, following hospitalization, older adults with HF are particularly susceptible to the "post-hospitalization syndrome."[12] Post-hospital syndrome is characterized by significant physical functional impairments beyond that expected in chronic stable HFrEF, leading to a period of high vulnerability for adverse clinical events, such as rehospitalization.[12] Rapid muscle loss and debility related to hospitalization, immobility, and acute illness likely contribute this syndrome,[13–16] and suggest opportunities for appropriately structured CR programs beginning early after discharge to improve physical function and potentially other important outcomes, including mortality, hospitalization, and quality of life.

Third, HF-ACTION, as well as most other CR studies to date, did not take into account the complexities of aging, such as frailty, multimorbidity, and polypharmacy, which are increasingly prevalent among older patients with HF. For example, the average age of patients enrolled in HF-ACTION was 59 years, whereas most patients hospitalized for HF are in their 60s, 70s, and 80s.[6] Although HF-ACTION enrolled 477 patients 70 years and older, the study may have selected for a relatively robust group able to perform maximal exercise testing to establish peak oxygen consumption and a 6-minute walk test as part of enrollment and with fewer comorbidities due to exclusion criteria. HF is a disease of aging, with incidence of HF increasing dramatically in the eighth and ninth decades of life.[17] Comorbidities frequently contribute to functional impairments and ability to participate in traditional endurance-based training modalities (eg, treadmill walking). Aging-related considerations may warrant a different approach than that of traditional CR, as discussed further later in this article.

Finally, HF-ACTION achieved only weak adherence to the exercise intervention despite tremendous efforts by the study investigators to promote regular participation.[18] Fewer than 50% of patients in the intervention arm of HF-ACTION reached their target number of exercise hours in a given week.[2] Nonadherence is common among patients with HF,[18] and issues of old age, multimorbidity, and debilitating symptoms are all relevant.[18] Such limitations in the current CR landscape will guide our discussion of the geriatric-specific complexities in CR for older adults with HF, and the clinical and research implications of those complexities.

GERIATRIC COMPLEXITIES AND CARDIAC REHABILITATION FOR OLDER ADULTS WITH HEART FAILURE

Frailty and Its Implications for Cardiac Rehabilitation

Frailty is the accumulation of deficits across multiple organ systems, leading to vulnerability in the face of stress (**Fig. 1**). Frailty is highly prevalent among patients with HF,

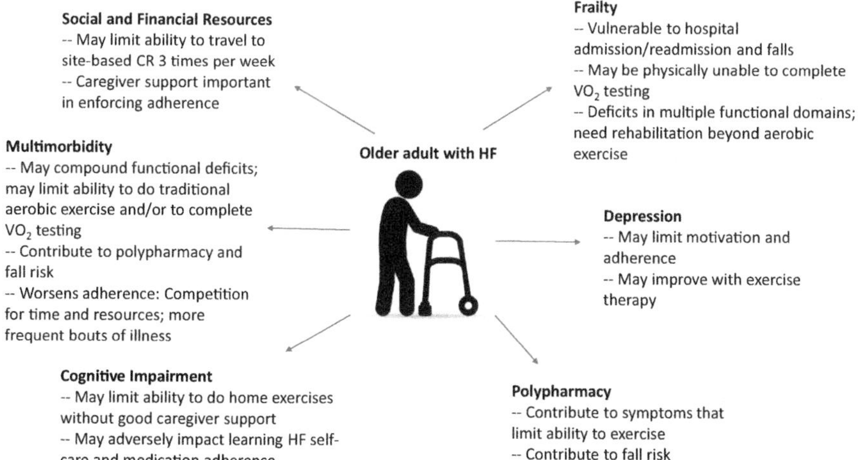

Fig. 1. Summary of the geriatric complexities often present among older adults with HF. VO$_2$, maximal oxygen uptake.

and even more prevalent among older adults hospitalized for HF.[19–21] Physical frailty is characterized by a phenotype of activity intolerance beyond what would be expected for aging or HF alone. Among older frail patients with HF, this manifests as severe physical function impairments across multiple domains (eg, balance, mobility) adversely affecting functional mobility.[20]

Frailty is an independent risk factor for adverse outcomes among older patients with HF, and exercise training has potential to mitigate the risk of all-cause and cardiovascular death associated with frailty.[22] Furthermore, CR is associated with better outcomes among frail older adults who suffered an acute myocardial infarction.[23] Therefore, frailty should not preclude structured exercise therapy; rather, it may help to identify a higher-risk population with greater potential to benefit from this intervention, especially if it can be structured to meet the specific needs of this patient population.

There is no clear "gold standard" for frailty measurement in HF. However, it would seem reasonable to choose frailty measure(s) based on which outcomes are most actionable or important to their patient population. Therefore, careful assessments of physical frailty, such as the Fried criteria,[24] Short Physical Performance Battery (SPPB; a well-validated measure of strength, mobility, and balance that predicts morbidity and mortality in older adults),[25] or individual measures, such as gait speed or handgrip strength, would seem appropriate options. The Clinical Frailty Scale[26] was proposed as a sensitive and specific screening tool for frailty in HF,[27] and may help identify patients who warrant closer evaluation for significant barriers to conventional CR participation. Frail patients also are at risk for loss of functional independence. Maintaining or regaining functional independence is often an important goal for most older adults that may be addressed through rehabilitation interventions or other components of a comprehensive CR program. Assessment of basic and instrumental activities of daily living in conjunction with frailty assessments may be helpful in structuring a rehabilitation intervention that may be particularly meaningful to the participant, potentially improving adherence and having a greater impact on quality of life.

CR clinicians must be innovative in designing an exercise program for patients with deficits across multiple physical domains and associated loss of functional independence, as these patients may not tolerate conventional CR strategies. In fact, many frail patients will have rehabilitation needs that exceed resources typically available (or reimbursed) in contemporary CR. Further study of alternative CR delivery models is needed to establish an evidence base for such comprehensive rehabilitation care.

Multimorbidity and Its Implications for Cardiac Rehabilitation

Multimorbidity is pervasive among older patients with HF, many of whom have at least 5 or more comorbid illnesses, a large portion of which are noncardiovascular conditions.[20,28] This geriatric ailment is associated with reduction in adherence to CR among patients with HF,[18] complicating CR participation in a number of ways. Even when chronic and stable, comorbid conditions can "compete" for patients' attention and resources.[29] Multimorbidity may also increase patients' risk for polypharmacy, which has its own attendant adverse outcomes. Furthermore, multimorbidity increases risk of acute illness and hospitalization, both non-HF and HF-related,[30] which may prevent participation. Comorbid illnesses also contribute to more severe functional impairments, which may further limit participation. For example, chronic conditions, such as chronic kidney disease and chronic obstructive pulmonary disease contribute to muscle wasting, weakness, and exertional intolerance.[31,32] Orthopedic and neurologic conditions in particular may affect patients' ability to participate in traditional CR modalities, such as treadmill walking. CR clinicians must be alert to these conditions and be prepared to alter exercise prescriptions accordingly.

Polypharmacy and Its Implications for Cardiac Rehabilitation

Polypharmacy may contribute to symptoms of fatigue, cognitive impairment, and depression. Alleviating these medication side effects may improve patients' adherence to CR. Therefore, a thoughtful protocol for reviewing patients' medications as part of CR may be beneficial. For example, stopping beta blockers in patients with HFpEF and no coronary artery disease may improve fatigue or orthostatic hypotension. Medications on the Beers list should receive close scrutiny, as many of these may cause symptoms that interfere with meaningful CR participation.[33] Multidisciplinary review, including a clinical pharmacist, can also be helpful in identifying drug-drug interactions and dosing adjustments related to declining renal or liver function. Any de-prescribing should be done (1) under the guidance of a qualified clinician who is trained in geriatrics, cardiology, and the medication management of HF in older adults, and (2) either by or in consultation with the prescribing provider. This team-based approach is necessary to avoid miscommunications and ensure referring providers maintain control over their patients' medication regimen.

Cognitive Impairment and Its Implications for Cardiac Rehabilitation

Cognitive impairment is common in HF, with an estimated prevalence of 43% to 80% depending on HF population (eg, acute vs chronic) and sensitivity of the instrument used.[20,34] Cognitive impairment is often mild and commonly unrecognized in clinical practice. However, even when recognized, cognitive impairment alone should not preclude CR participation; cognitive impairment did not diminish adherence to a supervised exercise program designed for community-dwelling older adults with impaired mobility.[35] Caregiver support can be especially important for older adults with HF and cognitive impairment. For example, patients who are unable to remember instructions for safe exercise participation or who have processing impairments will likely not be appropriate for a home-based program without sufficient caregiver support. All patients with cognitive impairment will be at risk for medication errors and poorer HF self-care; therefore, caregiver support can be helpful in these areas as well. In addition, direct communication of any newly identified cognitive impairment to the patient's cardiovascular and/or primary care provider is important for long-term management.

Depression and Its Implications for Cardiac Rehabilitation

Depression is present in approximately 22% of patients with HF,[36] and prevalence of depressive symptoms are nearly twice that among older adults hospitalized for HF.[20] Depression may complicate CR by reducing patients' motivation and adherence,[18] and can masquerade as cognitive impairment. Fortunately, exercise improves depressive symptoms in HF[37]; therefore, depression alone should not preclude CR participation. In fact, the social aspect of site-based CR may improve a patient's mood. As with cognitive impairment, patients' cardiovascular and/or primary care clinicians should always be notified of a positive depression screen in patients in whom depression has previously not been identified.

Social and Financial Resources and Their Implications for Cardiac Rehabilitation

Involvement, or bolstering, of the patient's social support network and use of community-based resources is integral to encouraging CR participation and long-term exercise adherence. The support of caregivers, formal and/or informal, may be required for transportation and supporting continued exercise adherence at home, both during and after completion of the CR program. Patients with cognitive impairment and/or depression will require significant support from a caregiver(s) when it comes to attending sessions regularly and retaining information taught by the CR staff. Patients who do not have a mode of transportation to the CR center are particularly challenged, and connecting patients with community-based resources may be necessary. There is a growing interest in home-based or hybrid CR programs in part because they reduce or obviate the need for transportation. However, patients should be carefully assessed for fall risk, poor physical function, and potential need for physical or occupational therapy (ie, home health or outpatient therapy) as a bridge to commencing either a home-based or outpatient CR program.

THE FUTURE IS BRIGHT: ONGOING OR FUTURE STUDIES OF CARDIAC REHABILITATION IN OLDER ADULTS WITH HEART FAILURE

Older adults hospitalized for HF have severe deficits in strength, balance, mobility, and endurance, likely as a result of geriatric complexities, such as frailty, multimorbidity, and polypharmacy.[20] However, as discussed previously, such patients are currently not immediately eligible for CR based on CMS criteria and lack of evidence. Even if these patients were eligible for CR, their rehabilitation needs immediately after hospitalization would frequently exceed the resources typically available at conventional CR. The REHAB-HF study is currently testing a rehabilitation intervention in this patient population. The intervention arm receives an individualized, progressive, multidomain exercise intervention that addresses strength, balance, mobility, and endurance among patients ≥60 years old who are hospitalized for HF.[38,39] Akin to traditional CR, patients attend exercise sessions at the study site 3 times per week for 12 weeks.[38] The REHAB-HF intervention in the pilot study was well tolerated and feasible when enrolling patients who were living independently before hospitalization and were discharged home without home health rehabilitation.[40]

The REHAB-HF protocol differs significantly from traditional CR in that investigators are not relying on maximal or sub-maximal exercise testing to guide exercise prescription; rather, investigators are relying on a functional assessment[25] to guide exercise prescription. This is because in patients with profound impairments in strength, mobility, or balance, exercise testing aimed at assessing aerobic capacity/anaerobic threshold may not be possible or may not yield valuable information. Targeting endurance (walking) training without also addressing deficits in balance, mobility, and strength may increase risk of falls. Furthermore, patients can track their progress through attainment of independence in activities of daily living, which may improve adherence, and clinicians can observe progress through serial objective measurements, such as the SPPB and the 6-Minute Walk Test.

A novel CR program tailored to the older adult with cardiovascular disease (including, but not limited to HF) is being tested in the NIH-sponsored Modified Application of Cardiac Rehabilitation for Older Adults (MACRO) study (ClinicalTrials.gov: NCT03922529). This trial will test the a comprehensive intervention that will specifically (1) broaden risk assessment of older patients with cardiovascular disease with functional, psychosocial, and cardiac domains; (2) enhance CR care transitions (eg, inpatient CR to home-based CR, with outpatient options then including site-based, home-based, and hybrid models of care); (3) assess the home environment for home exercise safety; (4) augment motivation with a novel behavioral strategy; and (5) integrate de-prescribing of medications that impede functional recovery. The MACRO study results may be anticipated in the next 3 to 5 years.

The COMPASS trial is testing a multidimensional intervention designed to identify and meet the postacute care needs of patients hospitalized for stroke.[41] The COMPASS intervention is centered around the patient and caregiver, and attempts to organize the various components of the patient's care (ie, stroke specialist, primary care, home health care) around their needs. COMPASS investigators are now working to develop a similar intervention for patients hospitalized for HF. Incorporating the physical rehabilitation needs into a comprehensive, patient- and caregiver-centered intervention for patients hospitalized for HF is another promising approach for meeting the unique needs of older adults hospitalized for HF.

GUIDANCE FOR THE CARDIAC REHABILITATION CLINICIAN

While CR clinicians await the results of the previously described studies, they may still apply these geriatric principles to current practice based on existing data (**Fig. 2**). Home-based CR for patients meeting traditional CR criteria is considered safe and effective,[42] therefore CR programs could consider incorporating a hybrid or home-based CR program for patients with barriers to transportation. Routine screening for all the geriatric complexities discussed previously should be considered in CR programs currently. However, programs must carefully plan for the care coordination required for handling new diagnoses of depression and cognitive impairment and for addressing polypharmacy.

CR programs also could consider routine testing of multiple domains of physical function (eg, SPPB), rather than simply assessing aerobic capacity. In addition to prognosis, such assessments can help inform prescription of multidomain exercise interventions, which have shown benefit in frail older patients in general. For example, the LIFE study tested a supervised, multidomain exercise intervention for sedentary adults aged 70 to 89 years at risk for mobility-disability (defined as SPPB score ≤10; scores range from 0 to 12, with lower scores indicating worse function). The LIFE study physical activity domains included walking as the primary intervention (target 30 min/d), supplemented with strength training targeting most major muscle

Traditional CR Model for HF
Site-based
Moderate intensity aerobic exercise
Exercise prescription based on VO_2 testing
Strict inclusion criteria:
• EF ≤ 35%
• No hospitalization within 6 wk
• No procedures within 6 mo
Novel CR Model for Older Adults with HF
Implement Now:
Hybrid or home-based models for patients meeting traditional inclusion criteria
Routine screening:
• Frailty
• Multimorbidity
• Polypharmacy
• Cognitive impairment
• Depression
• Poor social support
Multi-domain exercises
• Guided by SPPB or other physical performance assessments
• Strength
• Balance
• Mobility (eg, start/stop, turns, pace)
• Endurance (eg, walking)
Requires further study:
In patients recently hospitalized and/or with HFpEF:
• Hybrid or Home-based CR
• Multi-domain exercise prescription based on multi-domain physical function
In all older adults with HF:
• Novel methods for seamlessly incorporation lifestyle and geriatric-specific interventions into CR

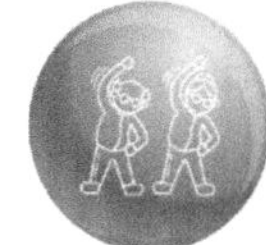

Fig. 2. Comparison of current, traditional CR programs and the potential direction CR programs can take currently, and changes that soon may be supported by evidence. EF, ejection fraction.

groups and balance training, each done 3 times per week for 10 minutes. The intervention was successful in delaying major mobility-disability (defined as inability to complete a 400-m walk test without stopping or assistance) after 1 year (hazard ratio 0.72; 95% confidence interval [CI] 0.57–0.91) and was safe (risk ratio of adverse events in intervention vs control arms 1.08; 95% CI 0.98–1.20).[43] A systematic review of frail older adults also supported the choice of a multidomain exercise intervention[44] like the one prescribed in the LIFE study and the ongoing REHAB-HF study. Therefore, CR clinicians may consider designing exercise prescriptions for older adults with HF with multiple physical domains in mind. Initial physical assessment tools, such as the SPPB, can help inform whether patients have greater deficit in strength, mobility, or balance, therefore guiding which domain(s) should receive the most emphasis, primarily early on in the CR program.

SUMMARY

Exercise has tremendous potential to improve mortality, hospitalization, and quality of life among older adults with HF. Traditional CR may be appropriate for robust older adults with HF; however, important modifications are needed to accommodate the age-related intricacies that typically occur. Although CR clinicians can make important modifications for this patient population now, additional research, including results of ongoing trials, is needed to implement evidenced-based novel CR models designed to meet the specific needs of this population.

REFERENCES

1. Anderson L, Oldridge N, Thompson DR, et al. Exercise-based cardiac rehabilitation for coronary heart disease: Cochrane Systematic Review and meta-analysis. J Am Coll Cardiol 2016;67(1):1–12.
2. O'Connor CM, Whellan DJ, Lee KL, et al. Efficacy and safety of exercise training in patients with chronic heart failure: HF-ACTION randomized controlled trial. JAMA 2009;301(14):1439–50.
3. Ambrosy AP, Cerbin LP, DeVore AD, et al. Aerobic exercise training and general health status in ambulatory heart failure patients with a reduced ejection fraction-findings from the Heart Failure and A Controlled Trial Investigating Outcomes of Exercise Training (HF-ACTION)trial. Am Heart J 2017;186:130–8.
4. Flynn KE, Pina IL, Whellan DJ, et al. Effects of exercise training on health status in patients with chronic heart failure: HF-ACTION randomized controlled trial. JAMA 2009;301(14):1451–9.
5. Long L, Mordi IR, Bridges C, et al. Exercise-based cardiac rehabilitation for adults with heart failure. Cochrane Database Syst Rev 2019;(1):CD003331.
6. Steinberg BA, Zhao X, Heidenreich PA, et al. Trends in patients hospitalized with heart failure and preserved left ventricular ejection fraction: prevalence, therapies, and outcomes. Circulation 2012;126(1):65–75.
7. Cheng RK, Cox M, Neely ML, et al. Outcomes in patients with heart failure with preserved, borderline, and reduced ejection fraction in the Medicare population. Am Heart J 2014;168(5):721–30.
8. Owan TE, Hodge DO, Herges RM, et al. Trends in prevalence and outcome of heart failure with preserved ejection fraction. N Engl J Med 2006;355(3):251–9.
9. Lang CC, Smith K, Wingham J, et al. A randomised controlled trial of a facilitated home-based rehabilitation intervention in patients with heart failure with preserved ejection fraction and their caregivers: the REACH-HFpEF Pilot Study. BMJ Open 2018;8(4):e019649.

10. Kitzman DW, Brubaker P, Morgan T, et al. Effect of caloric restriction or aerobic exercise training on peak oxygen consumption and quality of life in obese older patients with heart failure with preserved ejection fraction: a randomized clinical trial. JAMA 2016;315(1):36–46.
11. Pandey A, Kitzman DW, Brubaker P, et al. Response to endurance exercise training in older adults with heart failure with preserved or reduced ejection fraction. J Am Geriatr Soc 2017;65(8):1698–704.
12. Krumholz HM. Post-hospital syndrome–an acquired, transient condition of generalized risk. N Engl J Med 2013;368(2):100–2.
13. Welch C, K Hassan-Smith Z, A Greig C, et al. Acute sarcopenia secondary to hospitalisation—an emerging condition affecting older adults. Aging Dis 2018;9(1): 151–64.
14. Martinez-Velilla N, Casas-Herrero A, Zambom-Ferraresi F, et al. Effect of exercise intervention on functional decline in very elderly patients during acute hospitalization: a randomized clinical trial. JAMA Intern Med 2019;179(1):28–36.
15. Kanach FA, Pastva AM, Hall KS, et al. Effects of structured exercise interventions for older adults hospitalized with acute medical illness: a systematic review. J Aging Phys Act 2018;26(2):284–303.
16. Benjamin EJ, Virani SS, Callaway CW, et al. Heart disease and stroke statistics-2018 update: a report from the American Heart Association. Circulation 2018; 137(12):e67–492.
17. Mahmood SS, Wang TJ. The epidemiology of congestive heart failure: the Framingham Heart Study perspective. Glob Heart 2013;8(1):77–82.
18. Conraads VM, Deaton C, Piotrowicz E, et al. Adherence of heart failure patients to exercise: barriers and possible solutions: a position statement of the study group on exercise training in heart failure of the Heart Failure Association of the European Society of Cardiology. Eur J Heart Fail 2012;14(5):451–8.
19. Vidan MT, Blaya-Novakova V, Sanchez E, et al. Prevalence and prognostic impact of frailty and its components in non-dependent elderly patients with heart failure. Eur J Heart Fail 2016;18(7):869–75.
20. Warraich HK DJ, Duncan PW, Mentz RJ, et al. Physical function, frailty, cognition, depression and quality-of-life in hospitalized adults >60 years with acute decompensated heart failure with preserved versus reduced ejection fraction: insights from the REHAB-HF Trial. Circ Heart Fail 2018;11:e005254.
21. Denfeld QE, Winters-Stone K, Mudd JO, et al. The prevalence of frailty in heart failure: a systematic review and meta-analysis. Int J Cardiol 2017;236:283–9.
22. Higueras-Fresnillo S, Cabanas-Sanchez V, Lopez-Garcia E, et al. Physical activity and association between frailty and all-cause and cardiovascular mortality in older adults: population-based prospective cohort study. J Am Geriatr Soc 2018;66(11):2097–103.
23. Flint K, Kennedy K, Arnold SV, et al. Slow gait speed and cardiac rehabilitation participation in older adults after acute myocardial infarction. J Am Heart Assoc 2018;7(5) [pii:e008296].
24. Fried LP, Tangen CM, Walston J, et al. Frailty in older adults: evidence for a phenotype. J Gerontol A Biol Sci Med Sci 2001;56(3):M146–56.
25. Guralnik JM, Ferrucci L, Pieper CF, et al. Lower extremity function and subsequent disability: consistency across studies, predictive models, and value of gait speed alone compared with the short physical performance battery. J Gerontol A Biol Sci Med Sci 2000;55(4):M221–31.
26. Rockwood K, Song X, MacKnight C, et al. A global clinical measure of fitness and frailty in elderly people. CMAJ 2005;173(5):489–95.

27. Sze S, Pellicori P, Zhang J, et al. Identification of frailty in chronic heart failure. JACC Heart Fail 2019;7(4):291–302.
28. Manemann SM, Chamberlain AM, Boyd CM, et al. Multimorbidity in heart failure: effect on outcomes. J Am Geriatr Soc 2016;64(7):1469–74.
29. Flint KM, Forman DE. Lessons from the first 202 REHAB-HF participants. Circ Heart Fail 2018;11(11):e005611.
30. Braunstein JB, Anderson GF, Gerstenblith G, et al. Noncardiac comorbidity increases preventable hospitalizations and mortality among medicare beneficiaries with chronic heart failure. J Am Coll Cardiol 2003;42(7):1226–33.
31. Jones SE, Maddocks M, Kon SS, et al. Sarcopenia in COPD: prevalence, clinical correlates and response to pulmonary rehabilitation. Thorax 2015;70(3):213–8.
32. Moorthi RN, Avin KG. Clinical relevance of sarcopenia in chronic kidney disease. Curr Opin Nephrol Hypertens 2017;26(3):219–28.
33. By the American Geriatrics Society 2015 Beers Criteria Update Expert Panel. American Geriatrics Society 2015 updated Beers criteria for potentially inappropriate medication use in older adults. J Am Geriatr Soc 2015;63(11):2227–46.
34. Cannon JA, Moffitt P, Perez-Moreno AC, et al. Cognitive impairment and heart failure: systematic review and meta-analysis. J Card Fail 2017;23(6):464–75.
35. Reid KF, Walkup MP, Katula JA, et al. Cognitive performance does not limit physical activity participation in the lifestyle interventions and independence for elders pilot study (LIFE-P). J Prev Alzheimers Dis 2017;4(1):44–50.
36. Rutledge T, Reis VA, Linke SE, et al. Depression in heart failure: a meta-analytic review of prevalence, intervention effects, and associations with clinical outcomes. J Am Coll Cardiol 2006;48(8):1527–37.
37. Blumenthal JA, Babyak MA, O'Connor C, et al. Effects of exercise training on depressive symptoms in patients with chronic heart failure: the HF-ACTION randomized trial. JAMA 2012;308(5):465–74.
38. Reeves GR, Whellan DJ, Duncan P, et al. Rehabilitation therapy in older acute heart failure patients (REHAB-HF) trial: design and rationale. Am Heart J 2017; 185:130–9.
39. Pastva AM, Duncan PW, Reeves GR, et al. Strategies for supporting intervention fidelity in the rehabilitation therapy in older acute heart failure patients (REHAB-HF) trial. Contemp Clin Trials 2018;64:118–27.
40. Reeves GR, Whellan DJ, O'Connor CM, et al. A novel rehabilitation intervention for older patients with acute decompensated heart failure: the REHAB-HF pilot study. JACC Heart Fail 2017;5(5):359–66.
41. Bushnell CD, Duncan PW, Lycan SL, et al. A person-centered approach to post-stroke care: the COMprehensive post-acute stroke services model. J Am Geriatr Soc 2018;66(5):1025–30.
42. Zwisler AD, Norton RJ, Dean SG, et al. Home-based cardiac rehabilitation for people with heart failure: a systematic review and meta-analysis. Int J Cardiol 2016;221:963–9.
43. Pahor M, Guralnik JM, Ambrosius WT, et al. Effect of structured physical activity on prevention of major mobility disability in older adults: the LIFE study randomized clinical trial. JAMA 2014;311(23):2387–96.
44. de Labra C, Guimaraes-Pinheiro C, Maseda A, et al. Effects of physical exercise interventions in frail older adults: a systematic review of randomized controlled trials. BMC Geriatr 2015;15:154.

Peripheral Arterial Disease

Supervised Exercise Therapy Through Cardiac Rehabilitation

Scott G. Thomas, PhD[a,*], Susan Marzolini, PhD[b], Edward Lin, MSc[b], Cindy H. Nguyen, MSc[a], Paul Oh, MD[b]

KEYWORDS

- Peripheral vascular disease • Lower extremity arterial disease
- Intermittent claudication

KEY POINTS

- Peripheral arterial disease (PAD) occurs in 10% to 20% of individuals older than 65 years.
- As only one-third of patients demonstrate classic intermittent claudication symptoms, diagnosis should be based on the ankle-brachial index.
- Strong evidence supports routine use of supervised exercise therapy for PAD patients as a primary intervention and in conjunction with endovascular interventions.
- Cardiac rehabilitation programs are well suited to providing comprehensive effective care and should be routinely undertaken.

INTRODUCTION

Peripheral arterial disease (PAD) is a chronic condition that is often underdiagnosed and undertreated.[1,2] PAD-associated atherosclerosis limits blood flow to the lower limbs and reduces functional capacity, lowers quality of life, and increases the risk of morbidity and mortality.[3,4] When nearly 7000 primary care patients, age 65 years and older, were assessed, approximately 20% of men and 17% of women were demonstrated to have PAD.[5] Several studies confirm a high prevalence of PAD globally and particularly in older populations.[6,7]

Underdiagnosis of PAD may occur because older adults, especially women, lack awareness of PAD and symptoms are often nonspecific.[4,8] Only approximately one-third of patients with PAD have the classic intermittent claudication (IC) symptoms,[9]

[a] Faculty of Kinesiology and Physical Education, Department of Exercise Sciences, University of Toronto, 55 Harbord Street, Toronto M5S 2W6, Canada; [b] Cardiovascular Prevention and Rehabilitation Program, KITE, University Health Network, 347 Rumsey Road, Toronto M4G 1R7, Canada
* Corresponding author.
E-mail address: scott.thomas@utoronto.ca

Clin Geriatr Med 35 (2019) 527–537
https://doi.org/10.1016/j.cger.2019.07.009

and in many cases the primary symptom is mobility limitation.[10] Even for patients with identified PAD, there is a treatment gap with underuse of lifestyle and medication interventions.[11] It remains an important opportunity to better identify PAD patients and implement care, as there are effective interventions that improve function and quality of life and reduce the risks of morbidity and mortality.[3] This article identifies specific subgroups within older adults more likely to develop PAD, describes how to diagnose PAD, and provides evidence in support of systematic referral to cardiac rehabilitation (CR) programs to enhance successful comprehensive management.

DIAGNOSIS AND PROGNOSIS

PAD is a progressive disease caused by atherosclerosis, which can involve partial or complete obstruction of one or more peripheral arteries. The term PAD is synonymous with peripheral vascular disease or peripheral arterial occlusive disease. The primary focus here is on PAD patients with lower extremity arterial disease. Atherosclerosis is a systemic condition, and those with vessel damage in one location may have it at other sites.

Patients with PAD are generally classified into 1 of 4 categories depending on symptoms: (1) asymptomatic; (2) IC; (3) chronic limb ischemia; and (4) acute limb ischemia.[12] Around 50% of PAD patients are asymptomatic, but still carry a 60% increased risk of stroke and a 20% to 60% increased risk of myocardial infarction, and typically have reduced walking capacity.[13] IC is characterized by classic symptoms of muscle cramps, fatigue, and pain in the lower legs induced by walking and relieved by rest, and is present in approximately one-quarter of persons with PAD.[14] The discomfort of IC is caused by insufficient blood supply to muscles distal to the level of arterial involvement. Chronic limb ischemia or chronic limb-threatening ischemia (European designation[14]) is characterized by pain at rest and is associated with a high mortality rate.[15] Almost 25% of patients with chronic limb ischemia require amputation within 1 year of diagnosis.[16] Early detection and treatment are required to prevent limb loss and further progression of the disease. Acute limb ischemia involves sudden decreases of blood supply to the lower limbs, which threatens limb viability. Unfortunately, acute limb ischemia also results in amputation 10% to 15% of the time and is associated with a 1-year mortality rate of 20%.[16] Progression of the disease does not necessarily follow predictably in an order of severity. A patient with asymptomatic disease can progress immediately to acute limb ischemia without progressing through IC.

Prevalence of PAD increases with age, with estimates of approximately 5% to 6% for ages 50 to 54 and climbing to almost 20% at age 90 years.[6] Prevalence is similar between men and women, although clinical presentation may differ.[17] Current and former smoking and other cardiovascular disease both double the odds of PAD.[6] The presence of diabetes significantly raises the odds ratio to 1.7 and hypertension to approximately 1.5.[6]

PAD can be most readily diagnosed in general practice with the ankle-brachial index (ABI), the ratio of systolic blood pressure at the ankle to systolic blood pressure at the brachial artery.[14] The test can be performed with a blood pressure cuff, standard sphygmomanometer, and a Doppler instrument to detect pulses. PAD is considered present if the ABI is 0.9 or less. This threshold value has an approximate sensitivity of 80% and specificity of 95%.[18,19] Additional testing using postexercise ABI assessment can improve the sensitivity of the measure.[20,21] Other methods of diagnosis include physical examination findings such as arterial bruits and decreased capillary refill, and imaging techniques such as angiography and ultrasonography, although these are no not part of the guidelines.[3,14]

ABI remains the most simple and noninvasive tool for the diagnosis of PAD. An ABI of 0.9 or less indicates significantly greater risk of cardiovascular and all-cause mortality and should initiate intervention.[22,23] Visual guidance in performing the ABI measure is available on YouTube (https://www.youtube.com/watch?v=0_0VILSTAAE).

Symptom severity and functional status can be assessed using exercise testing. Treadmill tests can be used to determine pain-free walking distance/time, maximal walking distance/time, and peak aerobic capacity, which are responsive measures of changes in walking ability.[14] The most often recommended treadmill protocol is the Strandness, in which speed is set at 3 km per hour and grade at 10%.[14] However, other progressive standardized protocols have successfully been used to characterize aerobic capacity.[24]

The 6-minute walk test (6MWT) is used to assess walking performance and has the advantages of not requiring expensive equipment, with very good reliability and sensitivity.[24] In addition, some argue that the 6MWT better characterizes walking in daily life compared with treadmill testing, and normative values are available.[25] Beyond generic questionnaires such as Short-Form 12 (SF-12),[26] PAD-specific instruments such as the Walking Impairment Questionnaire (WIQ),[27] the Vascular Quality of Life Questionnaire(VascuQoL),[28] and the Peripheral Arterial Disease Questionnaire (PAQ)[29] can be used to assess functional status and health-related quality of life.

CLINICAL MANAGEMENT AND TREATMENT OUTCOMES

Several types of intervention may be used for patients with PAD: pharmacotherapy, health behavior change, and endovascular and supervised exercise. Patients with PAD are at high cardiovascular risk, and each person should receive an individualized and comprehensive program including structured exercise, and behavioral and lifestyle modification, along with pharmacotherapies to address risk factors, reduce cardiovascular ischemic events, and improve functional status.[3,14] Smoking cessation is a vital component of care for patients with PAD who continue to smoke, and the full range of options including supportive counseling combined with use of nicotine replacement, bupropion, and varenicline as appropriate should be applied. Optimization of lipids, blood pressure, and glucose control using individualized medication interventions is critical. Often there are readily identifiable opportunities to improve these risk factors especially in the PAD population.[3,14] Further medication considerations include appropriate use of antiplatelet and antithrombotic therapies, which are often suboptimally used in PAD.[2]

Specific endovascular interventions (ie, surgical bypass, angioplasty, and stenting) are important aspects of care. However, those who undergo endovascular therapy without supervised exercise therapy do not improve to the same degree.[30] Two systematic reviews of randomized clinical trials found that combined therapy led to greater improvements in pain-free and maximal walking distance and some aspects of health-related quality of life.[30,31] Indeed there is support (class of recommendation I and level of evidence A) for considering supervised exercise before revascularization.[3]

Exercise has been recommended by the major guidelines on PAD management (class of recommendation I, level of evidence A) as a first-line treatment and should be incorporated in all treatment plans for patients with all types of PAD.[3,14,32]

The traditional exercise program for patients with IC involves walking at a moderate pace to the point of near-maximal pain, followed by rest and repetition. The pace should be able to elicit claudication within 5 minutes and severe pain within 10 minutes with rests and repeats to a total session duration of 30 minutes, with minimum frequency of 3 times per week.[32,33] This method was originally validated by an early meta-analysis[34] and has been cited by exercise interventions and clinical guidelines since.[12,35]

Nonetheless, adherence to exercise in PAD patients is far from ideal,[36] which may be explained in part by the high levels of pain experienced by some patients during exercise. More recent reviews have indicated that walking to near-maximal pain may not be necessary in inducing significant functional improvements.[33,37] Furthermore, there is some evidence that repeated walking beyond the onset of claudication pain can create a catabolic state and skeletal muscle wasting.[38]

In addition, alternative modalities of exercise have been identified, and studies report equivalent effectiveness.[37] These modalities include pain-free treadmill exercise,[39–42] lower limb aerobic exercise,[43] polestriding,[44,45] arm ergometry,[46–48] circuit training,[49,50] and resistance training. The authors' recent systematic review demonstrated higher adherence and completion rates for low pain and alternative exercises.[51]

Resistance training (RT) can improve walking distance, capillary density, strength, and quality of life among individuals with symptomatic and asymptomatic PAD.[52,53] RT should be included with aerobic exercise in PAD exercise prescriptions. An inspection of the literature reveals that studies that include higher-intensity, progressive RT of the lower extremity, are more likely to result in positive outcomes.[52,53] Of note, a seminal study of 156 people with PAD, conducted by McDermott et al. in 2009,[53] included an RT program that did not result in substantive improvements. RT in that study included only 3 sets of a heel raises, with 8 repetitions and no progression, and was considered of insufficient intensity for benefit. Reinforcing the importance of high RT intensity, a randomized controlled study of progressive RT prescribed at a weight load of up to 80% of 1 repetition maximum resulted in superior 6MWT distances compared with low-intensity nonprogressive RT (30% of 1 repetition maximum) and with nonexercise controls in symptomatic PAD patients.[54]

Comorbidities are common among adults with PAD. In some cases PAD is the primary disease but often other conditions are identified first. For example, people with a history of ischemic stroke are at heightened risk of PAD and other vascular diseases. In 2 studies of systematically screened patients following stroke/transient ischemic attack (TIA), 51%[55] and 33.5%[56] had PAD (low ABI) with only 10% reported symptoms of PAD. Moreover, coexisting stroke/TIA and PAD place persons at greater cardiovascular risk for stroke, myocardial infarction, and cardiovascular death than for those with coexisting stroke/TIA and coronary artery disease (CAD).[57] Exercise can also help reduce common risk factors for a population that often carries multiple comorbidities.[58]

Numerous studies and reviews have consistently demonstrated the efficacy and effectiveness of exercise rehabilitation for patients with PAD.[3,32,33,58–62] Supervised exercise therapy has also been shown to be cost effective.[63]

A Cochrane systematic review of randomized controlled trials including patients with stable leg pain demonstrated that exercise training improved maximal walk distance on a treadmill by 5 minutes more than usual care.[32] Significant improvements are observed in aerobic fitness[64] and quality of life in the domains of physical functioning,[53,65] physical and emotional roles, and vitality.[65,66] The mechanisms underlying improvement in physical function include reduced blood viscosity, reduced systemic inflammation, improved endothelial function, improved mitochondrial function, and increased muscle mass.[67,68] Surprisingly, little improvement in ABI and little change in collateral flow are observed.[67,69]

Exercise therapy can be carried out in various settings including hospitals, community centers, and patients' homes. A systematic review comparing supervised with home-based walking programs and walking advice found significantly larger gains in maximal walking distance/time with supervised exercise programs.[70] Exercise trials investigating the efficacy of home-based programs have found significant improvements in claudication onset time and walking times (peak walking time,[71] maximal treadmill,[61] 6MWT distance,[61] and walking speed[45]).

Adverse events are rarely reported for structured community and home-based programs with one report of exercise-induced dyspnea[61] and 11 undisclosed adverse events leading to 6 discontinuations of a 12-week home-based program.[71] Although supervised exercise programs in clinical settings have been shown to have greater benefit and are more strongly recommended,[3,33] community and home-based programs have been shown to have the benefit of greater accessibility, convenience, and lower cost for patients.[61,62,72]

General recommendations by clinicians to patients to increase their walking are rarely efficacious.[72] A recent accelerometer study found that among treated symptomatic PAD patients less than 4% met activity recommendations.[73] Patients with IC frequently reported that physical activity was limited by other disease, fear of falling or worsening the disease, obstacles that exacerbate leg pain, and lack of places to sit when feeling leg pain.[73] Community- or institution-based programs can be efficacious but must consider these barriers and include behavioral support.[3]

CARDIAC REHABILITATION FOR PERIPHERAL ARTERIAL DISEASE

The efficacy of CR for patients with PAD has been demonstrated through several exercise trials with improvements in function in several measures (6MWT, maximal treadmill walking distance, and walking time). Furthermore, CR in clinical settings has been demonstrated to reduce cardiovascular risk factors and improve fitness.[68,74,75] CR improves quality of life in the domains of physical capacity, psychological functioning, negative mood, and social functioning,[74] and the domains of bodily pain and vitality.[76] The evidence demonstrates that CR programs are beneficial for patients with PAD and should be an option for providing access to supervised exercise and enhanced medical care for these patients.

Whether CR occurs in the hospital, community, or home-based settings, it has established efficacy and is consistently recommended in practice guidelines.[3,14] Despite such proven value, few older patients with PAD are identified in typical CR settings, and most of those who do are there because of a primary cardiac problem and their PAD is regarded as more of a comorbidity.[77] Yet patients with PAD are often those who benefit the most from CR. Patients with PAD who join CR programs are more likely to smoke, have type 2 diabetes, and have greater limitations in physical function in comparison with patients with CAD.[77] However, PAD patient characteristics overlap with those of CAD patients and they can both be successfully treated in CR programs.[76]

Given the overwhelming evidence supporting exercise therapy, one may wonder why is it not more frequently used. There are several possible explanations for the treatment gaps originating with the physician, the patient, and health care system levels. Referral and access to CR programs for persons with PAD remains low.[68,78] Survey data of 291 vascular surgeons from the Midwestern Vascular Surgical Society revealed that less than half of those surveyed recognized exercise and activity level as highly important risk factors.[79] Advice to "walk more" was considered as sufficient management, essentially overlooking a body of evidence that such general exercise advice is less effective than supervised exercise programs for improvements in walking ability, symptoms, and quality of life.[80,81] A survey of vascular units in the

United Kingdom found that only 40% of respondents even understood that they had access to a structured exercise program.[82]

Another barrier to access appears to be a lack of consensus on who in the circle of care should be responsible for referring patients to exercise training programs. Only 10% of vascular surgeons surveyed think that they should be responsible for risk factor modification, the majority believing it to be the primary care physician's responsibility.[79] Communication about referral between vascular surgeons and primary care physicians is deficient. A seamless automatic referral process to CR programs for PAD patients may help to overcome such embedded problems.[83]

Patients with PAD may not believe in the efficacy of exercise and may feel even more disinclined when exercise is uncomfortable and/or painful.[84,85] As reviewed earlier, adherence and participation can be better achieved and maintained with low pain and alternative modes of exercise.[51]

System-level problems often relate to inadequate funding, infrequent referrals, and lack of access. A priority in the management of persons with PAD should be to adopt a model of care whereby the first line of strategy is referral to a supervised exercise program (National Institute for Health and Care Excellence, 2012: https://www.nice.org.uk/Guidance/CG147). Indeed, to this end several campaigns to influence stakeholders in the Netherlands led to a 6% reduction in the cost of IC treatment over a 2-year period.[86]

CR is a setting wherein PAD patients can undergo structured exercise (aerobic training and RT) as well as comprehensive secondary prevention. PAD patients also benefit from CR's standards of cardiac screening, psychosocial support, nutrition, education, and risk factor modification. In Canada, this has led to the formation of an organization called CorHealth Ontario, where strategic priorities have been developed to harmonize secondary prevention services for patients with heart disease, stroke, and PAD (https://www.corhealthontario.ca/). In the United States, the Center for Medicare and Medicaid Services (CMS) will reimburse for 12 weeks (36 sessions) or more of Supervised Exercise Therapy (SET) for Symptomatic Peripheral Artery Disease (https://www.cms.gov/Outreach-and-Education/Medicare-Learning-Network-MLN/MLNMattersArticles/Downloads/MM10295.pdf) under a physician's direction and delivered by qualified auxiliary personnel who are trained in exercise therapy for PAD https://www.cms.gov/Regulations-and-Guidance/Guidance/Transmittals/2018-Transmittals-Items/R204NCD.html?DLPage=1&DLEntries=10&DLFilter=peripheral&DLSort=1&DLSortDir=ascending.

A toolkit developed jointly by the Vascular Disease Foundation and the American Association of Cardiovascular and Pulmonary Rehabilitation is available online (http://vasculardisease.org/files/pad-exercise-training-toolkit.pdf). In Europe, funding is available through most government-supported health care systems.

SUMMARY

PAD is underdiagnosed and undertreated, and as clinicians we can do better. Routine referral to CR programs involving supervised exercise therapy would substantially improve health outcomes for patients, including improved physical function, reduced risks of additional cardiovascular morbidity and mortality, and reduced costs for the health care system. Collaboration between health care professionals and CR programs is imperative to bridge the treatment gap for patients with PAD.

REFERENCES

1. Shu J, Santulli G. Update on peripheral artery disease: epidemiology and evidence-based facts. Atherosclerosis 2018;275:379–81.

2. Hiatt WR, Rogers RK. The treatment gap in peripheral artery disease. J Am Coll Cardiol 2017;69(18):2301–3.
3. Gerhard-Herman MD, Gornik HL, Barrett C, et al. 2016 AHA/ACC guideline on the management of patients with lower extremity peripheral artery disease: executive summary: a report of the American College of Cardiology/American Heart Association Task Force on Clinical Practice Guidelines. Circulation 2017;135:e686.
4. Lovell M, Harris K, Forbes T, et al. Peripheral arterial disease: lack of awareness in Canada. Can J Cardiol 2009;25:39–45.
5. Diehm C, Schuster A, Jens R, et al. High prevalence of peripheral arterial disease and co-morbidity in 6880 primary care patients: cross-sectional study. Atherosclerosis 2004;172:95–105.
6. Fowkes FG, Rudan D, Rudan I, et al. Comparison of global estimates of prevalence and risk factors for peripheral artery disease in 2000 and 2010: a systematic review and analysis. Lancet 2013;382:1329–40.
7. Fowkes FG, Aboyans V, Fowkes FJ, et al. Peripheral artery disease: epidemiology and global perspectives. Nat Rev Cardiol 2017;14:156–70.
8. Bush RL, Kallen MA, Liles DR, et al. Knowledge and awareness of peripheral vascular disease are poor among women at risk for cardiovascular disease. J Surg Res 2008;145:313–9.
9. Hirsch AT, Criqui MN, Treat-Jacobson D, et al. Peripheral arterial disease detection, awareness and treatment in primary care. JAMA 2001;286:1317–24.
10. McDermott MM, Fried L, Simonsick E, et al. Asymptomatic peripheral arterial disease is independently associated with impaired lower extremity functioning: The Women's Health and Aging Study. Circulation 2000;101:1007–12.
11. Berger JS, Ladapo JA. Underuse of prevention and lifestyle counseling in patients with peripheral artery disease. J Am Coll Cardiol 2017;69(18):2293–300.
12. Hirsch AT, Haskal ZJ, Hertzer NR, et al. ACC/AHA 2005 practice guidelines for the management of patients with peripheral arterial disease (lower extremity, renal, mesenteric, and abdominal aortic): a collaborative report from the American Association for Vascular Surgery/Society for Vascular Surgery, Society for Cardiovascular Angiography and Interventions, Society for Vascular Medicine and Biology, Society of Interventional Radiology. Circulation 2006;113(11): e463–654.
13. Olesen JB, Lip GY, Lane DA, et al. Vascular disease and stroke risk in atrial fibrillation: a nationwide cohort study. Am J Med 2012;125(8):826.e13-23.
14. Aboyans V, Ricco J-B, Bartelink M-L, et al. 2017 ESC guidelines on the diagnosis and treatment of peripheral arterial diseases, in collaboration with the European Society for Vascular Surgery (ESVS). Eur Heart J 2017. https://doi.org/10.1093/eurheartj/ehx095.
15. Dormandy J, Heeck L, Vig S. The fate of patients with critical leg ischemia. Semin Vasc Surg 1999;12(2):142–7.
16. Earnshaw JJ, Whitman B, Foy C. National Audit of Thrombolysis for Acute Leg Ischemia (NATALI): clinical factors associated with early outcome. J Vasc Surg 2004;39(5):1018–25.
17. Srivaratharajah K, Abramson BL. Women and peripheral arterial disease: a review of sex differences in epidemiology, clinical manifestations, and outcomes. Can J Cardiol 2018;34:356–61.
18. Clairotte C, Retout S, Potier L, et al. Automated ankle-brachial pressure index measurement by clinical staff for peripheral arterial disease diagnosis in nondiabetic and diabetic patients. Diabetes Care 2009;32(7):1231–6.

19. Dachun X, Jue L, Liling Z, et al. Sensitivity and specificity of the ankle–brachial index to diagnose peripheral artery disease: a structured review. Vasc Med 2010;15(5):361–9.
20. Stein R, Hriljac I, Halperin JL, et al. Limitation of the resting ankle-brachial index in symptomatic patients with peripheral arterial disease. Vasc Med 2006;11:29–33.
21. Tehan PE, Barwick AL, Sebastian M, et al. Diagnostic accuracy of the postexercise ankle-brachial index for detecting peripheral artery disease in suspected claudicants with and without diabetes. Vasc Med 2018;23(2):116–25.
22. Aboyans V, Ho E, Denenberg JO, et al. The association between elevated ankle systolic pressures and peripheral occlusive arterial disease in diabetic and nondiabetic subjects. J Vasc Surg 2008;48:1197–203.
23. Criqui MH, McClelland RL, McDermott MM, et al. The ankle-brachial index and incident cardiovascular events in the MESA (Multi-Ethnic Study of Atherosclerosis). J Am Coll Cardiol 2010;56(18):1506–12.
24. McDermott MM, Ades PA, Dyer A, et al. Corridor-based functional performance measures correlate better with physical activity during daily life than treadmill measures in persons with peripheral arterial disease. J Vasc Surg 2008;48:1231–7.
25. McDermott MM, Guralnik JM, Criqui MH, et al. Six-minute walk is a better outcome measure than treadmill walking tests in therapeutic trials of patients with peripheral artery disease. Circulation 2014;130(1):61–8.
26. Ware JE Jr, Kosinski M, Keller SD. A 12-Item Short-Form Health Survey: construction of scales and preliminary tests of reliability and validity. Med Care 1996;34(3):220–33.
27. Regensteiner JG, Steiner JF, Panzer RJ, et al. Evaluation of walking impairment by questionnaire in patients with peripheral arterial disease. J Vasc Med Biol 1990;23:104–15.
28. Morgan MBF, Crayford T, Murrin B, et al. Developing the Vascular Quality of Life Questionnaire: a new disease-specific quality of life measure for use in lower limb ischemia. J Vasc Surg 2001;33(4):679–87.
29. Spertus J, Jones P, Poler S, et al. The Peripheral Artery Questionnaire: a new disease-specific health status measure for patients with peripheral arterial disease. Am Heart J 2004;147(2):301–8.
30. Fakhry F, Fokkenrood HJP, Spronk S, et al. Endovascular revascularisation versus conservative management for intermittent claudication. Cochrane Database Syst Rev 2018;(3):CD010512.
31. Meneses A, Ritti-Dias R, Parmenter BJ, et al. Combined lower limb revascularisation and supervised exercise training for patients with peripheral arterial disease: a systematic review of randomised controlled trials. Sports Med 2016;47(5). https://doi.org/10.1007/s40279-016-0635-5 2016.
32. Lane R, Harwood A, Watson L, et al. TI: exercise for intermittent claudication. Cochrane Database Syst Rev 2017;(12):CD000990.
33. Fakhry F, van de Luijtgaarden KM, Bax L, et al. Supervised walking therapy in patients with intermittent claudication. J Vasc Surg 2012;56:1132–42.
34. Gardner AW, Poehlman ET. Exercise rehabilitation programs for the treatment of claudication pain: a meta-analysis. JAMA 1995;274:975–80.
35. Norgren L, Hiatt WR, Dormandy JA, et al. Inter-society consensus for the management of peripheral arterial disease (TASC II). J Vasc Surg 2007;45:S5–67.
36. Harwood A-E, Smith GE, Cayton T, et al. A systematic review of the uptake and adherence rates to supervised exercise programs in patients with intermittent claudication. Ann Vasc Surg 2016;34:280–9.

37. Parmenter BJ, Raymond J, Dinnen P, et al. A systematic review of randomized controlled trials: walking versus alternative exercise prescription as treatment for intermittent claudication. Atherosclerosis 2011;218(1):1–12.
38. Delaney CL, Miller MD, Chataway TK, et al. A randomised controlled trial of supervised exercise regimens and their impact on walking performance, skeletal muscle mass and calpain activity in patients with intermittent claudication. Eur J Vasc Endovasc Surg 2014;47(3):304–10.
39. Mika P, Spodaryk K, Cencora A, et al. Red blood cell deformability in patients with claudication after pain-free treadmill training. Clin J Sport Med 2006;16(4): 335–40.
40. Mika P, Spodaryk K, Cencora A, et al. Experimental model of pain-free treadmill training in patients with claudication. Am J Phys Med Rehabil 2005;84(10):756–62.
41. Mika P, Wilk B, Mika A, et al. The effect of pain-free treadmill training on fibrinogen, haematocrit, and lipid profile in patients with claudication. Eur J Cardiovasc Prev Rehabil 2011;18(5):754–60.
42. Barak S, Stopka CB, Archer Martinez C, et al. Benefits of low-intensity pain-free treadmill exercise on functional capacity of individuals presenting with intermittent claudication due to peripheral arterial disease. Angiology 2009;60(4):477–86.
43. Tisi PV, Hulse M, Chulakadabba A, et al. Exercise training for intermittent claudication: does it adversely affect biochemical markers of the exercise-induced inflammatory response? Eur J Vasc Endovasc Surg 1997;14(5):344–50.
44. Bulinska K, Kropielnicka K, Jasinski T, et al. Nordic pole walking improves walking capacity in patients with intermittent claudication: a randomized controlled trial. Disabil Rehabil 2016;38(13):1318–24.
45. Collins EG, Oconnell S, McBurney C, et al. Comparison of walking with poles and traditional walking for peripheral arterial disease rehabilitation. J Cardiopulm Rehabil Prev 2012;32(4):210–8.
46. Saxton JM, Zwierska I, Blagojevic M, et al. Upper- versus lower-limb aerobic exercise training on health-related quality of life in patients with symptomatic peripheral arterial disease. J Vasc Surg 2011;53(5):1265–73.
47. Bronas UG, Treat-Jacobson D, Leon AS. Comparison of the effect of upper body-ergometry aerobic training vs treadmill training on central cardiorespiratory improvement and walking distance in patients with claudication. J Vasc Surg 2011;53(6):1557–64.
48. Zwierska I, Walker RD, Choksy SA, et al. Upper- vs lower-limb aerobic exercise rehabilitation in patients with symptomatic peripheral arterial disease: a randomized controlled trial. J Vasc Surg 2005;42(6):1122–30.
49. Beckitt TA, Day J, Morgan M, et al. Calf muscle oxygen saturation and the effects of supervised exercise training for intermittent claudication. J Vasc Surg 2012; 56(2):470–5.
50. Mockford KA, Gohil RA, Mazari F, et al. Effect of supervised exercise on physical function and balance in patients with intermittent claudication. Br J Surg 2014; 101(4):356–62.
51. Lin E, Nguyen CH, Thomas SG. Completion and adherence rates to exercise interventions in intermittent claudication: traditional exercise versus alternative exercise – a systematic review. European Journal of Preventive Cardiology. [Epub ahead of print].
52. McGuigan MRM, Bronks R, Newton RU, et al. Resistance training in patients with peripheral arterial disease: effects on myosin isoforms, fiber type distribution, and capillary supply to skeletal muscle. J Gerontol A Biol Sci Med Sci 2001; 56a:B302–10.

53. McDermott MM, Ades PA, Guralnik JM, et al. Treadmill exercise and resistance training in patients with peripheral arterial disease with and without intermittent claudication: a randomized controlled trial. JAMA 2009;301:165–74.
54. Parmenter BJ, Raymond J, Dinnen P, et al. High-intensity progressive resistance training improves flat-ground walking in older adults with symptomatic peripheral arterial disease. J Am Geriatr Soc 2013;61(11):1964–70.
55. Weimar C, Goertler M, Röther J, et al. Systemic risk score evaluation in ischemic stroke patients (SCALA): a prospective cross sectional study in 85 German stroke units. J Neurol 2007;254:1562–8.
56. Agnelli G, Cimminiello C, Meneghetti G, et al. Polyvascular Atherothrombosis Observational Survey (PATHOS) Investigators. Low ankle-brachial index predicts an adverse 1-year outcome after acute coronary and cerebrovascular events. J Thromb Haemost 2006;4:2599–606.
57. Uchiyama S, Goto S, Matsumoto M, et al. Cardiovascular event rates in patients with cerebrovascular disease and atherothrombosis at other vascular locations: results from 1-year outcomes in the Japanese REACH Registry. J Neurol Sci 2009;287:45–51.
58. Leng GC, Lee AJ, Fowkes FG, et al. Incidence, natural history and cardiovascular events in symptomatic and asymptomatic peripheral arterial disease in the general population. Int J Epidemiol 1996;25:1172–81.
59. Aggarwal S, Moore RD, Arena R, et al. Rehabilitation therapy in peripheral arterial disease. Can J Cardiol 2016;32(10):S374–81.
60. McDermott MM. Exercise rehabilitation for peripheral artery disease: a review. J Cardiopulm Rehabil Prev 2018;38(2):63–9.
61. McDermott MM, Liu K, Guralnik JM, et al. Home-based walking exercise intervention in peripheral artery disease: a randomized clinical trial. JAMA 2013;310:57–65.
62. Treat-Jacobson D, McDermott MM, Bronas UG, et al. Optimal exercise programs for patients with peripheral artery disease: a scientific statement from the American Heart Association. Circulation 2019;139(4):e10–33.
63. van Asselt AD, Nicolai SP, Joore MA, et al. Cost-effectiveness of exercise therapy in patients with intermittent claudication: supervised exercise therapy versus a 'go home and walk' advice. Eur J Vasc Endovasc Surg 2011;41:97–100.
64. Parmenter BJ, Dieberg G, Smart NA. Exercise training for management of peripheral arterial disease: a systematic review and meta-analysis. Sports Med 2015;45(2):231–44.
65. Mazari FA, Gulati S, Rahman MN, et al. Early outcomes from a randomized, controlled trial of supervised exercise, angioplasty, and combined therapy in intermittent claudication. Ann Vasc Surg 2010;24(1):69–79.
66. Rejeski WJ, Spring B, Domanchuk K, et al. A group-mediated, home-based physical activity intervention for patients with peripheral artery disease: effects on social and psychological function. J Transl Med 2014;12:29.
67. Hamburg NM, Balady GJ. Exercise rehabilitation in peripheral artery disease functional impact and mechanisms of benefits. Circulation 2011;123:87–97.
68. Martin B, Hauer T, Austford LD, et al. Cardiac rehabilitation in subjects with peripheral arterial disease: a higher risk patient population who benefit from attendance. Can J Cardiol 2016;32(10):S110.
69. Szuba A, Oka RK, Harada R, et al. Limb hemodynamics are not predictive of functional capacity in patients with PAD. Vasc Med 2006;11:155–63.
70. Hageman D, Fokkenrood HJP, Gommans LNM, et al. Supervised exercise therapy versus home-based exercise therapy versus walking advice for intermittent

claudication. Cochrane Database Syst Rev 2018;(4):CD005263. https://doi.org/10.1002/14651858.CD005263.pub4.

71. Gardner AW, Parker DE, Montgomery PS, et al. Efficacy of quantified home-based exercise and supervised exercise in patients with intermittent claudication: a randomized controlled trial. Circulation 2011;123(5):491–8.
72. Mays RJ, Rogers RK, Hiatt WR, et al. Community walking programs for treatment of peripheral artery disease. J Vasc Surg 2013;58(6):1678–87.
73. Souza SA, Adilson S, Correia M, et al. Barriers and levels of physical activity in symptomatic peripheral artery disease patients: comparison between women and men. J Aging Phys Act 2019. https://doi.org/10.1123/japa.2018-0206.
74. Jeger RV, Rickenbacher P, Pfisterer ME, et al. Outpatient rehabilitation in patients with coronary artery and peripheral arterial occlusive disease. Arch Phys Med Rehabil 2008;89(4):618–21.
75. Nguyen CH, Marzolini S, Oh P, et al. Comparing health outcomes following cardiac rehabilitation: peripheral artery disease, coronary artery disease and concomitant disease. Canadian Society for Exercise Physiology. Appl Physiol Nutr Metab 2018;43(10 Suppl 2):S85.
76. Stauber S, Guéra V, Barth J, et al. Psychosocial outcome in cardiovascular rehabilitation of peripheral artery disease and coronary artery disease patients. Vasc Med 2013;18(5):257–62.
77. Nguyen C, Marzolini S, Oh P, et al. Characteristics of Patients entering Cardiac Rehabilitation: peripheral artery disease, coronary artery disease, and concomitant disease. Canadian Cardiovascular Conference. Can J Cardiol 2018;34(10 Suppl 1):S84.
78. Ambrosetti M, Temporelli PL, Faggiano P, et al. Lower extremities peripheral arterial disease among patients admitted to cardiac rehabilitation: the THINKPAD registry. Int J Cardiol 2014;171:192–8.
79. Leon LR Jr, Labropoulos N, Lebda P, et al. The vascular surgeon's role in risk factor modification: results of a survey. Perspect Vasc Surg Endovasc Ther 2005;17:145–53.
80. Gommans L, Saarloos R, Scheltinga M, et al. The effect of supervision on walking distance in patients with intermittent claudication: a meta-analysis. J Vasc Surg 2014;60:535–6.
81. Bermingham SL, Sparrow K, Mullis R, et al. The cost-effectiveness of supervised exercise for the treatment of intermittent claudication. Eur J Vasc Endovasc Surg 2013;46:707–14.
82. Harwood A, Smith G, Broadbent E, et al. Access to supervised exercise services for peripheral vascular disease patients. Bull Roy Coll Surg Engl 2017;99:207–11.
83. Grace SL, Chessex C, Arthur H, et al. Systematizing inpatient referral to cardiac rehabilitation 2010. Can J Cardiol 2011;27:192–9.
84. Sharath SE, Kougias P, Barshes NR. The influence of pain-related beliefs on physical activity and health attitudes in patients with claudication: a pilot study. Vasc Med 2017;22:378–84.
85. Cavalcante BR, Farah BQ, Barbosa JPdA, et al. Are the barriers for physical activity practice equal for all peripheral artery disease patients? Arch Phys Med Rehabil 2015;96:248–52.
86. Hageman D, Fokkenrood HJP, Essers PPM, et al. Improved adherence to a stepped-care model reduces costs of intermittent claudication treatment in The Netherlands. Eur J Vasc Endovasc Surg 2017;54(1). https://doi.org/10.1016/j.ejvs.2017.04.011.

Cardiac Rehabilitation for Transcatheter Aortic Valve Replacement

Franco Tarro Genta, MD

KEYWORDS

• TAVR • Cardiac rehabilitation • Assessment • Exercise capacity • Disability

KEY POINTS

- Patients with transcatheter aortic valve replacement (TAVR) are often very old, disabled, frail, and have low exercise capacity.
- Cardiac rehabilitation for TAVR has only low referral for residential and ambulatory formats. Still, it seems likely to grow as use of TAVR becomes more widespread.
- Evidence for cardiac rehabilitation–induced improvement in disability, frailty, quality of life, anxiety, exercise capacity, and survival in patients with TAVR is still in its early stages, but there is a signal of efficacy.
- A minimal data set (demarcating disability, frailty, anxiety, depression, exercise capacity score/measures to evaluate) is needed to better clarify the benefits achieved by cardiac rehabilitation in patients with TAVR.
- Suitable powered randomized studies are need to better define the role of cardiac rehabilitation in patients with TAVR compared with usual care.

INTRODUCTION

Since the first experience in 2002,[1] more than 300,000 patients worldwide have undergone transcatheter aortic valve replacement (TAVR)[2,3] for severe aortic stenosis (AS). The rise in TAVR as a treatment option is driven in large part by evidence showing its benefits compared with medical treatment in patients with symptomatic severe AS who were too ill to undergo surgical aortic valve replacement (sAVR),[4,5] and the recognition of TAVR as a valid alternative to sAVR in patients at high surgical risk.[6,7] Furthermore, improving operators' experience, evolution of devices, and advancing techniques have reinforced patterns of expanded use of TAVR.[8] Cardiac rehabilitation (CR) is recommended after valvular cardiac surgery[9,10] for improving exercise capacity,[11] with data also now showing its utility to improve quality of life (QOL), moderate frailty,[12] and increase survival.[13] This review describes the state of the art of CR for TAVR.

Department of Cardiology, Istituti Clinici Scientifici Maugeri SpA SB, Presidio Major Via Santa Giulia 60, Torino 10124, Italy
E-mail address: franco.tarrogenta@icsmaugeri.it

Clin Geriatr Med 35 (2019) 539–548
https://doi.org/10.1016/j.cger.2019.07.007
0749-0690/19/

CARDIAC REHABILITATION AFTER TRANSCATHETER AORTIC VALVE REPLACEMENT: BODY OF EVIDENCE

General Considerations

Despite the expanding use of TAVR worldwide,[2,3] literature reporting results of CR after TAVR is still scarce. Indeed, a recent Danish survey shows that having a TAVR was associated with a lower probability of both CR referral and participation.[14] The common characteristics of frailty and high comorbidity among patients with TAVR, and the absence of experience of administering CR in a such vulnerable patients may have accounted for these patterns.

The overall number of patients reported in the main CR literature[13,15–22] totals approximately 1500 (**Table 1**), of whom more than 1000 are from a single study.[13] Four studies[15–17,21] compared CR after TAVR with CR after sAVR. Of these, 2[16,17] were retrospective. All studies, except 2,[19,22] report results from an average 3-week residential CR setting starting soon after discharge for the incident valve replacement hospitalization. One pilot study[19] compared ExCap (exercise capacity) measured as increase in peak oxygen uptake at cardiopulmonary exercise test (CPET) and QOL differences between patients with TAVR admitted to ambulatory CR compared with TAVR usual care enrolled after up to 6 months from inpatient 2-week to 3-week CR program discharge. Another pilot study[22] assessed the feasibility of a 6-week ambulatory CR in patients admitted 1 month after TAVR compared with usual care. The largest study[13] prospectively compared 6-month survival in patients with TAVR refusing to participate in CR with patients participating in CR or Geriatric rehabilitation.

Patients admitted to CR were very old (average age >80 years), mainly women, and up to one-third were frail, but this was seldom assessed.[18,19,22] Moderate to high malnutrition was common, that is, up to 30%.[18] In one study, disability was evaluated by the functional independence measure (FIM)[17] and in 3 other studies, disability was evaluated by the Barthel Index (BI).[15,18,21] Submaximal ExCap was assessed by the 6-minute walking test (6MWT) in the studies but one.[13] There were substantial differences in the disability profile at CR admission (BI from 67 $\pm$ 24 to 84 $\pm$ 21) and ExCap at 6MWT (from 147.5 $\pm$ 101.7 to 278.8 $\pm$ 118.9 m) in CR inpatients between different studies. In studies with patients who had relatively lower disability and/or higher exercise capacity, a large proportion tolerated a symptom-limited cycle test[16,20] or a cardiopulmonary exercise test (CPET)[15] as part of CR. In studies enrolling patients who were more disabled and who had low ExCap, few patients could even sustain a 6MWT.[21]

Cardiac Rehabilitation Components and Training Modality

The primary components of CR in most studies were supervised exercise training by a therapist and physician supervision (**Table 2**).[15,21] Generally, programs were structured 3 times a week for 8 weeks[19] or once a week for 6 weeks[22] in the ambulatory setting versus 4 to 6 days per week (2–3 sessions per day) for 3 weeks in a residential CR setting.[15–18,20,21] One study did not report the frequency and modality of exercise training.[13] Endurance exercise (at bicycle, treadmill, pedal exerciser, arm ergometer, or simple walking) was the primary training priority; it was administered in individualized programs up to 30 minutes per session. The initial intensity and its increase, when described, was set according to $\leq$70% predicted heart rate,[15] depending on the initial symptom-limited stress test exercise intensity,[16,20] starting and increasing workload from 40% to 70% $\dot{V}O_2$ peak performed at baseline CPET[19] or based on Borg Rating of Perceived Exertion Scale.[15,17,21,22] Strength training (for lower extremities[16] at weight machines[19,20] or as a sit-to-stand exercise[22]), calisthenics, respiratory, and a

Table 1
Main studies addressing cardiac rehabilitation for TAVR

Authors	Type of Study	Patients with TAVR	Age, y, Mean ± SD	Women, %	LVEF, %, Mean ± SD	Disability	Frailty	6MWT Admission, Mean ± SD
Russo et al,[15] 2014	Prospective, observational Compared with sAVR	78	83.3 ± 3.6	68.3	55.9 ± 11.3	BI 80.9 ± 24	NA	240.8 ± 94.9
Völler et al,[16] 2015	Retrospective Compared with sAVR	76	80.30 ± 6	68	57.1 ± 9.19	NA	NA	262.45 ± 90.44
Fauchère et al,[17] 2014	Retrospective Compared with sAVR	34	82 ± 5	62		FIM 95.8 ± 10.2	NA	147.5 ± 101.7
Zanettini et al,[18] 2014	Prospective, observational	60	83.5 ± 5.0	32		BI 84 ± 21	Separate domains[a]	210 ± 87
Pressler et al,[19] 2016	Prospective, randomized	30[b]	81 ± 6	44	58 ± 8	NA	NA	366 ± 93
Eichler et al,[20] 2017	Prospective observational	136	80.6 ± 5.0	52.2	56.1 ± 9.7	NA	36.9%[e]	278.8 ± 118.9
Tarro Genta et al,[21] 2017	Prospective, observational Compared with sAVR	65	82 ± 6	45	55.3 ± 9	BI 67 ± 2 4	NA	162 ± 87
Rogers et al,[22] 2018	Prospective, randomized	27[c]	82.04 ± 4.8	55.6	>50% in 77.8%	NA	20%[f]	325.2 ± 22.8
Butter et al,[13] 2018	Prospective, observational	1017[d]	80.7 ± 6	55.5	55 ± 10	NA	NA	NA
Total		1523						

Abbreviations: 6MWT, 6-minute walking test distance in meters; BI, Barthel Index at cardiac rehabilitation (CR) admission; FIM, functional independence measure; LVEF, left ventricle ejection fraction; NA, not available; sAVR, surgical aortic valve replacement; TAVR, transcatheter aortic valve replacement.

[a] Separate frailty domains (cognitive impairment, malnutrition, anxiety and depression, dependency on basic life activities) not aggregated in score.
[b] 15 no CR; 15 CR.
[c] 14 no CR; 13 CR.
[d] 366 no CR; 435 CR, 216 geriatric rehabilitation.
[e] Frailty score $\geq$3 following Schoenenberger frailty index.[24]
[f] Fried[25] score greater than 2.

Table 2
Cardiac rehabilitation components and training modality

Authors	CR Component	Training Modality	CR Setting, Frequency of Exercise Training, Healthcare Supervisor
Russo et al,[15] 2014	Exercise training	Endurance: 30 min bicycle low/medium intensity $\leq$70% predicted heart rate 30 min of calisthenic exercises 30 min respiratory workout Workload increase based on Borg scale	Inpatients 6 sessions/wk Physical therapists and physician
Völler et al,[16] 2015	Exercise training, education, psychological support	Endurance: Bicycle ergometer (W based on initial exercise intensity but nonspecifically described) Resistance training lower extremities Outdoor walking, gymnastic in group or single	Inpatients 4–5 sessions/wk Physical therapists
Fauchère et al,[17] 2014	Exercise training	Endurance: Low/medium-intensity aerobic exercise Gymnastics and respiratory workout Workload increase based on Borg scale	Inpatients 3 wk 2–3 sessions/d, 6 d/wk Not specified supervision type
Zanettini et al,[18] 2014	Exercise training, education, psychological support, nutrition intervention	Bed exercises, sitting calisthenics, and ambulatory training in bedridden/very disabled Endurance: interval or steady-state aerobic training with bicycle or treadmill and calisthenics in other patients Intensity not described	Inpatients 6 days/wk Not specified supervision type
Pressler et al,[19] 2016	Exercise training vs standard of care	Endurance at bicycle at moderate intensity with progressive workload from 40% to 70% VO_2Peak performed at baseline Resistance training on 5 different machines	Outpatients 8 wk 3 sessions/wk Not specified supervision type

Eichler et al,[20] 2017	Exercise training, education, psychological support, nutrition intervention	Endurance: bicycle training based on initial exercise intensity Strength training only in higher physical capacity patients Outdoor walking, gymnastic and aqua and spinal gymnastic as appropriate	Inpatients 3 wk 5 d/wk Not specified supervision type
Tarro Genta et al,[21] 2017	Exercise training, education, psychological support, nutrition intervention	Endurance training (bicycle or treadmill) Workload increase based on Borg scale Respiratory and calisthenics sessions Bed exercises, sitting calisthenics, daily session of up to 30 min walking, pedal exerciser (0 W) session in more disabled patients	Inpatients 3 wk 3 sessions/d, 5–6 d/wk Physical therapists and physician
Rogers et al,[22] 2018	Exercise training vs standard of care	Endurance: Individualized training program mainly based on treadmill and bicycle Exercise such as sit-to-stand Increased workload based on Borg scale	Outpatients 1/weekly 60–90-min session for 6 wk Not specified supervision type
Butter et al,[13] 2018	Multidimensional (patient health education, lifestyle and dietary advice, psychological support, and physical activity) but nonspecifically described both for CR and GR	Nonspecified	Inpatients 3 wk Nonspecified frequency

Abbreviations: CR, cardiac rehabilitation; GR, geriatric rehabilitation.

mix of other exercises (outdoor walking, gymnastic, and aqua and spinal gymnastic) were variously combined between studies (see **Table 2**).

Overall these reports underscore the absence of a standardized approach to assessment and care delivery for this vulnerable population. Similar variability also extends to other domains of CR, including psychological support, education, and nutrition for which the types of interventions are seldom detailed.[19] Of note, the larger TAVR CR study did not detail the component of CR and geriatric rehabilitation that distinguished an approach for patients with TAVR from a general description.[13]

Outcomes

The first important result derived from the cited studies and confirmed in recent meta-analysis[12] is the safety of exercise-based CR. No adverse events correlated to administration of multicomponent CR in either inpatient or outpatient settings. These data provide much reassurance regarding the safety of CR for very disabled, frail, and multimorbid patients with TAVR. Moreover, the significant adverse events that occurred during inpatient CR[18,21] were predominantly unrelated to the valve procedure and highlighted the value of CR in early recognition and treatment of severe and possibly fatal conditions.[2]

Disability significantly improved at discharge from residential CR (**Table 3**) both if assessed as FIM[17] (95.8 ± 10.2 to 106.8 ± 9.9; $P<.001$) or BI[15,18,21] (80.9 ± 24.3 to 90.3 ± 17.2, 84 ± 21 to 95 ± 10, and 67 ± 24 to 85 ± 1, respectively; $P<.05$) with similar improvements in patients with TAVR or sAVR.[17,21] Of note, risk of fall was significantly reduced at discharge from inpatients CR (Morse Fall Scale 30 ± 21 to 25 ± 17; $P<.05$).[21]

Table 3
Main outcomes in CR studies on TAVR

Authors	Outcomes
Russo et al,[15] 2014	Δ BI; Δ 6MWT
Völler et al,[16] 2015	Δ 6MWT; Δ ExCap
Fauchère et al,[17] 2014	Δ 6MWT, Δ FIM
Zanettini et al,[18] 2014	Δ BI; Δ 6MWT; Δ EQ-VAS
Pressler et al,[19] 2016	In TG Δ VO_2 peak Vo_2, Δ AT, Δ Test duration at CPET; Δ Muscular strength, Δ QOL (KCCQ); all the above significantly improved compared with UC TAVR
Eichler et al,[20] 2017	Δ 6MWT, Δ ExCap, Δ Frailty index, Δ SF-12 PCS and MCS; Δ HADS Anxiety
Tarro Genta et al,[21] 2017	Δ BI, Δ MFS, Δ 6MWT
Rogers et al,[22] 2018	Pilot study not powered to evaluate differences: nondifferences at follow-up between TG and UC
Butter et al,[13] 2018	6-mo reduced mortality (all-cause and non-CV death) in TR (CR and geriatric rehabilitation) vs UC. The result is driven by CR vs geriatric rehabilitation

Abbreviations: Δ, significant improvement between admission and discharge in patients with TAVR admitted to CR; 6MWT, 6-minute walk test distance in meters; AT, anaerobic threshold; BI, Barthel Index; CPET, cardiopulmonary exercise testing; CR, cardiac rehabilitation; CV, cardiovascular; EQ-VAS, EuroQol visual analogue scale; ExCap, exercise capacity in W at stress test; FIM, functional independence measure; HADS, Hospital Anxiety and Depression Scale; KCCQ, Kansas City Cardiomyopathy Questionnaire; MCS, mental component scale; MFS, Morse Fall Scale; PCS, physical component scale; QOL, quality of life; SF, short form; TAVR, transcatheter aortic valve replacement; TG, training group; TR, total rehabilitation setting; UC, usual care; Vo_2, oxygen uptake.

During inpatient stay, CR frailty significantly improved compared with admission (Frailty Index, points 2.1 ± 1.5 vs 1.7 ± 1.5, $P<.001$)[19] determined primarily by significant changes of cognition, nutrition, and subjective mobility and disability. No differences in frailty (as for anxiety and depression) at 3 and 6 months were found in patients with TAVR admitted to outpatient 6-week CR sessions compared with usual care TAVR in a randomized pilot trial, but the investigators emphasized their study was not powered to formally compare these outcomes within or between groups.[22]

There were significant benefits in QOL derived for both TAVR inpatient CR (EuroQol visual analogic scale from 54 ± 14 to 75 ± 11, $P<.001$[18]; Short Form 12 physical component scale and mental component scale 35.9 ± 8.8 to 38.3 ± 8.3, $P = .001$ and 47.3 ± 10.6 to 50.7 ± 10.0, $P = .003$, respectively[20]) and outpatient CR (Short Form 12 physical component 39.5 ± 10.0 improved to 45.9 ± 8.9, $P<.05$; Kansas City Cardiomyopathy Questionnaire, overall summary improved from 76.5 ± 16.1 to 81.9 ± 18.3, and clinical summary improved from 75.7 ± 15.6 to 83.9 ± 13.9, $P<.05$, determined predominantly by improvements in physical limitations and symptom burden domains[19]).

Data about effects of CR in TAVR on anxiety and depression are conflicting; Hospital Anxiety and Depression Scale (HADS) in the anxiety domain was significantly improved in prospective study on 122 patients with TAVR who attended a 3-week residential CR (5.2 ± 4.0 to 4.0 ± 3.6, $P<.001$),[20] whereas 2 retrospective studies did not find differences between admission and discharge.[16,17] No improvement in HADS in the depression domain occurred in all these studies.[16,17,20] Of note, percentages of patients with TAVR with severe depression (evaluated with Geriatric Depression Score) did not change over time at up to 24 months of follow-up after residential CR discharge.[18]

ExCap was reported in all[15–22] but one study,[13] mainly as submaximal test improvement at 6MWT distance. Overall, the investigators confirmed (with different extents in patients able to afford 6MWT both at CR admission and discharge) a net improvement in the distance covered at discharge compared with admission in the inpatient setting (from 240.8 ± 94.9 to 272.7 ± 107.8 m, $P<.001$[15]; 147.5 ± 101.7 to 231.7 ± 132.7 m, $P<.001$[17]; 210 ± 87 to 275 ± 97 m, $P<.001$[18]; 366 ± 93 to 392 ± 100 m, $P<.05$[19]; 278.8 ± 118.9 to 335.1 ± 133.0 m, $P<.001$[20]; 162 ± 87 to 240 ± 92 m, $P<.001$[21]) but with no difference compared with TAVR usual care in outpatient CR (366 ± 93 to 392 ± 100 m, vs 319 ± 104 to 330 ± 95, P = NS,[19] and 319.7 ± 24.5 vs 370.0 ± 33, P = NS[22]). ExCap measured at symptom-limited cycle test significantly improved during residential CR (+19.84% W from baseline test with 95% confidence interval 4.76% to 37.08%, $P<.05$[16]; 50.8 ± 20.3 to 58.9 ± 21.3 W, $P<.001$[20]) and also by CPET in outpatient CR (peak Vo_2 from 12.7 ± 3.0 mL/min per kg to 15.9 ± 5.0 mL/min per kg from admission to CR discharge, $P<.05$)[19]; symptom-limited ExCap also significantly improved compared with TAVR usual care (peak Vo_2 from 12.7 ± 3.0 to 15.9 ± 5.0 mL/min per kg vs 15.0 ± 3.3 to 14.5 ± 3.6 mL/min per kg, $P = .007$).[19] The improvement in 6MWT achieved in patients receiving TAVR CR was on average >50 m, a margin that represents a clinically significant change.[23] Still, no randomized controlled studies have compared CR with usual care in patients with TAVR, and TAVR outpatients starting CR with a range of 1 to 6 months after TAVR,[19,22] blurring the utility of the program. Furthermore, because the 6MWT failed to show improvement compared with usual care may signify that weeks after TAVR submaximal ExCap improves spontaneously, with little added benefit from CR, and/or that other indices with greater specificity are required.

Finally, residential rehabilitation (CR plus geriatric rehabilitation) reduced 6-month mortality in patients with TAVR compared with patients with TAVR who did not participate in rehabilitation (adjusted odds ratio 0.49; 95% confidence interval 0.25–0.94; $P = .032$).[13] This result was based on overall and noncardiovascular mortality. Notably, only CR was associated with reduced mortality (odds ratio 0.31; 95% confidence interval 0.14–0.71; $P = .006$), whereas geriatric rehabilitation was not (odds ratio 0.83; 95% confidence interval 0.37–1.85; $P = .65$). Patients referred to CR compared with geriatric rehabilitation were younger, with lower New York Heart Association class, logistic Euro Score I and shorter median hospitalization after TAVR, whereas patients refusing CR were more frequently diabetic, with higher body mass index and higher N terminal pro brain natriuretic peptide.[13] Despite the interesting results reported in this study, selection bias may have occurred, as patients in the group declining rehabilitation may have had advantages in their home environments and with unique resources.[13]

SUMMARY

The evolution of TAVR technology and techniques are contributing to the expansion of TAVR worldwide,[8] with a rise in the number of older adults receiving TAVR who are disabled, frail, multimorbid, and enfeebled. Whereas CR is a logical consideration in this population, application has lagged. Our review highlights data showing that residential and ambulatory CR is safe and effective, with metrics of reduced disability and frailty, improved ExCap, QOL, and short-term survival. Although overall efficacy is evident, many pertinent questions remain:

- Are improvements associated with CR after TAVR secondary to its multidimensional interventions or simply related to enhancements in left ventricular function and increased cardiac output?
- Do patients benefit most from residential CR immediately after valve replacement or benefit more if they are first discharged to home and participate in ambulatory CR thereafter?
- What is the best approach for standardized assessments for pertinent geriatric domains (eg, disability, frailty, anxiety, depression ExCap) to better assess benefits associated with CR?
- Should there be a minimal training for assessment and treatment of frail and disabled patients with TAVR?
- Does prehabilitation treatment have a role in patients deemed to undergo TAVR for a better recovery after implantation?

These questions warrant larger suitably powered randomized studies able to highlight the role of CR in this expanding aged and vulnerable population.

REFERENCES

1. Cribrier SG. The odyssey of TAVR from concept to clinical reality. Tex Heart Inst J 2014;41(2):125–30.
2. Goel K, Holmes DR. Transcatheter aortic valve replacement. Optimizing outcomes for healthy recovery. J Cardiopulm Rehabil Prev 2018;38:1–7.
3. Vilela FD, De Assumpção Cortes L, Ferreira Da Costa GB, et al. Transcatheter aortic valve replacement. Int Clin Pathol J 2017;4(4):98–102.
4. Leon MB, Smith CR, Mack M, et al, PARTNER Trial Investigators. Transcatheter aortic-valve implantation for aortic stenosis in patients who cannot undergo surgery. N Engl J Med 2010;363(17):1597–607.
5. Popma JJ, Adams DH, Reardon MJ, et al, AI for the CoreValve United States Clinical Investigators. Transcatheter aortic valve replacement using a self-expanding

bioprosthesis in patients with severe aortic stenosis at extreme risk for surgery. J Am Coll Cardiol 2014;63:1972–81.
6. Smith CR, Leon MB, Mack MJ, et al, PARTNER Trial Investigators. Transcatheter versus surgical aortic-valve replacement in high-risk patients. N Engl J Med 2011;364(23):2187–98.
7. Adams DH, PopmaJJ, Reardon MJ, et al, for the CoreValve United States Clinical Investigators. Transcatheter aortic-valve replacement with a self-expanding prosthesis. N Engl J Med 2014;370:1790–8.
8. Neylon A, Ahmed K, Mercanti F, et al. Transcatheter aortic valve implantation: status update. J Thorac Dis 2018;10(Suppl 30):S3637–45.
9. Butchart EG, Gohlke-Bärwolf C, Antunes MJ, et al, Working Groups on Valvular Heart Disease, Thrombosis and Cardiac Rehabilitation and Exercise Physiology, European Society of Cardiology. Recommendations for the management of patients after heart valve surgery. Eur Heart J 2005;26(22):2463–71.
10. Piepoli MF, Corra' U, Benzer W, et al. Secondary prevention through cardiac rehabilitation: from knowledge to implementation. A position paper from the Cardiac Rehabilitation Section of the European Association of Cardiovascular Prevention and Rehabilitation. Eur J Cardiovasc Prev Rehabil 2010;17:1–17.
11. Sibilitz KL, Berg SK, Tang LH, et al. Exercise-based cardiac rehabilitation for adults after heart valve surgery. Cochrane Database Syst Rev 2016;(3):CD010876.
12. Ribeiro GS, Melo RD, Deresz LF, et al. Cardiac rehabilitation programme after transcatheter aortic valve implantation versus surgical aortic valve replacement: systematic review and meta-analysis. Eur J Prev Cardiol 2017;24(7):688–97.
13. Butter C, Groß J, Haase-Fielitz A, et al. Impact of rehabilitation on outcomes after TAVI: a preliminary study. J Clin Med 2018;7:326.
14. Hansen TB, Berg SK, Sibilitz KL, et al. Availability of, referral to and participation in exercise-based cardiac rehabilitation after heart valve surgery: results from the national CopenHeart survey. Eur J Prev Cardiol 2015;22(6):710–8.
15. Russo N, Compostella L, Tarantini G, et al. Cardiac rehabilitation after transcatheter versus surgical prosthetic valve implantation for aortic stenosis in the elderly. Eur J Prev Cardiol 2014;21(11):1341–8.
16. Völler H, Salzwedel A, Nitardy A, et al. Effect of cardiac rehabilitation on functional and emotional status in patients after transcatheter aortic-valve implantation. Eur J Prev Cardiol 2015;22:568–74.
17. Fauchère I, Weber D, Maier W, et al. Rehabilitation after TAVI compared to surgical aortic valve replacement. Int J Cardiol 2014;173:564–6.
18. Zanettini R, Gatto G, Mori I, et al. Cardiac rehabilitation and mid-term follow-up after transcatheter aortic valve implantation. J Geriatr Cardiol 2014;11:279–85.
19. Pressler A, Christle JW, Lechner B, et al. Exercise training improves exercise capacity and quality of life after transcatheter aortic valve implantation: a randomized pilot trial. Am Heart J 2016;182:44–53.
20. Eichler S, Salzwedel A, Reibis R, et al. Multicomponent cardiac rehabilitation in patients after transcatheter aortic valve implantation: predictors of functional and psychocognitive recovery. Eur J Prev Cardiol 2017;24(3):257–64.
21. Tarro Genta F, Tidu M, Bouslenko Z, et al. Cardiac rehabilitation after transcatheter aortic valve implantation compared to patients after valve replacement. J Cardiovasc Med 2017;18:114–20.
22. Rogers P, Al-Aidrous S, Banya W, et al. Cardiac rehabilitation to improve health-related quality of life following trans-catheter aortic valve implantation: a

randomised controlled feasibility study. RECOVER–TAVI Pilot, ORCA 4, for the Optimal Restoration of Cardiac Activity Group. Pilot Feasibility Stud 2018;4:185.

23. Reibis RK, Treszl A, Wegscheider K, et al. Exercise capacity is the most powerful predictor of 2-year mortality in patients with left ventricular systolic dysfunction. Herz 2010;35:104–10.
24. Schoenenberger AW, Stortecky S, Neumann S, et al. Predictors of functional decline in elderly patients undergoing transcatheter aortic valve implantation (TAVI). Eur Heart J 2013;34:684–92.
25. Fried LP, Tangen CM, Walston J, et al. Frailty in older adults: evidence for a phenotype; Cardiovascular Health Study Collaborative Research Group. J Gerontol A Biol Sci Med Sci 2001;56(3):M146–56.

Cardiac Rehabilitation to Optimize Medication Regimens in Heart Failure

Parag Goyal, MD, MSc[a,b,*], Eiran Z. Gorodeski, MD, MPH[c], Zachary A. Marcum, PharmD, PhD[d], Daniel E. Forman, MD[e]

KEYWORDS

- Heart failure • Drug therapy • Cardiac rehabilitation • Inappropriate prescribing
- Medication adherence

KEY POINTS

- Given its comprehensive nature and patient-centered focus, cardiac rehabilitation (CR) presents a remarkable opportunity to address medication optimization in older adults with heart failure (HF) as a port of an expanded model of cardiac rehabilitation care.
- With additional training of personnel and potential collaboration with HF clinicians, CR has the potential to offer an adjunctive platform to ensure euvolemia and safe use of diuretics through careful monitoring and thoughtful decision making.

Continued

Disclosure Statement: Dr P. Goyal is supported by National Institute on Aging grant R03AG056446 and American Heart Association grant 18IPA34170185. Dr E.Z. Gorodeski is supported by The Hunnell Fund, a philanthropic fund at Cleveland Clinic, and has an unrestricted research grant from Abbott. Dr E.Z. Gorodeski is a consultant for Abbott. Dr Z.A. Marcum is supported by Agency for Healthcare Research and Quality grant K12HS022982. Dr D.E. Forman is supported by NIA R01 AG060499-01, R01AG058883, R01AG051376, R01AG053952, P30AG024827, and NIH UO1AR071130. The National Institute on Aging, American Heart Association, Agency for Healthcare Research & Quality, National Institute of Health, Hunnel Fund, and Abbot had no role in the preparation of this article. There are no conflicts of interest to report.

[a] Division of Cardiology, Department of Medicine, Weill Cornell Medicine, New York, NY, USA; [b] Division of General Internal Medicine, Department of Medicine, Weill Cornell Medicine, 420 East 70th Street, 3rd floor. LH340, New York, NY 10021, USA; [c] Department of Cardiovascular Medicine, Heart and Vascular Institute, Cleveland Clinic, Desk J3-4, 9500 Euclid Avenue, Cleveland, OH 44195, USA; [d] Department of Pharmacy, School of Pharmacy, University of Washington, 1959 Northeast Pacific Street Box 357630, Seattle, WA 98195, USA; [e] Section of Geriatric Cardiology, Cardiac Rehabilitation and GeroFit, VA Pittsburgh Healthcare System, University of Pittsburgh, 3471 Fifth Avenue, Suite 500, Kaufmann Medical Building, Pittsburgh, PA 15213, USA

* Corresponding author. 420 East 70th Street, 3rd Floor, LH 340, New York, NY 10021.

E-mail address: pag9051@med.cornell.edu

; @ParagGoyalMD (P.G.); @EiranGorodeski (E.Z.G.); @ZacharyAMarcum (Z.A.M.)

Clin Geriatr Med 35 (2019) 549–560
https://doi.org/10.1016/j.cger.2019.06.001
0749-0690/19/

Continued

- Utilizing CR to introduce nuance into the management of guideline-directed medical therapy for older adults with HF has the potential to alter the paradigm of HF medication management.
- CR offers a platform for conducting a detailed medication reconciliation to reduce the risk of medication errors and to eliminate agents that could cause harm.
- Through a team-based approach involving CR personnel, CR offers the opportunity to better understand patterns of medication adherence, to elicit barriers to adherence, and to implement strategies to improve adherence.

INTRODUCTION

Heart failure (HF) is a disease with high morbidity and mortality and high impact on function and quality of life.[1,2] Although numerous pharmacologic agents have demonstrated improvements in clinical outcomes among adults with HF,[1,2] the concept of an optimal medication regimen remains inherently ambiguous because clinical priorities can conflict with one another. For example, polypharmacy, commonly defined as the use of at least 5 medications,[3,4] is nearly universal in older adults with HF,[5] but it is associated with myriad adverse outcomes, including falls,[6–9] disability,[10–12] and hospitalizations.[13–15] The presence of polypharmacy reflects HF prescriptions as well as medications prescribed for the many other comorbid chronic conditions that are endemic in an older HF population.[16] Diuretics, neurohormonal antagonists, and vasodilators are commonly prescribed for pathophysiologic processes and symptoms related to HF,[1,2] and multiple noncardiovascular medications are almost always prescribed as well.

Although there is a rich tradition of evidence-based rationale for any one medication in HF, there is little evidence regarding the optimal administration of medications in aggregate. Moreover, it is not clear how to best balance divergent management priorities, especially in the broader context of noncardiovascular priorities. Important challenges remain with regard to optimizing medication regimens amidst such clinical complexity. Accordingly, there is an ongoing need to address the challenge of optimizing medication regimens in older adults with HF through novel patient-centered strategies and to establish platforms wherein medication optimization is actionable.

Cardiac rehabilitation (CR) was recently approved by the Centers for Medicare & Medicaid Services for management of HF patients and provides a multifaceted secondary prevention program that combines a supervised exercise program with education and counseling to encourage lifelong health and fitness, improve self-care, facilitate self-efficacy, and ultimately improve clinical outcomes and quality of life.[17] Given its comprehensive nature and patient-centered focus,[18] CR has the potential to enhance several other aspects of chronic disease management, such as diet, lifestyle, and stress management, and presents a remarkable opportunity to address medication optimization as a port of an expanded model of CR care. Because most CR programs target enrollment shortly after a cardiac event when changes in HF medications are common, CR provides an ideal platform for important medication management interventions.[17] In this review, 4 major challenges to optimizing medication regimens in HF are reviewed and strategies offered for leveraging CR toward addressing these important challenges (**Table 1**).

Table 1
Challenges and potential strategies for optimizing medication regimens in older adults with heart failure

Challenge	Potential Strategies	Cardiac Rehabilitation–Related Strategies
Diuretic management		
Chronic congestion and chronically elevated intracardiac pressures are common.	Maintain euvolemia, avoid hypovolemia.	Conduct history and physical examination to identify congestion or signs of over-diuresis. Titrate diuretic dose at CR or relay information to patients' physicians for dose titration. Co-localize HF program.
Electrolyte abnormalities can result from diuretic use and are associated with adverse outcomes.	Avoid and/or treat electrolyte abnormalities.	Check blood work routinely. Replete electrolytes at CR or relay information to patients' physicians for repletion. Develop algorithm to address electrolyte abnormalities.
Guideline-directed Medical Therapy (GDMT)		
GDMT is frequently under-prescribed. GDMT can cause adverse effects.	Initiate and/or up-titrate GDMT. Down-titrate and/or discontinue GDMT; reinitiate GDMT if can be tolerated at later date.	Introduce nuanced approach to GDMT with close monitoring for tolerance and adverse effects over course of CR.
Review and reconciliation of noncardiovascular medications		
An increasing number of medications is associated with increased risk of adverse drug reactions from drug-drug interactions, drug-disease interactions, and drug-patient interactions	Conduct medication review Identify potentially harmful prescribing patterns Discontinue/deprescribe potentially harmful agents	Provide comprehensive review of medications by CR personnel Utilize pharmacist to review and reconcile medications Apply implicit or explicit criteria to identify potentially harmful medications
Medication adherence		
Nonadherence is common, undermining the goals of pharmacotherapy.	Provide patient education Ensure safe medication regimen management Provide clinical pharmacist consultation Offer medication-taking reminders Award incentives to promote adherence	Incorporate medication adherence into usual educational program. Manage medications with close monitoring for tolerance and adverse effects Incorporate pharmacist into CR. Incorporate mobile health technologies. Provide tangible incentives for adherence at CR.

CHALLENGE #1: DIURETIC MANAGEMENT

State of the Problem

Patients with HF are at risk for episodes of congestion, defined as signs and symptoms of extracellular fluid accumulation from increased intracardiac filling pressures.[19] Congestion is associated with reduced quality of life, hospitalization, and death.[20] Accordingly, diuretics are a cornerstone in the management of HF, targeting congestion.[21] Loop diuretics are recommended in chronic HF and are used in more than 90% of patients[19]; thiazides may be used as adjunctive therapy for those with persistent congestion despite loop diuretic use; and mineralocorticoid receptor antagonists (MRAs) may be used to augment diuresis by modulating the expression and activity of sodium and potassium channels in the distal nephron[19,20] and to combat neurohormonal-mediated adverse remodeling.

To ensure diuretic effectiveness, titrating to doses that can maintain euvolemia is critically important. This is frequently a major challenge, however, for clinicians. Recent data suggest that a large proportion of adults hospitalized with HF is inadequately decongested by hospital discharge[22]; and among ambulatory patients, a significant proportion experiences chronically elevated intracardiac pressures.[23] Although under-diuresis is associated with adverse outcomes,[23] over-diuresis is also important because it can lead to hypovolemia and symptoms such as dizziness and lightheadedness, predisposing older adults to falls.[24] In addition, adverse effects from diuretics, including electrolytes abnormalities such as hypokalemia and hyperkalemia (which are both linked to adverse outcomes),[25] must be monitored. These issues highlight the importance of close monitoring when managing diuretics to achieve euvolemia without adverse effects.

Cardiac Rehabilitation as a Solution

CR constitutes a potential platform for both the recognition and management of congestion. CR personnel typically include capable exercise physiologists, physical therapists, and/or nurses under the direction of physician leadership. These personnel could be tasked with identifying congestion through history taking and physical examination, and such information could then be used to titrate diuretic dose. Many CR programs already assume a similar role in managing lipid lowering therapy. Although the effectiveness of CR clinical staff to titrate diuretics has not yet been explored, the concept represents an opportunity for future study. Alternatively, clinical data regarding volume status obtained during a CR session could be routinely relayed to patients' usual physicians for proper diuretic titration. Co-localizing HF programs with CR could also provide a potential strategy for leveraging CR toward improving diuretic management in this population. With increasing evidence to support the use of continuous ambulatory pulmonary artery pressure monitoring to ensure euvolemia and prevent HF hospitalizations,[26] incorporating this new technology into CR represents yet another strategy that warrants investigation.

Because CR occurs over several sessions across a span of several weeks, CR can facilitate repeat evaluations during diuretic titration to ensure both effectiveness and safety. Routinely eliciting symptoms of congestion like shortness of breath and conducting a physical examination to assess for signs of congestion could help to ensure the effectiveness of the diuretic regimen. At the same time, an assessment for hypovolemia could easily be achieved during CR sessions by routinely inquiring about suggestive symptoms like dizziness and lightheadedness and by obtaining a blood pressure (already routinely performed in CR). CR programs could also incorporate routine collection and review of blood work for patients taking diuretics to assess for electrolyte abnormalities. Algorithms could be developed to address electrolyte disturbances by supplementing electrolytes and/or communicating directly with patients' physicians about abnormal results. With additional training of personnel, CR has the potential to offer an adjunctive platform to ensure euvolemia through careful monitoring and thoughtful decision making.

CHALLENGE #2: GUIDELINE-DIRECTED MEDICAL THERAPY

State of the Problem

Several pharmacologic agents have demonstrated their potential to improve outcomes in HF. β-blockers, angiotensin-converting enzyme inhibitors (ACEIs), angiotensin receptor blockers (ARBs), angiotensin receptor–neprilysin inhibitors (ARNIs), MRAs, and vasodilators (hydralazine/nitrates) have robust data to indicate that they

Table 2
Guideline-directed medical therapy for heart failure and their potential adverse effects

Medication	Landmark Randomized Controlled Trial	Mean Age in Landmark Randomized Controlled Trial (y)	Target Dose	Potential Adverse Effects
β-Blockers				
Metoprolol succinate	MERIT-HF	64	200 mg daily	Hypotension, bradycardia, dizziness, fatigue, depressed mood, confusion, erectile dysfunction
Carvedilol	COPERNICUS	63	25–50 mg bid	
Bisoprolol	CIBIS II	61	10 mg daily	
ACEIs				
Enalapril	SOLVD	61	10–20 mg bid	Hypotension, dizziness, syncope, fatigue, hyperkalemia, acute kidney injury, cough
Lisinopril	ATLAS	64	20–40 mg daily	
Captopril	ELITE	74	50 mg tid	
ARBs				
Candesartan	CHARM	66	32 mg daily	Hypotension, dizziness, syncope, hyperkalemia, acute kidney injury
Losartan	ELITE	74	150 mg daily	
Valsartan	Val-HeFT	63	160 mg bid	
ARNI				
Valsartan-sacubitril	PARADIGM	64	97 mg/103 mg BID	Hypotension, dizziness, falling, hyperkalemia, acute kidney injury, cough
MRAs				
Spironolactone	RALES	65	25 mg daily	Dizziness, hyperkalemia, hyponatremia, acute kidney injury
Eplerenone	EMPHASIS	64	50 mg daily	
Vasodilators				
Hydralazine	V-HeFT	58	75 mg QID	Hypotension, dizziness, tachycardia, palpitations
Isosorbide dinitrate	V-HeFT	58	40 mg QID	Hypotension, dizziness

improve mortality, supporting their use in HF with reduced ejection fraction.[1,2] A summary of these agents is shown in **Table 2**. Although they are included in clinical practice guidelines as class I indications, many of these agents are under-prescribed, especially among older adults.[27,28] In response to low prescribing rates, national quality improvement programs, such as Get With The Guidelines,[29] were created to improve the use of guideline-directed medical therapy (GDMT) in adults with HF. Additionally, the Centers for Medicare & Medicaid Services have incorporated the use of GDMT into their quality metrics for hospitalized HF patients as part of a national effort to facilitate broader use of these disease-modifying mortality-reducing agents. Despite these efforts, GDMT use remains suboptimal—in a recent study from the Change the Management of Patients with Heart Failure registry, composed of 3518 ambulatory HF patients with a reduced ejection fraction from 150 primary care and cardiology practices across the United States, 33%, 27%, and 67% were not prescribed β-blocker, ACEI/ARB/ARNI, and MRA therapy, respectively.[30] Moreover, among those who were prescribed GDMT, few were taking the recommended target doses (β-blockers: 28%; ACEIs/ARBs/ARNIs: 17%; and MRAs: 67%). This is important because lower doses may not provide maximal benefit. Thus, there remains a need for strategies to combat issues like clinical inertia and a lack of prescriber awareness to optimize the use of GDMT among those who can tolerate it and ultimately improve outcomes.

Juxtaposed to under-prescribing and under-titration of GDMT is the observation that GDMT may be poorly tolerated in some individuals. For example, the Cardiac Insufficiency Bisoprolol Study in Elderly (CIBIS-ELD) trial, which specifically enrolled older adults aged at least 65 years, revealed that overall β-blocker tolerability was lower compared with the tolerability observed in prior β-blocker trials composed of younger participants. In addition, CIBIS-ELD showed that advanced age was associated with reduced tolerability.[31] These observations are likely the result of multiple factors, including age-related changes in cardiovascular structure and function,[32] and unpredictable alterations in pharmacokinetics and pharmacodynamics observed with aging, both of which can have an impact on medication effects.[33] Older adults frequently experience impairments in cognition and function,[34] which increase the risk for adverse drug reactions.[35,36] Given their exclusion from major clinical trials,[37,38] less is known about how older adults with impairments in cognition and/or function tolerate HF medications and how much benefit they derive. A recent study of adults with HF revealed that individuals with significant functional impairment (impairments in their activities of daily living) took the same number of medications as those without such impairments, suggesting that clinicians may not consider factors like function and cognition when prescribing medications.[5] Given that the risk-benefit ratio of HF medications for older adults with HF could vary based on several different factors, there is a rationale for implementing a nuanced approach to GDMT in which patients are closely monitored for untoward effects, and down-titration or even discontinuation (also known as deprescribing[39]) is strongly considered for those who develop concerning signs and symptoms like dizziness, postural instability, orthostatic hypotension, or even worsened fatigue.

Cardiac Rehabilitation as a Solution

CR offers an excellent opportunity to optimize GDMT. For those not yet on GDMT who do not have apparent contraindications, this is an opportune time to start evidence-based agents like β-blockers, ACEIs/ARBs/ARNIs, MRAs, and/or vasodilators. Given that CR typically occurs over the span of weeks, initiation and/or up-titration of GDMT during CR is sensible because it provides a platform for monitoring as doses are changed. Moreover, it provides opportunity to systematically inquire about symptoms like increased fatigue or dizziness and to objectively evaluate changes in function, balance, and/or gait that provide important insight into GDMT tolerance. Vital signs, which are routinely assessed during CR, also can provide important information about GDMT tolerability. For example, bradycardia or hypotension could prompt changes to GDMT. For scenarios where GDMT is either decreased or discontinued, CR should additionally offer the opportunity for restarting or increasing GDMT if/when there is an improvement in function. This notion may be especially relevant for post-hospitalization patients, whose balance and gait speed as well as symptoms of dizziness and fatigue may improve with CR.

Although implementation of this model represents an ambitious undertaking, leveraging CR to introduce nuance into the management of GDMT could substantially alter the paradigm of HF management. Given potential benefits, future studies should examine whether such a model is feasible, effective, and pragmatic.

CHALLENGE #3: REVIEWING AND RECONCILING NONCARDIOVASCULAR MEDICATIONS

State of the Problem

Multimorbidity, or the condition of having multiple chronic conditions,[40] is nearly universal in HF. Among Medicare beneficiaries, 90% have at least 3 other chronic conditions and more than 60% have at least 5 other chronic conditions.[16] Consequently, a large number of medications taken by adults with HF are frequently noncardiovascular in nature. This is important because as the number of medications increases, the risks for drug-drug interactions, drug-disease interactions, and drug-patient interactions increase.[41] In routine care, the process of optimizing medication regimens may be undermined by several factors, including limitations in the time and resources of clinicians to conduct a thorough review, the disease-specific focus of many clinicians where medications outside the scope of their expertise may be overlooked, and fragmentation of care where multiple clinicians prescribe multiple medications with suboptimal communication with one another. This supports the need for an improved process of medication reconciliation. Consequently, potentially harmful medications often remain even after a patient sees a clinician. In a recent study of adults with HF from National Health and Nutrition Examination Survey, almost half of ambulatory adults with HF took a medication that could potentially exacerbate HF; most were noncardiovascular medications.[42] These issues underscore the importance of conducting comprehensive reviews of all medications (not just those that pertain to HF or cardiovascular conditions) during patient encounters.

Cardiac Rehabilitation as a Solution

CR offers a platform for conducting a detailed medication reconciliation to reduce the risk of medication errors and to eliminate agents that could cause harm. Medication review using implicit and explicit criteria to identify harmful prescribing patterns[43] and medication reviews performed by pharmacists[44] have demonstrated improvements in medication prescribing quality. CR could be leveraged to provide these services. A thorough medication review could be performed where duplicate medications and medications for resolved indications are eliminated and potentially harmful interactions are identified through the aid of the electronic medical record, a checklist, and/or a pharmacist. Although there has been significant national focus on adding appropriate medications (GDMTs) that can improve outcomes in HF, eliminating agents that can cause harm in HF may be equally important.[42] Although this would

Box 1
List of major heart failure exacerbating medications

Therapeutic Class	Subclass/Drug
Analgesics	COX, nonselective inhibitors (NSAIDs; COX, selective inhibitors (COX-2 inhibitors)
Anesthesia medications	Desflurane; enflurane; halothane; isoflurane; sevoflurane; ketamine
Diabetes mellitus medications	Thiazolidinediones; saxagliptin; sitagliptin
Antiarrhythmic medications	Flecainide; disopyramide; sotalol; dronedarone
Antihypertensive medications	Diltiazem; verapamil; moxonidine
Anti-infective medications	Itraconazole; amphotericin B
Anticancer medications	Doxorubicin; daunorubicin; epirubicin; idarubicin; mitoxantrone; cyclophosphamide; ifosfamide; 5-FU; capecitabine; bevacizumab; interferon; interleukin-2; lapatinib; pertuzumab; trastuzumab; lenalidomide
Hematologic medications	Anagrelide; cilostazol
Neurologic and psychiatric medications	Carbamazepine; citalopram; bromocriptine; pergolide; pramipexole; clozapine; ergotamine; methysergide; lithium
Ophthalmologic medications	Topical β-blockers
Pulmonary medications	Albuterol; bosentan; epoprostenol
Rheumatologic agents	TNF-α inhibitors; chloroquine; hydroxychloroquine

Abbreviations: 5-FU, 5-fluorouracil; COX, cyclooxygenase; NSAID, nonsteroidal anti-inflammatory drug; TNF, tumor necrosis factor.

require additional resource allocation, CR could offer an opportunity to identify medications that can exacerbate HF[45] (**Box 1**), thereby facilitating discontinuation of agents that may contribute to adverse outcomes in this vulnerable population.

CHALLENGE #4: MEDICATION ADHERENCE

State of the Problem

Among the self-care behaviors required for HF treatment, medication adherence is critical for achieving positive health outcomes. Unfortunately, medication adherence in patients with HF is suboptimal. In a study of 178,000 Medicare beneficiaries, just 52% were considered adherent to HF medications.[46] Reasons for this observation are multifactorial. Patient-related factors include cognitive impairment, which can lead to forgetfulness about taking medications; low health literacy, which can lead to an underappreciation about the importance of taking medications; and low motivation, which can lead to disinterest in taking medications. Medication regimen–related factors contributing to nonadherence include pill burden, regimen complexity, medication intolerance, and cost.[47,48] Given the link between improvements in medication adherence and outcomes,[49,50] the need to address medication adherence persists for older adults with HF.

Several interventions aimed at improving adherence have been studied, demonstrating their potential for improving clinical outcomes.[49,50] A systematic review and meta-analysis of interventions to improve HF medication adherence revealed that they significantly reduced mortality risk (relative risk, 0.89; 95% CI 0.81–0.99) and decreased the likelihood for hospital readmission (odds ratio, 0.79; 95% CI 0.71–0.89).[49,50] Interventions to improve medication adherence may be grouped into 6 categories, each of which requires varying levels of time and resources: patient education, medication regimen management, clinical pharmacist consultation for chronic disease comanagement, cognitive behavioral therapies, medication-taking reminders, and incentives to promote adherence. To effectively implement medication adherence interventions, there is a need to appropriately measure adherence, understand the underlying reason(s) for nonadherence, and then subsequently tailor an intervention that can address the underlying issue. A major challenge for achieving these objectives is that although self-report is an inexpensive way to measure nonadherence, questions about adherence are infrequently asked in routine patient encounters. Another important challenge is that that the time and resources necessary to implement an effective intervention may not be available. These issues highlight the importance of developing novel strategies that can leverage preexisting infrastructure and resources to implement interventions that can improve adherence.

Cardiac Rehabilitation as a Solution

CR offers an excellent opportunity to improve medication adherence. The structure of CR, which includes episodic interactions with CR personnel over the course of several weeks, is particularly well-suited for multifaceted initiatives that frequently are required to change complex health behaviors.[18] Also, a key component of CR is tailored education and counseling to provide patient-centered care. This concept is directly aligned with the current literature on medication adherence interventions, which promotes a patient-tailored approach to address adherence barriers rather than one-size-fits-all.[51]

Through a team-based approach involving CR personnel, CR could offer the opportunity to better understand patterns of medication adherence and elicit barriers to adherence. Once these issues have been identified, CR personnel could potentially implement patient-centered interventions to improve medication adherence. Selection of the intervention may be drawn from several different intervention categories that may be applicable in the CR setting. Patient education about the importance of pharmacotherapy and medication adherence could be incorporated into the education already provided as part of the CR program. Nuanced approaches to medication regimen management, as described previously, could provide an additional strategy to improve medication adherence. Clinical pharmacist consultation could be incorporated into CR to ensure drug safety, as described previously, as well as to improve medication adherence. Medication-taking reminders, such as through the use of mobile health (mHealth) strategies (eg, text messaging), is currently being studied among patients enrolled in CR[52] and offers a novel avenue for improving adherence. Finally, incentives to promote adherence through recognition and/or financial reward also could be incorporated into CR. Given the number of possible strategies that could be adapted to the CR setting, leveraging CR toward maximizing medication adherence seems to be a fruitful area for further investigation, with great potential for improving the health outcomes of older adults with HF.

SUMMARY

CR is an inherently patient-centered program that provides holistic care to adults with cardiovascular conditions to promote lifelong health and fitness, facilitate self-care and self-efficacy, and ultimately improve clinical outcomes.[17] As described in this review, CR offers an excellent platform for patient-centered optimization of medication regimens for older adults with HF through its potential to address several aspects of care that have historically served as major challenges to clinicians—diuretic management, the use of GDMT, review and reconciliation of noncardiovascular medications, and medication adherence. Given the link between pharmacotherapy and outcomes in this vulnerable population, the effectiveness of CR may be greatly enhanced by incorporating formal processes, such as those discussed in this article, for optimizing medication regimens. Little is known about how best to incorporate these aspects into CR, and many challenges exist impeding potential benefits of medication management within CR programs. Given the degree of benefit that could result from optimizing medication regimens in HF patients, future work should explore how CR can pragmatically be leveraged toward this purpose and how CR can further maximize both clinical outcomes and quality of life for this highly vulnerable population.

REFERENCES

1. Yancy CW, Jessup M, Bozkurt B, et al. 2013 ACCF/AHA guideline for the management of heart failure: executive summary: a report of the American College of Cardiology Foundation/American Heart Association Task Force on practice guidelines. Circulation 2013;128(16):1810–52.
2. Yancy CW, Jessup M, Bozkurt B, et al. 2017 ACC/AHA/HFSA focused update of the 2013 ACCF/AHA guideline for the management of heart failure: a report of the American College of Cardiology/American Heart Association Task Force on clinical practice guidelines and the heart failure Society of America. J Am Coll Cardiol 2017;70(6):776–803.
3. Qato DM, Alexander GC, Conti RM, et al. Use of prescription and over-the-counter medications and dietary supplements among older adults in the United States. JAMA 2008;300(24):2867–78.
4. Rich MW. Pharmacotherapy of heart failure in the elderly: adverse events. Heart Fail Rev 2012;17(4–5):589–95.
5. Goyal P, Bryan J, Kneifati-Hayek J, et al. Association between functional impairment and medication burden in adults with heart failure. J Am Geriatr Soc 2019; 67(2):284–91.
6. Freeland KN, Thompson AN, Zhao Y, et al. Medication use and associated risk of falling in a geriatric outpatient population. Ann Pharmacother 2012;46(9):1188–92.
7. Kojima T, Akishita M, Nakamura T, et al. Polypharmacy as a risk for fall occurrence in geriatric outpatients. Geriatr Gerontol Int 2012;12(3):425–30.
8. Tromp AM, Pluijm SM, Smit JH, et al. Fall-risk screening test: a prospective study on predictors for falls in community-dwelling elderly. J Clin Epidemiol 2001;54(8): 837–44.
9. Ziere G, Dieleman JP, Hofman A, et al. Polypharmacy and falls in the middle age and elderly population. Br J Clin Pharmacol 2006;61(2):218–23.
10. Magaziner J, Cadigan DA. Community resources and mental health of older women living alone. J Aging Health 1989;1(1):35–49.
11. Crentsil V, Ricks MO, Xue QL, et al. A pharmacoepidemiologic study of community-dwelling, disabled older women: factors associated with medication use. Am J Geriatr Pharmacother 2010;8(3):215–24.
12. Jyrkka J, Enlund H, Lavikainen P, et al. Association of polypharmacy with nutritional status, functional ability and cognitive capacity over a three-year period in an elderly population. Pharmacoepidemiol Drug Saf 2011;20(5):514–22.
13. Akazawa M, Imai H, Igarashi A, et al. Potentially inappropriate medication use in elderly Japanese patients. Am J Geriatr Pharmacother 2010;8(2):146–60.
14. Marcum ZA, Amuan ME, Hanlon JT, et al. Prevalence of unplanned hospitalizations caused by adverse drug reactions in older veterans. J Am Geriatr Soc 2012;60(1):34–41.

15. Picker D, Heard K, Bailey TC, et al. The number of discharge medications predicts thirty-day hospital readmission: a cohort study. BMC Health Serv Res 2015;15:282.
16. Centers for Medicare & Medicaid Services. Chronic conditions among Medicare beneficiaries. Available at: https://www.cms.gov/Research-Statistics-Data-and-Systems/Statistics-Trends-and-Reports/Chronic-Conditions/Chartbook_Charts.html. Accessed February 18, 2019.
17. Schopfer DW, Forman DE. Cardiac rehabilitation in older adults. Can J Cardiol 2016;32(9):1088–96.
18. Schopfer DW, Forman DE. Growing relevance of cardiac rehabilitation for an older population with heart failure. J Card Fail 2016;22(12):1015–22.
19. Mullens W, Damman K, Harjola VP, et al. The use of diuretics in heart failure with congestion - a position statement from the Heart Failure Association of the European Society of Cardiology. Eur J Heart Fail 2019;21(2):137–55.
20. Ellison DH, Felker GM. Diuretic treatment in heart failure. N Engl J Med 2018; 378(7):684–5.
21. Brunner-La Rocca HP, Sanders-van Wijk S. Guiding heart failure therapy after GUIDE-IT: back to the drawing board. J Am Coll Cardiol 2018;72(21):2563–6.
22. Lala A, McNulty SE, Mentz RJ, et al. Relief and recurrence of congestion during and after hospitalization for acute heart failure: insights from diuretic optimization strategy evaluation in acute decompensated heart failure (DOSE-AHF) and cardiorenal rescue study in acute decompensated heart failure (CARESS-HF). Circ Heart Fail 2015;8(4):741–8.
23. Stevenson LW, Zile M, Bennett TD, et al. Chronic ambulatory intracardiac pressures and future heart failure events. Circ Heart Fail 2010;3(5):580–7.
24. Marcum ZA, Perera S, Newman AB, et al. Antihypertensive use and recurrent falls in community-dwelling older adults: findings from the health ABC study. J Gerontol A Biol Sci Med Sci 2015;70(12):1562–8.
25. Savarese G, Xu H, Trevisan M, et al. Incidence, predictors, and outcome associations of dyskalemia in heart failure with preserved, mid-range, and reduced ejection fraction. JACC Heart Fail 2019;7(1):65–76.
26. Dickinson MG, Allen LA, Albert NA, et al. Remote monitoring of patients with heart failure: a white paper from the heart failure Society of America Scientific Statements Committee. J Card Fail 2018;24(10):682–94.
27. Lee DS, Tu JV, Juurlink DN, et al. Risk-treatment mismatch in the pharmacotherapy of heart failure. JAMA 2005;294(10):1240–7.
28. Forman DE, Cannon CP, Hernandez AF, et al. Influence of age on the management of heart failure: findings from Get with the Guidelines-Heart Failure (GWTG-HF). Am Heart J 2009;157(6):1010–7.
29. Smaha LA, American Heart A. The American heart association Get with the guidelines program. Am Heart J 2004;148(5 Suppl):S46–8.
30. Greene SJ, Butler J, Albert NM, et al. Medical therapy for heart failure with reduced ejection fraction: the CHAMP-HF registry. J Am Coll Cardiol 2018; 72(4):351–66.
31. Dungen HD, Apostolovic S, Inkrot S, et al. Titration to target dose of bisoprolol vs. carvedilol in elderly patients with heart failure: the CIBIS-ELD trial. Eur J Heart Fail 2011;13(6):670–80.
32. Dai X, Hummel SL, Salazar JB, et al. Cardiovascular physiology in the older adults. J Geriatr Cardiol 2015;12(3):196–201.

33. Mangoni AA, Jackson SH. Age-related changes in pharmacokinetics and pharmacodynamics: basic principles and practical applications. Br J Clin Pharmacol 2004;57(1):6–14.
34. Gorodeski EZ, Goyal P, Hummel SL, et al. Domain management approach to heart failure in the geriatric patient: present and future. J Am Coll Cardiol 2018; 71(17):1921–36.
35. Larson EB, Kukull WA, Buchner D, et al. Adverse drug reactions associated with global cognitive impairment in elderly persons. Ann Intern Med 1987;107(2): 169–73.
36. Hanlon JT, Pieper CF, Hajjar ER, et al. Incidence and predictors of all and preventable adverse drug reactions in frail elderly persons after hospital stay. J Gerontol A Biol Sci Med Sci 2006;61(5):511–5.
37. Cherubini A, Oristrell J, Pla X, et al. The persistent exclusion of older patients from ongoing clinical trials regarding heart failure. Arch Intern Med 2011;171(6):550–6.
38. Skolnick AH, Alexander KP. Older adults in clinical research and drug development: closing the geriatric gap. Circ Cardiovasc Qual Outcomes 2015;8(6): 631–3.
39. Scott IA, Hilmer SN, Reeve E, et al. Reducing inappropriate polypharmacy: the process of deprescribing. JAMA Intern Med 2015;175(5):827–34.
40. Tinetti ME, Fried TR, Boyd CM. Designing health care for the most common chronic condition–multimorbidity. JAMA 2012;307(23):2493–4.
41. Maher RL, Hanlon J, Hajjar ER. Clinical consequences of polypharmacy in elderly. Expert Opin Drug Saf 2014;13(1):57–65.
42. Kneifati-Hayek J, Kennel P, Bryan J, et al. Use of heart failure-exacerbating medications among adults with heart failure. J Card Fail 2019;25(1):72–3.
43. Marcum ZA, Hanlon JT. Inappropriate medication Use and medication errors in the elderly. In: Wehling M, Burkhardt H, editors. Drug therapy in the elderly. 2nd edition. New York: Springer-Verlag; 2013. p. 43–50.
44. Hanlon JT, Weinberger M, Samsa GP, et al. A randomized, controlled trial of a clinical pharmacist intervention to improve inappropriate prescribing in elderly outpatients with polypharmacy. Am J Med 1996;100(4):428–37.
45. Page RL 2nd, O'Bryant CL, Cheng D, et al. Drugs that may cause or exacerbate heart failure: a scientific statement from the American heart association. Circulation 2016;134(6):e32–69.
46. Zhang Y, Wu SH, Fendrick AM, et al. Variation in medication adherence in heart failure. JAMA Intern Med 2013;173(6):468–70.
47. Gellad WF, Grenard JL, Marcum ZA. A systematic review of barriers to medication adherence in the elderly: looking beyond cost and regimen complexity. Am J Geriatr Pharmacother 2011;9(1):11–23.
48. Marcum ZA, Gellad WF. Medication adherence to multidrug regimens. Clin Geriatr Med 2012;28(2):287–300.
49. Nieuwlaat R, Wilczynski N, Navarro T, et al. Interventions for enhancing medication adherence. Cochrane Database Syst Rev 2014;(11):CD000011.
50. Ruppar TM, Cooper PS, Mehr DR, et al. Medication adherence interventions improve heart failure mortality and readmission rates: systematic review and meta-analysis of controlled trials. J Am Heart Assoc 2016;5(6) [pii:e002606].
51. Kini V, Ho PM. Interventions to improve medication adherence: a review. JAMA 2018;320(23):2461–73.
52. Maddison R, Stewart R, Doughty R, et al. Text4Heart II - improving medication adherence in people with heart disease: a study protocol for a randomized controlled trial. Trials 2018;19(1):70.

Cardiac Rehabilitation as Part of Management in Postacute Care

Opportunities for Improving Care

Mary Ann C. Podlogar, BSN, MAEd*, Mary A. Dolansky, RN, PhD

KEYWORDS

• Acute care • Cardiac rehabilitation • Disease management • Postacute care
• Secondary prevention

KEY POINTS

- Review the current state of Medicare reimbursement for cardiac rehabilitation.
- Identify gaps in services of cardiac rehabilitation in postacute care settings.
- Define opportunities to improve the use of cardiac rehabilitation for elderly patients across the postacute care continuum.
- Provide recommendations for future research.

INTRODUCTION: MEDICARE BARRIERS

Cardiac rehabilitation (CR) is an evidence-based intervention, yet only 20% of eligible patients attend, and the rate of attendance is even lower for patients discharged to postacute care.[1] Current standards for Medicare reimbursement limit the degree to which CR can positively affect outcomes for postacute patients. CR is traditionally broken into 3 stages of segmented delivery, each of which is reimbursed and recognized differently by Medicare. For the purposes of this article, we have included a fourth stage (phase IB)[2] to the CR continuum as it relates specifically to care received in postacute settings and constitutes a substantive aspect of care that impacts current underuse, and to opportunities for improvement. Current Medicare reimbursements for CR (**Fig. 1**) separates reimbursements for each phase of care. Phase I CR refers to the inpatient CR services received during a hospitalization and is not covered by Medicare. Phase IB[2] CR refers to subacute

Disclosure Statement: The authors have nothing to disclose.
Case Western Reserve University, Frances Payne Bolton School of Nursing, 2120 Cornell Road, Cleveland, OH 44106, USA
* Corresponding author.
E-mail address: mcp102@case.edu

Clin Geriatr Med 35 (2019) 561–569
https://doi.org/10.1016/j.cger.2019.07.010
0749-0690/19/Published by Elsevier Inc.

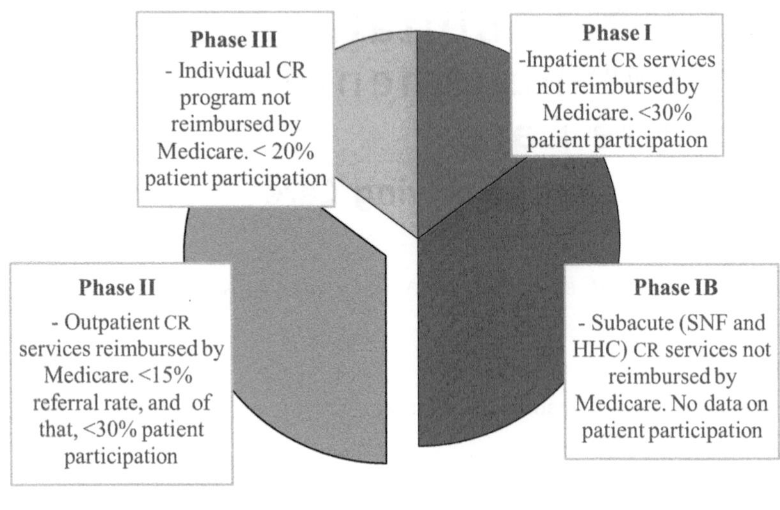

Fig. 1. Current trends in medicare reimbursement and participation for CR.

inpatient services delivered in skilled nursing facilities (SNFs), and it is also not covered by Medicare. Phase II CR refers to services received during supervised sessions at hospital-affiliated outpatient rehabilitation centers and is covered by Medicare. Phase III CR is composed of unmonitored and self-guided home exercise programs and is also not covered by Medicare. Notably, only phase II CR is covered under Medicare part B for the strict duration of 36 sessions (2–3 sessions per week for 12–18 weeks) in physician-directed outpatient settings, starting 1 to 3 weeks after discharge for conditions such as acute coronary syndrome, percutaneous coronary intervention, coronary artery bypass graft surgery, and stable heart failure (HF).[3] These reimbursement regulations leave major gaps in care opportunities for both acute inpatients who could benefit from immediate CR, as well as recently discharged patients who require additional postacute care services in either SNFs or home health care (HHC) settings. Medicare reimbursement regulations are preventing the receipt of the benefits of CR from much of the eligible population. As recently as 2014, the Centers for Medicare and Medicaid Services changed reimbursements to allow patients with an *International Classification of Diseases,* 9th edition, diagnosis of HF to be eligible for CR services.[4] Although this change opened many new avenues for patients with HF and medical providers, it remains restrictive in its application. Per the new Medicaid guidelines, CR is only approved for stable patients who have HF with a reduced ejection fraction of less than 35%, a New York Heart Association functional class II to IV diagnosis, and have remained without acute treatment for more than 6 weeks.[3,4] As a result, HF patients discharged from an inpatient hospital stay are not eligible for CR in the most crucial period of their recovery. This restriction would seem to be contradictory to standard discharge practices, as patients who have undergone cardiac surgery are recommended to begin CR exercises almost immediately after discharge.[3] Furthermore, the change neglects patients who have HF with a preserved ejection fraction, an expanding population composed of patients who are typically over 65 years of age and total more than one-half of the HF cases nationally.[5] Because the percent of the population with HF with a preserved ejection fraction is expected to double in the coming decade, with an estimated 30% of patients being discharged to SNFs,[2] it seems critical that reimbursement regulations for elderly cardiac patients be altered to match the growing demand. Significant changes to Medicare reimbursements are necessary to increase provider referral and patient participation and to improve the long-term health outcomes for postacute cardiac patients.

CURRENT TRENDS IN CARDIAC REHABILITATION REFERRAL

CR is an American Heart Association/American College of Cardiology class 1A indication for postacute heart attack recovery and is a class 1 indication for patients with HF,[6] yet referral rates and postacute use remain consistently low. Among physicians and hospitalists, the leading factor influencing a CR referral is the perceived benefit of the program among providers.[7] A distorted impression of providers that CR lacks value, relevance, or safety no doubt contributes to minimal referrals, especially for eligible elderly patients. A recent study of 105,619 cardiac patients found that a mere 10.4% of patients discharged from an inpatient hospitalization were referred for CR services.[8] The low referral rates are remarkable, because repeated studies[4,9–12] have indicated that participation in a CR program decreases total mortality, and rehospitalizations, and improves physical function and quality of life. Of further concern is the lack of use of inpatient CR as an opportunity for an initial evaluation of exercise tolerance and function capabilities, both prerequisites of CR as outlined by the American Association of Cardiovascular and Pulmonary Rehabilitation (AACVPR). A recent study of inpatient CR programs found that less than 50% of hospitals treating cardiac patients offered formal inpatient CR and, of those who provided services, only 30% of patients participated.[13] The underuse of outpatient CR programs might be a result of the lack of provider emphasis on the importance of inpatient CR services. It is estimated that outpatient CR participation would increase by up to 18% if providers scheduled a patient's first rehabilitation appointment before hospital discharge.[1] Per the AACVPR, patients should receive a physician-based rating of their cardiac risk for exercise (low, moderate, high) before beginning a CR program. This type of standardized assessment is both convenient and feasible in the inpatient setting and may alleviate delays in care after transfer. The implementation of the IMPACT Act (Improving Medicare Post-Acute Care Transformation Act) in 2014 brought about a new approach to postacute care management, which requires the use of the inpatient setting for discharge referral and evaluation. The IMPACT Act resulted in the creation of the Continuity Assessment Record and Evaluation (CARE) form that, as of 2018, is a requirement for all providers to complete before initiating a postacute care transfer.[7] The Continuity Assessment Record and Evaluation form is designed to be a standardized assessment tool that requires providers to review patient capabilities, goals, and functional status before discharge. The form is currently undergoing several tests and is due to be presented to congress for use in the coming years. If adopted, this form may provide an avenue for streamlined postacute care transfers that include immediate implementation of cardiac-specific care delivery. To this end, several health systems have been working to pilot and initiate automatic CR referrals upon discharge for eligible patients. The automated referral system developed by Grace and colleagues,[1] has the potential to not only triple referral rates, but also encompasses CR referral as a quality indicator for patient care plans. Nevertheless, for the time being, there is still no national standardized procedure to identify, evaluate, refer, and design cardiac-specific care for eligible CR patients. **Fig. 2** outlines considerations to improving both provider referrals to CR and patient transfer procedures to postacute care settings.

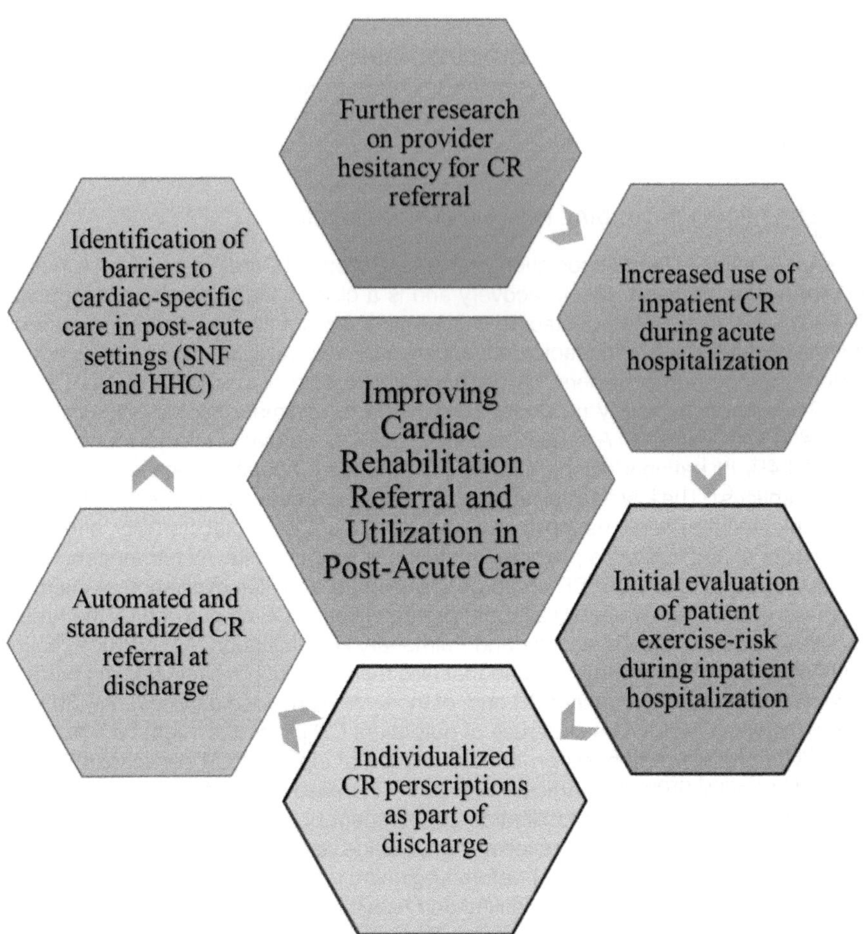

Fig. 2. Opportunities to improve CR referral and use in postacute care.

CARDIAC REHABILITATION IN POSTACUTE CARE SETTINGS

CR can be delivered in a variety of postacute settings including SNF and HHC settings. A recent publication surveying the nation's cardiac discharges of persons greater than 65 years of age noted that 30% of patients with a myocardial infarction, 25% of patients with HF, and a combined 31% of cardiac surgery patients were discharged to a SNF after a hospitalization.[14] The characteristics of postacute cardiac care delivery in SNFs differ greatly from facility to facility, and under changing reimbursement models, facilities receive varying levels of reimbursement for services provided. Medicare proposes reimbursement for 100% of skilled nursing rehabilitation services within the first 20 days of admission, if the patient is deemed medically eligible.[14] Remarkably, due to a lack of consistency in patient transfer procedures, provider continuity of care, and restrictive Medicare regulations many patients are not deemed eligible for services within this critical window of management. Furthermore, SNFs are often not equipped with the staff or resources necessary to deliver care specific to the unique needs of an older cardiac patient. The lack of cardiac specific care contributes to patterns wherein nearly 20% of patients discharged from SNFs seek acute medical care within 30 days of discharge.[15] The alarming rate at which cardiac patients are readmitted to the hospital from SNFs is not only an indication of inadequate care, but also a financial burden that is costing the United States nearly $4 billion annually.[9]

The delivery of care in SNFs becomes further complicated with the integration of CR services as a part of the daily regimen. The AACPVR defines cardiac-specific care as comprehensive disease management that includes risk modification, cardiac response to exercise, patient education, survival management, and recommendation of continued outpatient rehabilitation.[2,3] In contrast, the use of cardiac-specific care, specifically during CR, is ineffectively managed and underutilized in SNFs. In 1 study of patients receiving CR services at an SNF, only 5% of therapy records reported exercise tolerance monitoring during therapy, and cardiac responses were reported only if the patient became symptomatic.[2] Such underassessment is fundamentally unsafe. Likewise, components of comprehensive cardiac management that are regularly used as a part of traditional outpatient CR, such as patient education, medication reconciliation, emotional health, and dietary management, are not part of routine SNF standards of care.

CR as part of HHC is similarly underdeveloped, understructured, and not regularly documented. CR has been traditionally delivered through physician-supervised outpatient facilities after a hospital discharge. However, recent advances in technology as well as changes to accepted settings for CR allow for the possibility of a more streamlined and remote approach to service delivery that could be integrated into HHC. Several recent studies have attempted to examine telehealth as a mode to deliver CR services through home health settings. Telehealth for the delivery of CR in the home has been shown to be feasible and safe for younger cardiac patients[9]; however, there is little evidence surrounding the feasibility and safety of telehealth management for complex patients who are older. Interestingly, studies have indicated that patients display greater adherence to an at-home CR program than to an outpatient facility-based program.[16] Studies have identified several barriers to participation in facility-based CR, including a lack of transportation, patient's perceived benefit, personal schedule, and perceived program difficulty.[9,16,17] Furthermore, facility-based CR is often more difficult for many patients to access because approximately 20% of adults over the age of 65 do not have access to reliable transportation.[16] Participation is further affected by the constraints of limited available CR sessions, many of which coincide with traditional working hours. Many of the identified barriers to CR participation may be overcome using home-health care as an alternative delivery model. However, further research needs to be conducted to identify barriers and to CR feasibility for older adults in the home health care setting.

CARDIAC REHABILITATION AS A PART OF DISEASE MANAGEMENT

We have identified several opportunities to improve cardiac disease management using CR for elderly patients in postacute care settings. These suggested improvements (**Fig. 3**) are heavily influenced by the American Heart Association/American College of Cardiology's CR guidelines and the AACVPR's Million Hearts Initiative. Opportunities to improve disease management using CR services include (1) deliberate and structured patient care goals, (2) purposeful and relevant disease-specific patient education, (3) consistent monitoring and management of exercise related symptoms, and (4) the integration of secondary prevention guidelines.

Deliberate and Structured Patient Care Goals

Clinical success often depends on the perceived level of progress and benefit held by the patient.[17] Thus, it is imperative that patients set goals for recovery that are both

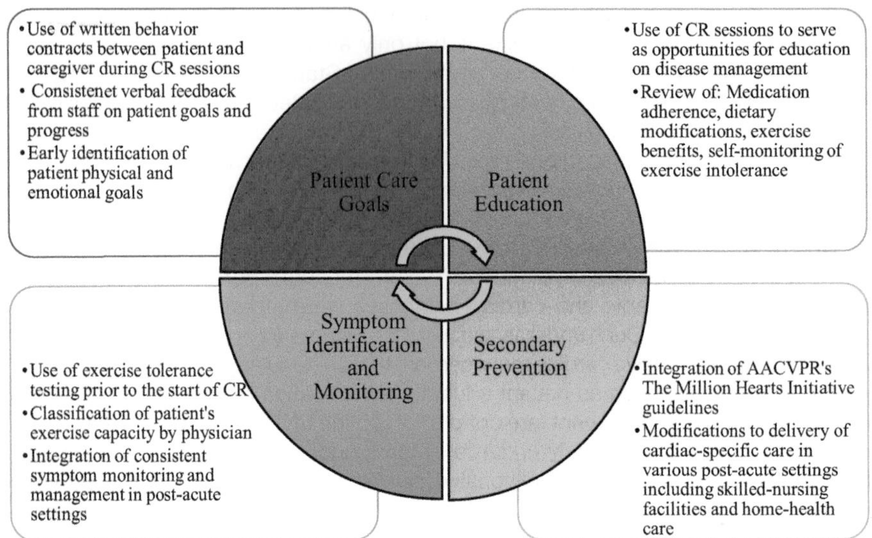

Fig. 3. Opportunities to integrate comprehensive disease management into CR in postacute care.

attainable and realistic. Reports from recent CR studies indicate that patients experience better outcomes in their level of physical activity when behavioral interventions are used.[10] Per the Million Hearts Initiative for improving standards of care, examples of behavioral intervention to increase physical activity during CR may range from the use of written behavior contracts, to consistent feedback, and even the use of incentives or rewards. Goal setting is especially beneficial for the elderly population, because the intended outcome of CR is increased functionality and independence.[10] The theme of CR as part of disease management presents several opportunities to integrate components of cardiac care including dietary modifications, exercise adherence, and medication review into CR sessions. Although heavily understudied, initial findings regarding the use of goal setting in CR has proven to be effective in not only promoting adherence to the exercise program, but also supports improved long-term functional outcomes specifically impacting dietary modifications and weight loss during CR.[18]

Purposeful and Relevant Disease-Specific Education

It is estimated that patients discharged from an acute setting retain approximately 20% of their discharge instructions.[19] This is often due to inconsistencies in the delivery method, present level of illness, and complexity of the disease treatment regimen. With this staggering lack of disease-specific knowledge, it is not surprising that 22% of patients discharged to a postacute facility are readmitted to the hospital within 6 days.[15] Even more problematic is the lack of education provided or required by postacute facilities, such as SNFs. To date, discharge teaching is not a requirement for SNFs. In a recent study of the use of comprehensive cardiac care management for SNF residents, less than 50% of nurses reported the use of disease-specific educational materials (ie, myocardial infarction, HF), and no nurses reported discussing outpatient rehabilitation options with patients before discharge.[2] The structured environment of CR should allow for the concurrent delivery of disease-specific education to patients without adding additional requirements to their care regimen. Doubling CR sessions as educational opportunities presents providers with adequate time to review topics, such as medication adherence, dietary modifications, exercise benefits, and self-monitoring of exercise intolerances.

Consistent Monitoring and Management of Exercise Related Symptoms

According to the recommendations from the AACVPR, patients who participate in CR should not only receive a specific exercise risk rating before beginning an exercise program, but should also receive continuous monitoring of exercise related symptoms throughout exercise training, as well as education on recognizing individual symptoms during therapy.[2,3] Unfortunately, these recommendations are not consistently integrated into practice, specifically in postacute settings such as SNFs, resulting in unsafe practices and misuse of CR therapies. In 1 study of SNF residents receiving exercise therapy, only 5% of medical records indicated the use of structured exercise tolerance monitoring, despite a documented 33% prevalence of patient symptoms (dizziness, fatigue) experienced during exercise.[2] It is critically important that medical staff incorporate consistent exercise tolerance monitoring in CR sessions specifically for elderly patients, because there are no data regarding the safety of CR in this population in an SNF or HHC setting.

Cardiac Rehabilitation as Secondary Prevention

The Million Hearts initiative developed in 2012 has challenged the medical field to increase CR use to 70% in the coming years.[6,18] Although daunting, this goal may be attainable by emphasizing CR programs as opportunities for secondary prevention. Secondary prevention is based on reducing modifiable risk factors that may trigger another cardiac event,[20,21] such as weight loss, dietary modifications, and emotional health regulation. The American Heart Association recommends that CR incorporate the principles of secondary prevention routinely into care. Although often used in outpatient CR facilities, the theme of secondary prevention is not well-understood in

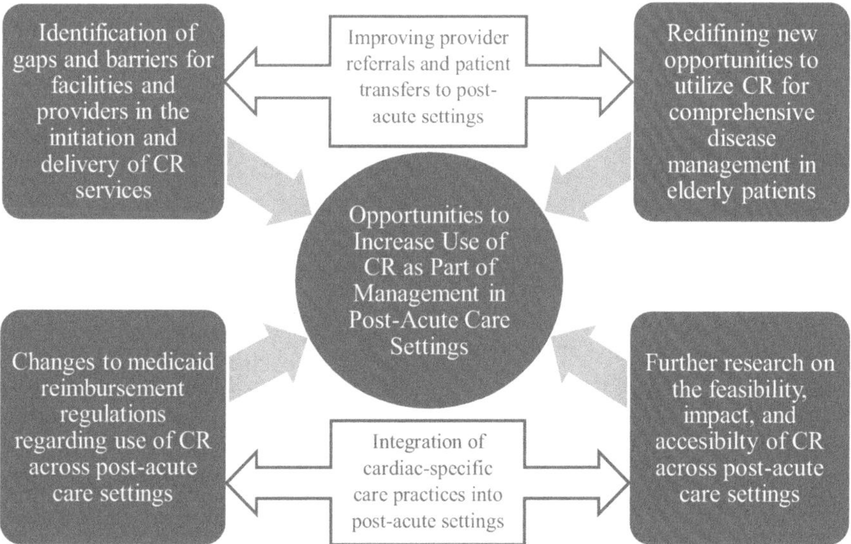

Fig. 4. Opportunities to increase use of CR in postacute care.

postacute facilities such as in SNFs and HHC. Elderly cardiac patients are most susceptible to rehospitalization due to exacerbations as a result of disease mismanagement. More than 50% of hospital readmission from a SNF are avoidable.[22,23] For this reason, the use of CR for secondary prevention is a vital adjunct to the safety, health, and decreased mortality of elderly cardiac patients.

RECOMMENDATIONS FOR FUTURE RESEARCH

Pragmatic trials demonstrating the effectiveness of integrating CR services into SNFs and HHC are needed (**Fig. 4**). Small pilot studies demonstrate beginning evidence for innovation in measuring the impact of services in this area.[12] Other CR models need to be tested in postacute care that start with chronic disease self-management classes[24] and transition to progressive exercise regimens or those who use navigators. Implementation studies are needed that test different system interventions that improve the uptake and adoption of integrating cardiac CR into existing SNF and HHC services.

SUMMARY

CR is an effective and necessary component of disease management for patients with HF. Although the current literature cites the benefits and importance of postacute CR for patients with all forms of HF, several barriers currently exist that are affecting referral rates and CR participation in this population. Current Medicare reimbursement regulations are limiting the degree to which CR can be effectively used as a standard of postacute HF care, especially for older patients. The routine integration of CR into SNFs and HHC present a vast opportunity to improve long-term outcomes for postacute patients. The authors have presented several suggestions to address barriers of CR including reimbursements, access and regulation for patients with HF; however, further research is needed to identify specific opportunities for improvements in CR access and delivery in postacute care settings.

REFERENCES

1. Ades PA, Keteyian SJ, Wright JS, et al. Increasing cardiac rehabilitation participation from 20% to 70%: a road map from the Million Hearts Cardiac Rehabilitation Collaborative. Mayo Clin Proc 2017;92(2):234–42.
2. Dolansky MA, Zullo MD, Hassanein S, et al. Cardiac rehabilitation in skilled nursing facilities: a missed opportunity. Heart Lung 2012;41(2):115–24.
3. Thomas RJ, King M, Lui K, et al. AACVPR/ACCF/AHA 2010 update: performance measures on cardiac rehabilitation for referral to cardiac rehabilitation/secondary prevention services endorsed by the American College of Chest Physicians, the American College of Sports Medicine, the American Physical Therapy Association, the Canadian Association of Cardiac Rehabilitation, the Clinical Exercise Physiology Association, the European Association for Cardiovascular Prevention and Rehabilitation, the inter-American Heart Foundation, the National Association of Clinical Nurse Specialists, the Preventive Cardiovascular nurses Association, and the Society of Thoracic Surgeons. J Am Coll Cardiol 2010;56(14):1159–67.
4. Forman DE. Rehabilitation practice patterns for patients with heart failure: the United States perspective. Heart Fail Clin 2015;11(1):89–94.
5. Schopfer DW, Forman DE. Cardiac rehabilitation in older adults. Can J Cardiol 2016;32(9):1088–96.

6. Burke RE, Cumbler E, Coleman EA, et al. Post-acute care reform: implications and opportunities for hospitalists. J Hosp Med 2017;12(1):46–51.
7. Golwala H, Pandey A, Ju C, et al. Temporal Trends and factors associated with cardiac rehabilitation referral among patients hospitalized with heart failure: findings from Get with the Guidelines-Heart Failure Registry. J Am Coll Cardiol 2015; 66(8):917–26.
8. Tomaselli GF, Harty MB, Horton K, et al. The American Heart Association and the Million Hearts Initiative: a presidential advisory from the American Heart Association. Circulation 2011;124(16):1795–9.
9. Rawstorn JC, Gant N, Direito A, et al. Telehealth exercise-based cardiac rehabilitation: a systematic review and meta-analysis. Heart 2016;102(15):1183–92.
10. Orr NM, Boxer RS, Dolansky MA, et al. Skilled nursing facility care for patients with heart failure: can we make it "heart failure ready?". J Card Fail 2016; 22(12):1004–14.
11. White M, Garbez R, Carroll M, et al. Is "teach-back" associated with knowledge retention and hospital readmission in hospitalized heart failure patients? J Cardiovasc Nurs 2013;28(2):137–46.
12. Dolansky MA, Zullo MD, Boxer RS, et al. Initial efficacy of a cardiac rehabilitation transition program: cardiac TRUST. J Gerontol Nurs 2011;37(12):36–44.
13. Pack QR, Priya A, Lagu T, et al. Cardiac rehabilitation utilization during an acute cardiac hospitalization: a national sample. J Cardiopulm Rehabil Prev 2019;39(1): 19–26.
14. Dolansky MA, Xu F, Zullo M, et al. Post-acute care services received by older adults following a cardiac event: a population-based analysis. J Cardiovasc Nurs 2010;25(4):342–9.
15. Jones CD, Cumbler E, Honigman B, et al. Hospital to post-acute care facility transfers: identifying targets for information exchange quality improvement. J Am Med Dir Assoc 2017;18(1):70–3.
16. United States. Federal Highway Administration. Our nation's highways. Washington, DC: U.S. Dept. of Transportation; 2014.
17. Anderson L, Sharp GA, Norton RJ, et al. Home-based versus centre-based cardiac rehabilitation. Cochrane Database Syst Rev 2017;(6):CD007130.
18. Melnyk BM, Orsolini L, Gawlik K, et al. The Million Hearts initiative: guidelines and best practices. Nurse Pract 2016;41(2):46–53 [quiz: 53–4].
19. Aspry K, Dunsiger S, Breault C, et al. Effect of case management with goal-setting on diet scores and weight loss in cardiac rehabilitation patients. J Cardiopulm Rehabil Prev 2018;38(6):380–7.
20. Nazir A, Smucker WD. Heart failure in post-acute and long-term care: evidence and strategies to improve transitions, clinical care, and quality of life. J Am Med Dir Assoc 2015;16(10):825–31.
21. Lavie CJ, Milani RV. Cardiac rehabilitation and exercise training in secondary coronary heart disease prevention. Prog Cardiovasc Dis 2011;53(6):397–403.
22. Frengley JD, Sansone GR, Alba A, et al. Influence of age on rehabilitation outcomes and survival in post-acute inpatient cardiac rehabilitation. J Cardiopulm Rehabil Prev 2011;31(4):230–8.
23. McMahon SR, Ades PA, Thompson PD. The role of cardiac rehabilitation in patients with heart disease. Trends Cardiovasc Med 2017;27(6):420–5.
24. Boxer RS, Dolansky MA, Bodnar CA, et al. A randomized trial of heart failure disease management in skilled nursing facilities: design and rationale. J Am Med Dir Assoc 2013;14(9):710.e5-11.

Prehabilitation

The Right Medicine for Older Frail Adults Anticipating Transcatheter Aortic Valve Replacement, Coronary Artery Bypass Graft, and Other Cardiovascular Care

Kevin F. Boreskie, MSc[a,b], Jacqueline L. Hay, MSc[a,b], D. Scott Kehler, PhD[c], Nicole M. Johnston, BKin[a,b], Alexandra V. Rose, BSc[a,b], Christopher J. Oldfield, BKin[a,b], Kanwal Kumar, MD[d], Olga Toleva, MD, MPH, CCFP, FRCPC[e], Rakesh C. Arora, MD, PhD, FRCSC[f,g], Todd A. Duhamel, PhD[a,b,g,*]

KEYWORDS

- Prehabilitation • Preoperative care • Frailty • Cardiac surgery
- Coronary artery bypass • Percutaneous valvular interventions
- Transcatheter aortic valve implantation • Transcatheter aortic valve replacement

KEY POINTS

- Strategies to improve postoperative outcomes after cardiac procedures are needed because older and frailer patients are being referred for surgery.

Continued

Disclosure Statement: R.C. Arora has received honoraria from Mallinckrodt Pharmaceuticals and Abbott Nutrition and an unrestricted educational grant from Pfizer Canada unrelated to this article. The other authors have nothing to disclose.

[a] Faculty of Kinesiology and Recreation Management, University of Manitoba, Winnipeg, Manitoba, Canada; [b] Institute of Cardiovascular Sciences, St. Boniface Hospital, Albrechtsen Research Centre, R4012-351 Tache Avenue, Winnipeg, Manitoba R2H 2A6, Canada; [c] Division of Geriatric Medicine, Dalhousie University, QEII Health Sciences Center, Room 1314, Camp Hill Veterans Memorial Building, 5955 Veterans' Memorial Lane, Halifax, Nova Scotia B3H 2E1, Canada; [d] Department of Surgery, Section of Cardiac Surgery, Max Rady College of Medicine, University of Manitoba, St. Boniface General Hospital, Y3500-409 Tache Avenue, Winnipeg, Manitoba R2H 2A9, Canada; [e] Department of Medicine, Section of Cardiology, Max Rady College of Medicine, University of Manitoba, Bergen Cardiac Centre, Y3400-409 Tache Avenue, Winnipeg, Manitoba R2H 2A6, Canada; [f] Institute of Cardiovascular Sciences, St. Boniface Hospital, Albrechtsen Research Centre, R3038-351 Tache Avenue, Winnipeg, Manitoba R2H 2A6, Canada; [g] Department of Surgery, Section of Cardiac Surgery, Max Rady College of Medicine, University of Manitoba, Winnipeg, Manitoba R2H 2A6, Canada
* Corresponding author. St-Boniface Hospital, Albrechtsen Research Centre, R4012-351 Tache Avenue, Winnipeg, Manitoba R2H 2A6, Canada.
E-mail address: todd.duhamel@umanitoba.ca

Clin Geriatr Med 35 (2019) 571–585
https://doi.org/10.1016/j.cger.2019.07.006
geriatric.theclinics.com
0749-0690/19/

Continued

- Prehabilitation improves the outcomes of patients awaiting cardiac surgery, while lowering health care costs through reductions in intensive care unit and hospital length of stay.
- Further high-quality research examining multimodal interventions in populations, such as those who are older, frail individuals, and women, is needed to provide additional evidence to support prehabilitation approaches in cardiac procedures.

INTRODUCTION

Improvements in medicine have led to increased longevity and an aging population.[1] In turn, the prevalence of chronic conditions, such as cardiovascular disease (CVD), is expected to rise,[2] posing health care challenges that will require an evolution of current practice. These challenges will be further complicated by the presence of frailty, which is a physiologic decline that increases vulnerability to adverse health outcomes in the face of a stressor.[3,4] Frailty increases with advancing age[5] and is associated with poor functional survival.[6] Increasingly, older and more frail patients are being referred for cardiac procedures, such as coronary artery bypass graft (CABG) and transcatheter aortic valve implantation (TAVI), but the characteristic physiologic decline seen in frail adults can lead to adverse surgical outcomes.[7] Consequently, strategies to improve postoperative outcomes for these surgical patients are of critical importance.

More recently, the recognition that changes are needed to improve surgical recovery led to the creation of multidisciplinary protocols designed to optimize outcomes of surgical patients through patient risk factor optimization in the preoperative period.[8] The preoperative period presents a critical opportunity to improve the resilience of those vulnerable patients awaiting cardiac surgery.[8] Preoperatively, frail patients are already deconditioned, undernourished, and depressed.[9–11] It is increasingly recognized that the time to act is before surgery, because the time spent waiting in advance of surgery and the postoperative period during recovery are often spent inactive,[12–14] which can further compound these declines. This review summarizes the past, current, and future research that demonstrate the benefit of implementing prehabilitation in the ever-growing population of older and more frail cardiac patients.

COMPLICATIONS OF FRAIL OLDER ADULTS IN CARDIAC SURGERY

The pathophysiology surrounding the development of frailty is not fully understood, but one line of inquiry is that the gradual accumulation of cellular or subclinical damage over one's lifetime gives rise to clinically observable health deficits,[15] such as CVD. Frailty has been shown to be associated with increased risk for developing CVD in longitudinal studies,[4,16] and those with known CVD risk have also been shown to be at increased risk for developing frailty.[17] The relationship between frailty and CVD seems to be bidirectional with each aggravating the risk for the other.[18] In consequence, studying the coexistence between frailty and CVD is important, especially when considering that the incidence of frailty and CVD will likely rise with increasing age.[19]

Frailty denotes a reduced physiologic capacity to adapt to a health stressor, such as cardiac surgery.[20] The advancing age of the typical cardiac surgery patient[21,22] represents a challenge to the health care system in that older patients (mean age, 75.8 $\pm$ 4.4 years) with frailty, as assessed by gait speed, have up to a three-fold likelihood of suffering postoperative morbidity and mortality.[23] These older, frailer adults are more likely to present with multiple comorbidities, further complicating their cases resulting in prolonged hospital length of stay,[24,25] and higher rates of postoperative morbidity[26] and mortality.[24–27] Systematic reviews examining the effect of preoperative frailty status on surgical outcomes in cardiac procedures (CABG, TAVI, and aortic valve replacement) have found that frailty measures were able to predict mortality at 6 months or longer postoperatively,[28] regardless of how invasive the procedure was, and the risk of major adverse cardiac and cerebrovascular events postoperatively (odds ratio, 4.89; 95% confidence interval [CI], 1.64–14.60).[29] Not only do these adverse outcomes influence the patients themselves, but they also create a further burden on the health care system. A recent study of Canadian CABG and heart valve surgery patients found that the median cost of frail patients was $32,742 (interquartile range, $23,221–$49,627) as compared with $23,370 (interquartile range, $19,977–$29,705) in nonfrail patients.[30]

IMPROVING RECOVERY FROM SURGERY

Cardiac rehabilitation is the accepted standard of care after surgery,[31,32] because evidence demonstrates that engaging in physical activity after cardiac surgery is key to enhancing health for patients postsurgery.[10,33] For example, cardiac rehabilitation serves as a means of promoting physical activity and healthy behaviors, which in turn reduces risk of hospital readmission, cardiac mortality, and all-cause mortality.[34–36] However, only 30% of cardiac patients enroll in cardiac rehabilitation programs postoperatively.[37,38] Cardiac patients with frailty are even less likely to complete or attend cardiac rehabilitation.[39] This is problematic because these are individuals who could potentially benefit the most from a health promotion program. Programs based on physical exercise are effective at reversing or preventing further functional decline in frail, older adults.[40,41] Cardiac rehabilitation programs cause a relative reduction in risk for all-cause morbidity and cardiac mortality,[29] but this does not help at-risk frail patients who are vulnerable in the earlier perioperative stage.

The Enhanced Recovery After Surgery (ERAS) group has developed enhanced recovery guidelines using evidence-based best practice to improve surgical recoveries for a variety of surgical subspecialties. A group of cardiac surgeons, cardiac anesthetists, and cardiac critical care specialists also recognizing these needs in their own field have created what is known as the ERAS Cardiac Society. The ERAS Cardiac Society has developed multiple expert recommendations aimed at improving patient recovery, addressing the preoperative, perioperative, and immediate postoperative time points through multimodal care,[8] as listed in **Table 1**.

Recently, the ERAS Cardiac Society added prehabilitation to their expert recommendations as a means of improving patient resilience preoperatively (class IIa, moderate strength recommendation).[8] The opportunity to intervene preoperatively is restricted by the length of preoperative period. Waitlists and urgency of the procedure can impact this length of time. For example, the average wait time for elective cardiac surgeries in Canada is 10 weeks.[42] This is the optimal period to intervene and increase patient resilience before the surgical intervention. Currently, frail individuals are at risk of further physiologic decline in this wait period, because patients on surgical waitlists often perform little physical activity while waiting for their intervention.[12–14,43] These reductions in physical fitness have the potential to result in further declines in frailty status. Furthermore, poor physical fitness preoperatively is associated with complications postoperatively.[44] The preoperative period can also be an anxiety-producing experience for patients awaiting surgery and there is evidence that support programs

Table 1
ERAS Cardiac Society expert recommendations

Before surgery	Alcohol and smoking cessation A_{1C}/albumin and correction of nutritional deficiency Avoidance of prolonged fasting Patient engagement technology Prehabilitation (nutrition optimization/exercise training/anxiety reduction)
During surgery	Antifibrinolytics Avoidance of hyperthermia Infection reduction bundle Optimization of sternal closure
After surgery	Avoidance of hypothermia Biomarkers for acute kidney injury Chest drain management Delirium screening Early extubation Glycemic control Goal-directed therapy Intensive care unit liberation bundle Multimodal analgesia Thromboprophylaxis

Data from Engelman DT, Ali WB, Williams JB, et al. Guidelines for Perioperative Care in Cardiac Surgery: Enhanced Recovery After Surgery Society Recommendations. JAMA Surg. Published online May 04, 2019.

can mitigate this vulnerability.[45] Despite this, there are currently no formalized preoperative interventions in place to promote healthy lifestyle behaviors in the health care system.

Described in a recent paper, this prehabilitation programming should use the "NEW" approach, which includes a focus on nutrition optimization (N), exercise training (E), and worry/anxiety reduction (W).[46] This approach is justified considering the wide-reaching effects of frailty across physiologic systems, and the finding that interventions involving physical activity and nutrition components have the most success reducing frailty status, improving resilience.[40]

COMPLETED CARDIAC PREHABILITATION TRIALS

The first seminal prehabilitation trial in cardiac patients was conducted by Arthur and colleagues[47] in 2000. The preoperative intervention included 249 patients waiting for elective CABG procedure and followed a traditional center-based cardiac rehabilitation model. Patients randomized to the intervention received education on risk factor modification, monthly support calls from a nurse, and two exercise sessions per week for a period of 8 weeks. Hospital length of stay postoperatively was 1 day shorter in the intervention group, and the intervention group also experienced a median 2.1-hour reduction in time spent in the intensive care unit, as compared with the standard of care group.[47] This related to savings of $133 per patient per day.[47] Although this trial did not improve the physical fitness of the intervention group, the prehabilitation group did report better quality of life in the 6-month period postoperatively compared with patients receiving standard care.

Unfortunately, there is still a paucity of research examining the feasibility and benefits of implementing prehabilitation into clinical practice for cardiac surgery patients. A systematic review and meta-analysis[48] of randomized and nonrandomized prehabilitation trials in patients awaiting nonurgent cardiac surgical procedures identified eight studies, including the seminal work of Arthur and colleagues,[47] examining postsurgical complications in adults. These trials used a variety of prehabilitation approaches including respiratory training techniques,[44,49–52] aerobic training,[47] combined aerobic and respiratory training,[53] and aerobic and strength training.[12] All of the trials were performed on patients awaiting CABG procedures[12,44,47,49–53] with one study also including patients awaiting mitral valve surgeries.[53]

Data from other surgical subspecialties[54] support the reductions in composite postsurgical complications (odds ratio, 0.41; 95% CI, 0.28–0.62; $P<.001$) found in the cardiac surgery–specific combined meta-analysis.[48] Maximal inspiratory pressure (standard mean difference, 0.66; 95% CI, 0.35–0.96; $P<.001$)[48] was also improved with prehabilitation. Although the meta-analysis identified a standard mean difference of −0.56 (95% CI, −1.13 to 0.01) days for length of stay for prehabilitation patients, this variable was not considered to have reached statistical significance because of the high heterogeneity ($I2$ = 93%) of the combined trials.[48]

These results are also supported by previous systematic reviews in cardiac surgery patients with such findings as reduced incidence of postoperative pulmonary complications (relative risk, 0.39; 95% CI, 0.23–0.66),[55] postoperative atelectasis (relative risk, 0.52; 95% CI, 0.32–0.87),[56] and pneumonia (relative risk, 0.45; 95% CI, 0.24–0.83).[56] Moreover, reduced length of hospital stay postoperatively was found in the Hulzebos and colleagues[56] systematic review (−3.21 days; 95% CI, −5.73 to −0.69) and in the Snowdon and colleagues[55] systematic review when trials composed of older adults were analyzed separately (−1.32; 95% CI, −2.36 to −0.28). These data suggest that older frail surgical patients may derive the most benefit from prehabilitation.

The potential for prehabilitation to improve cardiac surgery patient outcomes has been identified,[48,55,56] but there is a scarcity of high-quality research in larger sized trials, leading to high heterogeneity in results for a variety of important postoperative outcomes. Many of these past trials have been trials of feasibility and included only healthy surgical patients, specifically excluding those who are older and frailer. Furthermore, patients awaiting TAVI are traditionally high surgical risk or inoperable older adults who also have severe aortic stenosis,[57] which has led to the exclusion of these participants from prehabilitation trials. Additional studies examining higher intensity physical activity or resistance training interventions are needed because these may be necessary to elicit the optimal stimulus for physiologic adaptation and improved resilience.

ONGOING CARDIAC PREHABILITATION TRIALS

Table 2 summarizes eight prehabilitation clinical trials currently recruiting participants in cardiac populations found on the ClinicalTrials.gov Web site. Studies include participants from the United States,[58–61] Canada,[62–64] and Spain.[65] Patient populations include those awaiting transcatheter aortic valve replacement,[58,60,64] CABG,[62,65] thoracic aortic repair,[59] heart transplant,[63,65] or valve surgery,[62] and patients with vascular disease.[61] Mainly trials are recruiting adults 18[60,62,63,65] to 21[59] years and older, and only two studies are specifically recruiting adults older than the age of 60 years[58] and 70 years,[64] respectively. The projected sample sizes in each study ranges from 30[63] to 220[64] participants. Most of the interventions use a single component nutrition,[64] exercise,[58,60,62] or patient engagement approach.[59,61] Two studies are using a multimodal intervention approach.[63,65] One of these studies is combining high-intensity interval training with nutritional and stress management workshops,[63] and one of these studies personalized the resistance training intervention provided.[65]

Table 2
Ongoing prehabilitation trials in cardiac surgery

Name of Study	ClinicalTrials.gov Identifier	Country	Study Start Date	Condition/Disease	Trial Design	Participants	Primary Outcome	Intervention/Details
Prehabilitation to Improve Functional and Clinical Outcomes in Patients with Aortic Stenosis (TAVR-FRAILTY)	NCT02597985	United States	October 2015	Aortic stenosis Details: patients awaiting TAVR surgery	RCT	Age: ≥60 y Number of participants: 40	Change in SPPB	Intervention: 3 supervised exercise training sessions per week at an exercise intensity of RPE 12–14 for 4 wk at cardiac rehabilitation facility (treadmill walking or non–weight bearing if needed) Nonintervention group: usual care
Prehabilitation for Aortic Repair Patients (PREPARE)	NCT02767518	United States	February 2016	Aortic aneurysm Details: patients with thoracic aortic disease scheduled for repair	RCT	Age: ≥21 y Number of participants: 100	Feasibility of recruiting and enrolling (feedback from participants)	Intervention: self-directed Michigan Surgical & Health Optimization Program (participants receive an informational DVD, a pedometer, an incentive spirometer, and access to the program Web site to help promote healthful behaviors and improved well-being in the days leading up to surgery) Nonintervention group: follow preoperative instructions from surgical team

Prehabilitation for PAD Revascularization Patients	NCT02767895	United States	July 2016	Peripheral vascular disease Peripheral artery disease	RCT	Age: ≥40 y Number of participants: 40	Feasibility and acceptability (measured by recruiting numbers, drop-out rates, QOL surveys, pedometer use)	Intervention: self-directed Michigan Surgical & Health Optimization Program (participants receive an informational DVD, a pedometer, an incentive spirometer, and access to the program Web site to help promote healthful behaviors and improved well-being in the days leading up to surgery)
Prehabilitation for Patients Undergoing Transcatheter Aortic Valve Replacement (TAVR-Prehab)	NCT03107897	United States	August 2016	Aortic valve stenosis Details: patients awaiting TAVR surgery	RCT	Age: ≥18 y Number of participants: 70	Functional exercise capacity (measured by a change in 6-min-walk test)	Intervention: 8–12 visits to physical therapy before TAVR procedure Nonintervention group: preprocedure standard of care

(*continued on next page*)

Table 2
(continued)

Name of Study	ClinicalTrials.gov Identifier	Country	Study Start Date	Condition/Disease	Trial Design	Participants	Primary Outcome	Intervention/Details
Implementation of a Trimodal Prehabilitation Program as a Preoperative Optimization Strategy in Cardiac Surgery	NCT03466606	Spain	March 2018	Coronary artery disease Valvular heart disease Details: participants either (1) heart transplant candidates or (2) waiting for CABG	RCT	Age: $\geq$18 y Number of participants: 200	Incidence of postoperative complications (Clavien Dindo classification)	Intervention: 4–6 wk, personalized supervised resistance training program to promote physical activity and healthy lifestyles Nonintervention group: conventional treatment
PREHAB HTx Study (Cardiovascular Prehabilitation in Patients Awaiting Heart Transplantation)	NCT02957955	Canada	May 2018	Heart failure Details: participants are awaiting heart transplantation	RCT	Age: $\geq$18 y Number of participants: 30	Functional capacity (measured by 6-min-walk test)	Intervention: usual care + supervised exercise sessions (on-site high-intensity interval training 2 times weekly for 12 wk), nutritional workshop, stress management course Nonintervention group: standard of care including encouraging participants to remain active without structured training program

Prehabilitation in Elective Frail and Elderly Cardiac Surgery Patients (PERFECT)	NCT03399162	Canada	May 2018	Coronary artery disease Valvular heart disease Details: participants undergoing CABG, valve, or CABG + valve	RCT	Age: ≥18 y Number of participants: 130	Functional capacity (measured by 6-min-walk test)	Intervention: 8-wk exercise program, (2 times/wk of 60-min supervised exercise, plus 3 times/wk 30-min home-based exercise) Active comparator group: standard of care including a workshop and counseling
The PERFORM-TAVR Trial (PERFORM-TAVR)[a]	NCT03522454	Canada	May 2018	Frail patients Details: participants undergoing TAVR	RCT	Age: ≥70 y Number of participants: 220	SPPB	Intervention: 2 times/d consume a protein supplement for 4 wks presurgery Nonintervention group: lifestyle counseling in line with current AHA guidelines, which recommend patients engage in moderate intensity activity 5 times/wk for 30 min and eat a healthy diet

Abbreviations: AHA, American Heart Association; QOL, quality of life; RCT, randomized controlled trial; RPE, rate of perceived exertion; SPPB, short physical performance battery; TAVR, transcatheter aortic valve replacement.

[a] The PERFORM-TAVR trial is also implementing a postoperative physical activity and nutrition intervention.

The length of the exercise-based interventions range from 4 weeks[58,64,65] to 12 weeks[63,65] in duration. The primary outcomes in five of the studies are functional capacity measured by the 6-minute-walk test,[60,62,63] or short physical performance battery.[58,64] Two studies are feasibility and acceptability trials,[59,61] and one study is examining the incidence of postoperative complications.[65] The PERFORM-TAVR study[64] is performing a protein supplementation nutrition intervention preoperatively followed by an exercise intervention postoperatively.

THE FUTURE OF PREHABILITATION IN CARDIAC SURGERY

The emerging accumulation of evidence demonstrates that cardiac prehabilitation is the right medicine for patients undergoing cardiac procedures. Additional randomized controlled trials with larger cohorts in a wider variety of cardiac surgical procedure contexts, such as TAVI, are needed to further strengthen this evidence, and the inclusion of specific clinical outcomes, such as associated health care costs and surgical outcomes. These data are needed to inform future health care policy decisions related to preoperative cardiac care.

Certain patient populations, such as women and older, frailer adults, have been underrepresented in the literature, which is problematic because these populations are more likely to experience complications and secondary events postoperatively and could benefit the most from prehabilitation.[7,66–68] Furthermore, women are less likely to participate in such programs as cardiac rehabilitation.[69]

To begin addressing these disparities, women's-only prehabilitation approaches should be investigated, because improved cardiac rehabilitation attendance has been demonstrated using a women's-only tailored approach.[70,71] Researchers are also encouraged to analyze sex differences to understand if there are distinctions in response to prehabilitation interventions.[72] Similarly, given the barriers that many older frailer patients present with, patient-centered approaches are needed to improve the feasibility and efficacy of prehabilitation. For example, access to prehabilitation should not be limited by barriers, such as transportation, which has been reported as a common barrier to accessing rehabilitation programs.[73] Creative solutions are needed to increase the accessibility to prehabilitation programs, such as the home-based prehabilitation pilot applied by Waite and colleagues[74] or the home-based solution provided by Bruns and colleagues[75] with their computer-supported prehabilitation trial in patients awaiting colorectal cancer surgery. Applications of strategies to improve adherence and participation in cardiac rehabilitation, such as provisions through telemedicine,[76] require additional examination in a cardiac prehabilitation context.

Interventions for frail older adults awaiting cardiac surgery should be structured as multicomponent programs with an emphasis on physical activity to improve health in all systems affected by frailty.[40] Interventions aimed at increasing physical activity levels[77] and minimizing prolonged bouts of sedentary behavior[78] in frail patients may be able to improve the resilience of frail cardiac patients preoperatively. The efficacy of prehabilitation trials for improving frailty status should be assessed more often in future trials through the collection of frailty measures as outcome variables. Additional studies combining aerobic and resistance training, such as the recently completed trial described by Stammers and colleagues[79] awaiting publication, and studies incorporating higher intensities of physical activity, such as the ongoing trial by Reed and colleagues,[63] should be examined because these approaches may be required to see improved frailty status.[80] High-intensity interval training in cardiac rehabilitation has been found to be safe for individuals with CVD.[81] New guidelines have recently been developed to guide high-intensity interval training in clinical populations[82] and should be investigated in older frailer populations in advance of cardiac procedures.

SUMMARY

The implementation of prehabilitation programs in advance of surgery will become increasingly vital in the ever-growing population of older, frailer cardiac patients. The effects of prehabilitation extend beyond improved patient outcomes and are economically impactful. Moreover, prehabilitation programs build on the strength of existing postoperative cardiac rehabilitation infrastructure through the initiation of similar care earlier in the patient journey. High-quality, creative research conducted in larger and varied patient populations will lend the additional evidence needed to implement prehabilitation into clinical practice as the right medicine for older frail adults anticipating cardiovascular care.

REFERENCES

1. WHO | World report on ageing and health. 2015. Available at: http://www.who.int/ageing/events/world-report-2015-launch/en/. Accessed November 29, 2018.
2. Canada PHA of, Canada PHA of. Executive summary: tracking heart disease and stroke in Canada 2009. 2009. Available at: https://www.canada.ca/en/public-health/services/reports-publications/2009-tracking-heart-disease-stroke-canada/executive-summary.html. Accessed February 7, 2019.
3. Fried LP, Ferrucci L, Darer J, et al. Untangling the concepts of disability, frailty, and comorbidity: implications for improved targeting and care. J Gerontol A Biol Sci Med Sci 2004;59(3):255–63.
4. Fried LP, Tangen CM, Walston J, et al. Frailty in older adults: evidence for a phenotype. J Gerontol A Biol Sci Med Sci 2001;56(3):M146–56.
5. Kehler DS, Ferguson T, Stammers AN, et al. Prevalence of frailty in Canadians 18-79 years old in the Canadian health measures survey. BMC Geriatr 2017;17(1):28.
6. Lytwyn J, Stammers AN, Kehler DS, et al. The impact of frailty on functional survival in patients 1 year after cardiac surgery. J Thorac Cardiovasc Surg 2017;154(6):1990–9.
7. Brown NA, Zenilman ME. The impact of frailty in the elderly on the outcome of surgery in the aged. Adv Surg 2010;44(1):229–49.
8. Expert recommendations - ERAS. Available at: https://www.erascardiac.org/recommendations/expert-recommendations. Accessed February 8, 2019.
9. Torpy JM, Lynm C, Glass RM. JAMA patient page. Frailty in older adults. JAMA 2006;296(18):2280.
10. Horne D, Kehler DS, Kaoukis G, et al. Impact of physical activity on depression after cardiac surgery. Can J Cardiol 2013;29(12):1649–56.
11. Horne D, Kehler S, Kaoukis G, et al. Depression before and after cardiac surgery: do all patients respond the same? J Thorac Cardiovasc Surg 2013;145(5):1400–6.
12. Sawatzky J-AV, Kehler DS, Ready AE, et al. Prehabilitation program for elective coronary artery bypass graft surgery patients: a pilot randomized controlled study. Clin Rehabil 2014;28(7):648–57.
13. Nery RM, Barbisan JN. Effect of leisure-time physical activity on the prognosis of coronary artery bypass graft surgery. Rev Bras Cir Cardiovasc 2010;25(1):73–8.

14. Mooney M, Fitzsimons D, Richardson G. "No more couch-potato!" Patients' experiences of a pre-operative programme of cardiac rehabilitation for those awaiting coronary artery bypass surgery. Eur J Cardiovasc Nurs 2007;6(1):77–83.
15. Afilalo J, Alexander KP, Mack MJ, et al. Frailty assessment in the cardiovascular care of older adults. J Am Coll Cardiol 2014;63(8):747–62.
16. Sergi G, Veronese N, Fontana L, et al. Pre-frailty and risk of cardiovascular disease in elderly men and women. The Pro.V.A. Study. J Am Coll Cardiol 2015; 65(10):976–83.
17. Gale CR, Cooper C, Sayer AA. Framingham cardiovascular disease risk scores and incident frailty: the English longitudinal study of ageing. Age (Dordr) 2014; 36(4):9692.
18. Flint K. Which came first, the frailty or the heart disease?: exploring the vicious cycle. J Am Coll Cardiol 2015;65(10):984–6.
19. Afilalo J, Karunananthan S, Eisenberg MJ, et al. Role of frailty in patients with cardiovascular disease. Am J Cardiol 2009;103(11):1616–21.
20. Fulop T, Larbi A, Witkowski JM, et al. Aging, frailty and age-related diseases. Biogerontology 2010;11(5):547–63.
21. Buth KJ, Gainer RA, Legare J-F, et al. The changing face of cardiac surgery: practice patterns and outcomes 2001-2010. Can J Cardiol 2014;30(2):224–30.
22. Pierri MD, Capestro F, Zingaro C, et al. The changing face of cardiac surgery patients: an insight into a Mediterranean region. Eur J Cardiothorac Surg 2010; 38(4):407–13.
23. Afilalo J, Eisenberg MJ, Morin J-F, et al. Gait speed as an incremental predictor of mortality and major morbidity in elderly patients undergoing cardiac surgery. J Am Coll Cardiol 2010;56(20):1668–76.
24. Green P, Woglom AE, Genereux P, et al. The impact of frailty status on survival after transcatheter aortic valve replacement in older adults with severe aortic stenosis: a single-center experience. JACC Cardiovasc Interv 2012;5(9):974–81.
25. Lee DH, Buth KJ, Martin B-J, et al. Frail patients are at increased risk for mortality and prolonged institutional care after cardiac surgery. Circulation 2010;121(8): 973–8.
26. Singh M, Rihal CS, Lennon RJ, et al. Influence of frailty and health status on outcomes in patients with coronary disease undergoing percutaneous revascularization. Circ Cardiovasc Qual Outcomes 2011;4(5):496–502.
27. Sündermann S, Dademasch A, Rastan A, et al. One-year follow-up of patients undergoing elective cardiac surgery assessed with the Comprehensive Assessment of Frailty test and its simplified form. Interact Cardiovasc Thorac Surg 2011;13(2):119–23 [discussion: 123].
28. Kim DH, Kim CA, Placide S, et al. Preoperative frailty assessment and outcomes at 6 months or later in older adults undergoing cardiac surgical procedures: a systematic review. Ann Intern Med 2016;165(9):650–60.
29. Sepehri A, Beggs T, Hassan A, et al. The impact of frailty on outcomes after cardiac surgery: a systematic review. J Thorac Cardiovasc Surg 2014;148(6): 3110–7.
30. Goldfarb M, Bendayan M, Rudski LG, et al. Cost of cardiac surgery in frail compared with nonfrail older adults. Can J Cardiol 2017;33(8):1020–6.
31. Wenger NK. Current status of cardiac rehabilitation. J Am Coll Cardiol 2008; 51(17):1619–31.
32. Leon AS, Franklin BA, Costa F, et al. Cardiac rehabilitation and secondary prevention of coronary heart disease: an American Heart Association scientific statement from the Council on Clinical Cardiology (Subcommittee on Exercise,

Cardiac Rehabilitation, and Prevention) and the Council on Nutrition, Physical Activity, and Metabolism (Subcommittee on Physical Activity), in collaboration with the American Association of Cardiovascular and Pulmonary Rehabilitation. Circulation 2005;111(3):369–76.

33. Lavie CJ, Thomas RJ, Squires RW, et al. Exercise training and cardiac rehabilitation in primary and secondary prevention of coronary heart disease. Mayo Clin Proc 2009;84(4):373–83.
34. Heran BS, Chen JM, Ebrahim S, et al. Exercise-based cardiac rehabilitation for coronary heart disease. Cochrane Database Syst Rev 2011;(7):CD001800.
35. Martin B-J, Hauer T, Arena R, et al. Cardiac rehabilitation attendance and outcomes in coronary artery disease patients. Circulation 2012;126(6):677–87.
36. Taylor RS, Brown A, Ebrahim S, et al. Exercise-based rehabilitation for patients with coronary heart disease: systematic review and meta-analysis of randomized controlled trials. Am J Med 2004;116(10):682–92.
37. Dafoe W, Arthur H, Stokes H, et al. Canadian Cardiovascular Society Access to Care Working Group on Cardiac Rehabilitation. Universal access: but when? Treating the right patient at the right time: access to cardiac rehabilitation. Can J Cardiol 2006;22(11):905–11.
38. Grace SL, Chessex C, Arthur H, et al. Systematizing inpatient referral to cardiac rehabilitation 2010: Canadian Association of Cardiac Rehabilitation and Canadian Cardiovascular Society Joint Position Paper: Endorsed by the Cardiac Care Network of Ontario. Can J Cardiol 2011;27(2):192–9.
39. Kimber DE, Kehler DS, Lytwyn J, et al. Pre-operative frailty status is associated with cardiac rehabilitation completion: a retrospective cohort study. J Clin Med 2018;7(12). https://doi.org/10.3390/jcm7120560.
40. Apóstolo J, Cooke R, Bobrowicz-Campos E, et al. Effectiveness of interventions to prevent pre-frailty and frailty progression in older adults: a systematic review. JBI Database System Rev Implement Rep 2018;16(1):140.
41. Puts MTE, Toubasi S, Andrew MK, et al. Interventions to prevent or reduce the level of frailty in community-dwelling older adults: a scoping review of the literature and international policies. Age Ageing 2017;46(3):383–92.
42. Barua B. Waiting your turn: wait times for health care in Canada, 2017 report. Vancouver (BC): Fraser Institute; 2017. Available at: http://bit.ly/2AtqqSx. Accessed February 20, 2019.
43. Kehler DS, Stammers AN, Tangri N, et al. Systematic review of preoperative physical activity and its impact on postcardiac surgical outcomes. BMJ Open 2017; 7(8):e015712.
44. Valkenet K, van de Port IGL, Dronkers JJ, et al. The effects of preoperative exercise therapy on postoperative outcome: a systematic review. Clin Rehabil 2011; 25(2):99–111.
45. McHugh F, Lindsay G, Hanlon P, et al. Nurse led shared care for patients on the waiting list for coronary artery bypass surgery: a randomised controlled trial. Heart 2001;86(3):317–23.
46. Arora RC, Brown CH, Sanjanwala RM, et al. "NEW" prehabilitation: a 3-way approach to improve postoperative survival and health-related quality of life in cardiac surgery patients. Can J Cardiol 2018;34(7):839–49.
47. Arthur HM, Daniels C, McKelvie R, et al. Effect of a preoperative intervention on preoperative and postoperative outcomes in low-risk patients awaiting elective coronary artery bypass graft surgery. A randomized, controlled trial. Ann Intern Med 2000;133(4):253–62.

48. Marmelo F, Rocha V, Gonçalves D. The impact of prehabilitation on post-surgical complications in patients undergoing non-urgent cardiovascular surgical intervention: systematic review and meta-analysis. Eur J Prev Cardiol 2018;25(4):404–17.
49. Savci S, Degirmenci B, Saglam M, et al. Short-term effects of inspiratory muscle training in coronary artery bypass graft surgery: a randomized controlled trial. Scand Cardiovasc J 2011;45(5):286–93.
50. Hulzebos EHJ, van Meeteren NLU, van den Buijs BJWM, et al. Feasibility of preoperative inspiratory muscle training in patients undergoing coronary artery bypass surgery with a high risk of postoperative pulmonary complications: a randomized controlled pilot study. Clin Rehabil 2006;20(11):949–59.
51. Hulzebos EHJ, Helders PJM, Favié NJ, et al. Preoperative intensive inspiratory muscle training to prevent postoperative pulmonary complications in high-risk patients undergoing CABG surgery: a randomized clinical trial. JAMA 2006; 296(15):1851–7.
52. Sobrinho MT, Guirado GN, Silva MA, et al. Preoperative therapy restores ventilatory parameters and reduces length of stay in patients undergoing myocardial revascularization. Braz J Cardiovasc Surg 2014;29(2):221–8.
53. Tung H-H, Shen S-F, Shih C-C, et al. Effects of a preoperative individualized exercise program on selected recovery variables for cardiac surgery patients: a pilot study. J Saudi Heart Assoc 2012;24(3):153–61.
54. Santa Mina D, Clarke H, Ritvo P, et al. Effect of total-body prehabilitation on postoperative outcomes: a systematic review and meta-analysis. Physiotherapy 2014; 100(3):196–207.
55. Snowdon D, Haines TP, Skinner EH. Preoperative intervention reduces postoperative pulmonary complications but not length of stay in cardiac surgical patients: a systematic review. J Physiother 2014;60(2):66–77.
56. Hulzebos EHJ, Smit Y, Helders PPJM, et al. Preoperative physical therapy for elective cardiac surgery patients. Cochrane Database Syst Rev 2012;(11):CD010118.
57. Cao C, Liou KP, Pathan FK, et al. Transcatheter aortic valve implantation versus surgical aortic valve replacement: meta-analysis of clinical outcomes and cost-effectiveness. Curr Pharm Des 2016;22(13):1965–77.
58. Prehabilitation to improve functional and clinical outcomes in patients with aortic stenosis - full text view. Available at: ClinicalTrials.gov https://clinicaltrials.gov/ct2/show/NCT02597985. Accessed February 22, 2019.
59. Prehabilitation for aortic repair patients - full text view. Available at: ClinicalTrials.gov https://clinicaltrials.gov/ct2/show/NCT02767518. Accessed February 26, 2019.
60. Prehabilitation for patients undergoing transcatheter aortic valve replacement - full text view. Available at: ClinicalTrials.gov https://clinicaltrials.gov/ct2/show/NCT03107897. Accessed February 26, 2019.
61. Prehabilitation for PAD revascularization patients - full text view. Available at: ClinicalTrials.gov https://clinicaltrials.gov/ct2/show/NCT02767895. Accessed February 26, 2019.
62. PRehabilitiation in elective frail and elderly cardiac surgery PaTients - full text view. Available at: ClinicalTrials.gov https://clinicaltrials.gov/ct2/show/NCT03399162. Accessed February 26, 2019.
63. Cardiovascular prehabilitation in patients awaiting heart Transplantation (PREHAB HTx study) - full text view. Available at: ClinicalTrials.gov https://clinicaltrials.gov/ct2/show/NCT02957955. Accessed February 26, 2019.
64. The PERFORM-TAVR trial - full text view. Available at: ClinicalTrials.gov https://clinicaltrials.gov/ct2/show/NCT03522454. Accessed March 1, 2019.

65. Implementation of a Trimodal prehabilitation program as a preoperative optimization Strategy in cardiac surgery - full text view. Available at: ClinicalTrials.gov https://clinicaltrials.gov/ct2/show/NCT03466606. Accessed February 22, 2019.
66. Heart report. Heart and Stroke Foundation of Canada. Available at: https://www.heartandstroke.ca:443/what-we-do/media-centre/heart-report. Accessed February 21, 2019.
67. Chung J, Stevens L-M, Ouzounian M, et al. Sex-related differences in patients undergoing thoracic aortic surgery: evidence from the Canadian thoracic aortic collaborative. Circulation 2019. https://doi.org/10.1161/CIRCULATIONAHA.118.035805.
68. Vaccarino V, Lin ZQ, Kasl SV, et al. Gender differences in recovery after coronary artery bypass surgery. J Am Coll Cardiol 2003;41(2):307–14.
69. Oosenbrug E, Marinho RP, Zhang J, et al. Sex differences in cardiac rehabilitation adherence: a meta-analysis. Can J Cardiol 2016;32(11):1316–24.
70. Beckie TM, Beckstead JW. Predicting cardiac rehabilitation attendance in a gender-tailored randomized clinical trial. J Cardiopulm Rehabil Prev 2010; 30(3):147–56.
71. Gunn E, Bray SR, Mataseje L, et al. Psychosocial outcomes and adherence in a women's only exercise and education cardiac rehabilitation program. J Cardiopulm Rehabil Prev 2007;27(5):345.
72. Heidari S, Babor TF, De Castro P, et al. Sex and gender equity in research: rationale for the SAGER guidelines and recommended use. Res Integr Peer Rev 2016;1(1):2.
73. Neubeck L, Freedman SB, Clark AM, et al. Participating in cardiac rehabilitation: a systematic review and meta-synthesis of qualitative data. Eur J Prev Cardiol 2012;19(3):494–503.
74. Waite I, Deshpande R, Baghai M, et al. Home-based preoperative rehabilitation (prehab) to improve physical function and reduce hospital length of stay for frail patients undergoing coronary artery bypass graft and valve surgery. J Cardiothorac Surg 2017;12(1):91.
75. Bruns ERJ, Argillander TE, Schuijt HJ, et al. Fit4SurgeryTV at-home prehabilitation for frail elderly planned for colorectal cancer surgery: a pilot study. Am J Phys Med Rehabil 2018. https://doi.org/10.1097/PHM.0000000000001108.
76. Rawstorn JC, Gant N, Direito A, et al. Telehealth exercise-based cardiac rehabilitation: a systematic review and meta-analysis. Heart 2016;102(15):1183–92.
77. Kehler DS, Clara I, Hiebert B, et al. The association between bouts of moderate to vigorous physical activity and patterns of sedentary behavior with frailty. Exp Gerontol 2018;104:28–34.
78. Kehler DS, Hay JL, Stammers AN, et al. A systematic review of the association between sedentary behaviors with frailty. Exp Gerontol 2018;114:1–12.
79. Stammers AN, Kehler DS, Afilalo J, et al. Protocol for the PREHAB study—pre-operative Rehabilitation for reduction of Hospitalization after coronary Bypass and valvular surgery: a randomised controlled trial. BMJ Open 2015;5(3):e007250.
80. Theou O, Stathokostas L, Roland KP, et al. The effectiveness of exercise interventions for the management of frailty: a systematic review. J Aging Res 2011;2011: e569194.
81. Wewege MA, Ahn D, Yu J, et al. High-intensity interval training for patients with cardiovascular disease-is it safe? A systematic review. J Am Heart Assoc 2018; 7(21):e009305.
82. Taylor JL, Holland DJ, Spathis JG, et al. Guidelines for the delivery and monitoring of high intensity interval training in clinical populations. Prog Cardiovasc Dis 2019. https://doi.org/10.1016/j.pcad.2019.01.004.

Gender Disparities in Cardiac Rehabilitation Among Older Women

Key Opportunities to Improve Care

Bianca W. Yoo, MD[a], Nanette K. Wenger, MD[b,*]

KEYWORDS

• Cardiac rehabilitation • Women • Geriatric • Elderly • Home-based

KEY POINTS

- Despite its documented benefits, older adults underutilize cardiac rehabilitation (CR) and older women underutilize it disproportionately relative to men. Lack of awareness by patients and providers regarding the value of CR, competing caregiver responsibilities, limited accessibility, and lifetime patterns of sedentariness are common contributors to underutilization of CR among women.
- Alternative CR models may help attract more older women. Although data are limited, small studies demonstrate that home-, mobile-, and community-based CR programs achieve benefits that are similar to traditional programs.
- More extensive education may help providers, including primary care and PM&R clinicians, better appreciate and promote CR.

BACKGROUND

Although advances in pharmacologic treatment and technology for patients with coronary heart disease (CHD) and heart failure (HF) have evolved over the past half century, cardiac rehabilitation (CR) has still been demonstrated to reduce morbidity and mortality in patients with CHD and HF and remains a class I recommendation by the American College of Cardiology, American Heart Association, and European Society of Cardiology. Patients are eligible for CMS-based reimbursement for CR following myocardial infarction (MI), percutaneous coronary intervention, coronary

Disclosure: The authors have nothing do disclose.

[a] Division of Cardiology, Department of Medicine, Emory University School of Medicine, 101 Woodruff Circle Suite, Atlanta, GA 30322, USA; [b] Division of Cardiology, Department of Medicine, Emory University School of Medicine, 49 Jesse Hill Jr. Drive, Southeast, Atlanta, GA 30303, USA

* Corresponding author.

E-mail address: nwenger@emory.edu

https://doi.org/10.1016/j.cger.2019.07.012

artery bypass graft surgery (CABG), stable angina, heart valve repair or replacement, and heart transplantation. More recently, Medicare expanded CR approval to patients with systolic HF and symptomatic peripheral artery disease. Despite an aging population and evidence of CR's improvement in cardiac mortality rates, quality of life, physiologic risk factors, and functional capacity,[1,2] CR remains substantially underutilized in older adults, particularly older women.

Older patients are highly vulnerable to the morbidities and mortality associated with CHD, especially as older adults tend to have more baseline comorbidities and reduced fitness relative to younger adults. Advanced age also increases the risk of complications of MI and coronary revascularization, with resultant longer hospitalizations, compounding deconditioning, and increased psychosocial and financial strains.[2] Women tend to develop cardiovascular disease at relatively older ages than men and tend to be more susceptible to frailty and disability, adding to their risks.

CR referral, participation, and completion rates are remarkably low in older women, especially among ethnic minorities and economically constrained subgroups.[3–6] Although older women account for a large percentage of the patients eligible for CR, physicians are less aggressive in referring them to CR and in treating their disease than for men. In addition, women tend to have more transportation barriers and are more likely to have caregiving responsibilities to dependents at home,[7] eroding CR participation even further.

In older patients with CHD, CR and exercise training have been demonstrated to advance cognitive improvements,[8] functional capacity,[9] quality of life,[10] and survival. A study of 30,161 Medicare patients (average age 74 years) demonstrated that CR participation over 36 sessions was associated with a 47% lower risk of death (hazard ratio [HR], 0.53; 95% confidence interval [CI], 0.48–0.59) compared with those who attended one session and a 14% lower risk of death (HR, 0.86; 95% CI, 0.77–0.97) compared with those who attended 24 sessions, suggesting a dose-response relationship.[11] Likewise, the same study reported a 31% lower risk of MI (HR, 0.69; 95% CI, 0.58–0.81) in those who attended 24 sessions than in those who attended one session and a 12% lower risk of MI (HR, 0.88; 95% CI, 0.83–0.93).[11] Notably, older women who participated in resistance training demonstrated increased work capacity, balance, endurance, coordination, and flexibility.[12] Furthermore, these programs fostered independence and a sense of community through socialization after health events with the potential to otherwise be overwhelming and demoralizing.[13]

Among older adults aged 60 to 79 years, women experience CAD, MI, and HF at lower rates than men, and angina at nearly equivalent rates, but the relative prevalence of disease among women increases as age advances as women outlive men. Data from the National Health and Nutrition Examination Survey from 2013 to 2016 showed the prevalence of HF was 4.6% in women versus 6.9% in men in those aged 60 to 79 years. In the same age strata, prevalence for CAD and MI was 12.6% and 4.2% in women and 19.7% and 11.5% in men, respectively. Angina occurred at similar rates between women and men (7.3% vs 7.1%) in this age strata. However, among women and men greater than 79 years, prevalence of HF increased to 12.0% in women and 12.8% in men. Similarly, the prevalence of CAD and MI in women and men was 25.4% versus 31.0% and 12.7% versus 17.3%. Prevalence of angina in the same age group was higher in women than men (12.4% vs 11.2%). Despite higher prevalence of disease and symptoms, referral of older women to CR was substantially lower. Furthermore, older adults with HF with preserved ejection fraction (HFpEF) are generally older and more likely to be women,[14] HFpEF is not currently a reimbursable category by CMS indications. Thus, it also stands out that underreferral of HFpEF to CR affects women disproportionately.

Although most of the patients eligible for CR are older than 65 years, geriatric patients, especially older women, are significantly less likely to participate, despite the documented benefits. In a study of 267, 427 Medicare beneficiaries (65 years old and older) admitted for acute MI or CABG, who survived at least 30 days following hospital discharge, only 13.9% of patients with acute MI and 31% of patients with CABG participated in CR. In the same study, only 13% of patients older than 79 years attended CR.[15] Similarly, CR referral and completion were significantly lower in women (adjusted odds ratio [OR] 0.74, 95% CI, 0.69–0.79 and OR 0.73, 95% CI, 0.66–0.81, respectively), even though the female cohort demonstrated reduced mortality and greater relative benefit from CR compared with their male counterparts.[16]

BARRIERS TO CARDIAC REHABILITATION REFERRAL AND PARTICIPATION

Despite CR's demonstrated benefits and guideline recommendations, up to 80% of eligible patients are not referred.[17] Women face unique social and societal barriers that undercut referral rates and participation, including competing caregiver obligations and common perception that it is a male-dominated program. Women usually tend to have lower enrollment, poorer adherence, and higher dropout rates than their male counterparts.[18] Similarly, older patients have unimpressive rates of referral and participation.

Patient Barriers

Several patient barriers limit referral rates and participation and are especially common among older women. Women often assume the role of caretakers of spouses and grandchildren, limiting their capacities to attend CR. In addition, older adults are at higher risk for cognitive, physical, and visual impairments and poor health literacy that interferes with coordination of care. Patients must be able to interpret appointment slips, understand educational material provided by the program, and have adequate executive function skills to orchestrate the attendance of 3 appointments weekly (calendar planning, coordinating transportation).[18] Older adults often have financial limitations because many are retired or unable to work, adding to the limitations in CR access.

Underreferrals also add to many patients' lack of perceived need for CR. Women typically increase their physical activity levels sooner than men after a coronary event by resuming household chores at an earlier stage in their recovery. Many develop a false impression that their increased activity level provides similar benefit to a time-intensive CR program.[14] When paired with other barriers such as home responsibilities, appointments for other comorbidities, lack of education and physician encouragement to attend, and insecurities concerning group exercise, the priority to attend CR often wanes.

Medical Barriers

As adults age, susceptibility to multiple diseases tends to increase. CHD, HF, chronic obstructive pulmonary disease, osteoarthritis, peripheral artery disease (PAD), and diabetes all accumulate leading to patterns of shortness of breath, fatigue, and pain, which can significantly impair an older adult's functional status.[1] These symptoms deter not only patient attendance but also physician referrals. In addition, older patients often have multiple subspecialty appointments that diminish capacities and enthusiasm for the traditional CR thrice weekly schedule especially in the context of high copayments and poor access. When these deterrents are superimposed onto other factors, such as home responsibilities, debilitating symptoms, and lack of educations on CR benefits, older women often disregard CR.

Older patients are particularly vulnerable to deconditioning, frailty, and disability, which often complicate the initiation of an exercise program. Patients, providers, and family members often perceive muscle weakness, joint instability, cognitive impairment, sensory deficits (hearing, vision, proprioception), and polypharmacy (beta-blockers, diuretics, sleep aids, analgesics) as prohibitive to CR or a threat to safety. Older women also have the highest risk of osteoporosis, which can further limit mobility and perceived safety. Yet, often these patients benefit the most from CR.[19] Physicians are often reluctant to refer their older patients due to fall risk, yet exercise therapy has demonstrated a reduction in falls in vulnerable senior adults.[13]

Older patients still benefit from CR because the program provides opportunities to develop safe activity routines and care plans by addressing specific medical and social complexities, all while improving mobility, strength, and balance.[13] Studies have shown that older patients attending CR are not at increased risk for complications or adverse events.[20] Moreover, older patients have comparable benefits to those who are younger, usually with only modest modification in training technique.

Fitness levels in older adults vary widely, and for many older women, frailty also influences the intensity and type of exercise training that may be tolerated. This highlights the importance of individualized prescriptive exercise by certified specialists such as that provided through CR.[21] Moreover, women may be reluctant to even start an exercise program due to the lack of prior physical activity experience.[18] Therefore, an individualized care plan under the supervision of a skilled and attentive CR team provides an important opportunity to incorporate important lifestyle changes through exercise education and social support.

Depression is independently associated with increased cardiovascular morbidity and mortality in older adults,[22,23] and it is more prevalent in women than in men. Although age alone is not a risk factor for depression, older cardiovascular patients commonly experience multiple depression risk factors, such as having multiple medical comorbidities, cognitive impairment, living in nursing facilities, bereavement, and experiencing major life transitions.[24,25] Thus, older women with cardiovascular disease are particularly vulnerable to mood disorders. Depression may also interfere with patients' ability to manage their medical issues (ie, medication adherence, follow-up appointment attendance). CR moderates these detrimental patterns. In one study, patients older than 65 years were significantly less likely to be depressed after CR, and a meta-analysis showed decreased depression in older patients who paired exercise therapy with psychosocial interventions versus usual depression care.[13]

Health Care System Barriers

Multiple barriers affect our health care system and prevent older women from attending CR. Clinicians commonly underrefer patients, particularly older women. Cardiothoracic surgeons are often the most likely to refer their patients as part of a standardized recovery process after surgery, but cardiologists widely underrefer for CHD, HF, and PAD. Although it is possible that internists and hospitalists might take a more active role to also refer patients to CR, there remains widespread perception that this is primarily the responsibility of a cardiologist. Furthermore, most of these noncardiologist clinician groups often remain unaware of the CR's benefits and its value, especially for older patients with physical disability, frailty, and cognitive impairment.

Many hospitals have implemented automated referral systems to increase referral rates, with some success. However, Medicare does not reimburse for CR in patients residing in postacute care rehabilitation facilities. Therefore, the subset of older patients with CVD referred to skilled nursing facilities or other postacute care after hospitalization (most often older, frail, multimorbid women) commonly miss referral to CR, as there is no reliable mechanism to refer after such postacute care.

Program Availability and Characteristics

Characteristics innate to CR programs also affect enrollment of older women. Limited accessibility (most centers are associated with health care organizations located in urban settings) and costs (to both patients and the health care system) all contribute to underutilization.[17] Geographic location, participant capacity, proximity to public transportation, and parking availability are all relevant factors because many older women do not drive due to visual or cognitive impairments or the costs associated with owning a vehicle. Some older women rely on spouses and family members for transportation, implicitly linking CR to the burden that a family member must be involved with their participation. Furthermore, some women do not feel comfortable participating in what many perceive as male-dominated programs.[18]

Home-based cardiac rehabilitation programs

Option to complete CR at home or in the community potentially allows such patients to overcome many of the barriers that otherwise preclude CR. Home-based CR, albeit only in its early stages, is recognized by professional societies for their potential to increase utilization and participation. The American Association of Cardiovascular and Pulmonary Rehabilitation, the American Heart Association, and the American College of Cardiology recently published a scientific statement that identified home-based CR as a possible strategy to overcome various barriers contributing to underutilization and as a potentially reasonable alternative option for stable patients,[26] particularly those with low and intermediate cardiovascular risk.[18,27] A 2017 Cochrane review, which included 2890 participants with CR with acute MI, coronary revascularization, or HF across 23 trials, demonstrated that home-based programs have similar efficacy as facility-based programs. There was no significant difference in total mortality, exercise capacity, or health-related quality of life in patients attending home- versus facility-based CR.[28]

Smartphone-based cardiac rehabilitation programs

Over the past decade, the smartphone has revolutionized ability to communicate, share information, and track health. Although use of this technology is commonly associated with younger-aged populations, older patients also embrace daily use of smartphones, and this may offer particular value for older women CR candidates. In 2019, 53% of Americans older than 65 years owned smartphones, with slightly higher rates in men than women (84% compared with 79%).[29] Smartphones contain several built-in features to facilitate home-based CR programs such as messaging and two-way video capabilities and accelerometers to track steps and flights that are conducive to many exciting health care application (ie, "app") platforms. Through apps, patients can log meals, monitor vital signs, track activity, and stream educational videos. Home blood pressure cuffs, pulse oximeters, and glucometers can also be linked with smartphones, allowing patients and providers to monitor trends.[30] Ideally, this information is displayed on a user-friendly interface to better display progress and expectations.[31]

More women use social media than men (78% compared with 65%) and may find CR apps to be especially appealing. Use of social media by people older than or equal to 65 years has increased 5 fold in the past decade (8% in 2009–40% in 2019).[32]

Women are more likely than men to use social media for sharing and self-help.[33] Therefore, options for women-only environments with motivational messages and social support that is personal and appealing remain compelling considerations that merit further investigation.

Although data from smartphone-based CR programs are limited, outcomes from small studies are promising. In a randomized controlled trial comparing a mobile phone–based CR model to a traditional model in 120 participants (mostly middle-aged men), the mobile-based group demonstrated increased program completion (80% vs 47%) and improved psychological well-being, while maintaining similar improvement in functional capacity, depression, and dietary discretion.[34] Similarly, Harzand and colleagues[35] reported significant improvement in functional capacity, systolic blood pressure, and increased confidence in self-care. Although Harzand's study included only 13 participants, nearly half were older than 65 years and/or smartphone naïve and suggested feasibility and utility of such technology-based care that is particularly useful to older women.

SUMMARY

CR has been demonstrated to reduce morbidity and mortality and to improve functional capacity, mood, and quality of life in an expanding population of patients with cardiovascular disease. Older adults and especially older women underutilize this valuable component of therapy, undercutting recovery and quality of care. Alternative models of CR may help overcome underuse in older women, including home-based CR and technology-based CR applications. Further testing and validation are needed to address issues of safety, efficacy, and feasibility particularly for older women who are eligible for CR but who are also frail, disabled, multimorbid, and who have other age-related health complexities.

REFERENCES

1. Menezes AR, Lavie CJ, Forman DE, et al. Cardiac rehabilitation in the elderly. Progress in cardiovascular diseases. Prog Cardiovasc Dis 2014;57(2):152–9.
2. Menezes AR, Lavie CJ, Milani RV, et al. Cardiac rehabilitation and exercise therapy in the elderly: should we invest in the aged? J Geriatr Cardiol 2012;9:68–75.
3. Doll JA, Hellkamp A, Ho PM, et al. Participation in cardiac rehabilitation programs among older patients after acute myocardial infarction. JAMA Intern Med 2015; 175(10):1700–2.
4. Thomas RJ, King M, Lui K, et al. AACVPR/ACC/AHA 2007 performance measures on cardiac rehabilitations for referral to and delivery of cardiac rehabilitation/secondary prevention services endorsed by the American College of chest physicians, American College of Sports Medicine, American Physical Therapy Assoiation, Canadian Association of Cardiac Rehabilitation, European Association for Varfiovascular Prevention and Rehabilitation, Inter-American Heart Foundation, National Association of Clinical Nurse Specialists. Preventive Cardiovascular Nurses Association, and the Society of Thoracic Surgeons. J Am Coll Cardiol 2007;50:1400–33.
5. Suaya JA, Sherpard DS, Normand ST, et al. Use of cardiac rehabilitation by medicare beneficiaries after myocardial infarction or coronary bypass surgery. Circulation 2007;116:1653–62.
6. Arena R, Williams M, Forman DE, et al. Increasing referral and participation rates to outpatient cardiac rehabilitation: the valuable role of healthcare professionals in the inpatient and home health settings. Circulation 2012;125:1321–9.

7. Pasquali SK, Alexander KP, Peterson ED. Cardiac rehabilitation in the elderly. Am Heart J 2001;142:748–55.
8. Suaya JA, Stason WB, Ades PA, et al. Cardiac rehabilitation and survival in older coronary patients. J Am Coll Cardiol 2009;54(1):25–33.
9. Lavie CJ, Milani RV. Effects of Cardiac Rehab programs on exercise capacity, coronary risk factors, behavioral characteristics and qil in a large elderly cohort. Am J Cardiol 1995;76:177–9.
10. Ståhle A, Mattsson E, Rydén L, et al. Improved physical fitness and quality of life following training of elderly patients after acute coronary events. A 1 year follow-up randomized controlled study. Eur Heart J 1999;20(20):1475–84.
11. Hammill BG, Curtis LH, Schulman KA, et al. Relationship between cardiac rehabilitation and long-term risks of death and myocardial infarction among elderly Medicare beneficiaries. Circulation 2010;121:63–70.
12. Ades PA, Savage P, Cress ME, et al. Resistance training on physical performance in disabled older female cardiac patients. Med Sci Sports Exerc 2003;35: 1265–70.
13. Schopfer DW, Forman DE. Cardiac rehabilitation in older adults. Can J Cardiol 2016;32(9):1088–96.
14. Benjamin EJ, Muntner P, Alonso A, et al. Heart disease and stroke statistics-2019 update: a report from the American Heart Association. Circulation 2019;139(10): e56–528.
15. Lavie CJ, Milani RV, Littman AE. Benefits of cardiac rehabilitation and exercise training in secondary coronary prevention in the elderly. J Am Coll Cardiol 1993;22:678–83.
16. Colbert JD, Haykowsky MJ, Hauer TL, et al. Cardiac rehabilitation referral, attendance and mortality in women. Eur J Prev Cardiol 2015;22(8):979–86.
17. Sandesara PB, Lambert CT, Gordon NF, et al. Cardiac rehabilitation and risk reduction. J Am Coll Cardiol 2015;65(4):389–95.
18. Balady GJ, Ades PA, Bittner VA, et al, American Heart Association Science Advisory and Coordinating Committee. Referral, enrollment, and delivery of cardiac rehabilitation/secondary prevention programs at clinical centers and beyond: a presidential advisory from the American Heart Association. Circulation 2011; 124:2951–60.
19. Flint K, Kennedy K, Arnold SV, et al. Slow gait speed and cardiac rehabilitation participation in older adults after acute myocardial infarction. J Am Heart Assoc 2018;7(5):e008296.
20. Wenger NK. Current Status of cardiac rehabilitation. J Am Coll Cardiol 2008; 51(17):1619–31.
21. Vigorito C, Abreu A, Ambrosetti M, et al. Frailty and cardiac rehabilitation: a call to action from the EAPC Cardiac Rehabilitation Section. Eur J Prev Cardiol 2017; 24(6):577–90.
22. Whooley MA, de Jonge P, Vittinghoff E, et al. Depressive symptoms, health behaviors, and risk of cardiovascular events in patients with coronary heart disease. JAMA 2008;300(20):2379–88.
23. Ariyo AA, Haan M, Tangen CM, et al. Depressive symptoms and risks of coronary heart disease and mortality in elderly Americans. Circulation 2000;102:1773–9.
24. Cole MG, Dendukuri N. Risk factors for depression among elderly community subjects: a systematic review and meta-analysis. Am J Psychiatry 2003;160(6): 1147–56.

25. Hoover DR, Siegel M, Lucas J, et al. Depression in the first year of stay for elderly long-term nursing home residents in the USA. Int Psychogeriatr 2010;22(7): 1161–71.
26. Thomas RJ, Beatty AL, Beckie TM, et al. Home-based cardiac rehabilitation: a scientific statement from the American association of cardiovascular and pulmonary rehabilitation, the American Heart Association, and the American College of Cardiology. Circulation 2019;140(1):e69–89.
27. Sandesara PB, Dhindsa D, Khambhati J, et al. Cardiac rehabilitation to achieve panvascular prevention: new care models for a new world. Can J Cardiol 2018; 34(10):S231–9.
28. Anderson L, Sharp GA, Norton RJ, et al. Home-based versus centre-based cardiac rehabilitation. Cochrane Database Syst Rev 2017;(1):CD007130.
29. Department of Internet & Technology. "Who owns cellphones and smartphones." Mobile fact sheet. Washington, DC: Pew Research Center; 2019.
30. Walters DL, Sarela A, Fairfull A, et al. A mobile phone-based care model for outpatient cardiac rehabilitation: the care assessment platform (CAP). BMC Cardiovasc Disord 2010;10:5.
31. Pfaeffli L, Maddison R, Jiang Y, et al. Measuring physical activity in a cardiac rehabilitation population using a smartphone-based questionnaire. J Med Internet Res 2013;15(3):e61.
32. Department of Internet & Technology. "Who uses social media" social media fact sheet. Washington, DC: Pew Research Center. 2005–2019.
33. The Neilson Company. The female/male digital divide. Available at: https://www.nielsen.com/us/en/insights/article/2014/the-female-male-digital-divide/. Accessed July 1, 2019.
34. Varnfield M, Karunanithi M, Lee C, et al. Smartphone-based home care model improved use of cardiac rehabilitation in postmyocardial infarction patients: results from a randomised controlled trial. Heart 2014;100:1770–9.
35. Harzand A, Witbrodt B, Davis-Watts ML, et al. Feasibility of a smartphone-enabled cardiac rehabilitation program in male veterans with previous clinical evidence of Coronary Heart Disease. Am J Cardiol 2018;122(9):1471–6.

UNITED STATES POSTAL SERVICE®

Statement of Ownership, Management, and Circulation (All Periodicals Publications Except Requester Publications)

1. Publication Title	2. Publication Number	3. Filing Date
CLINICS IN GERIATRIC MEDICINE	000 – 704	9/18/2019
4. Issue Frequency	5. Number of Issues Published Annually	6. Annual Subscription Price
FEB, MAY, AUG, NOV	4	$286.00

7. Complete Mailing Address of Known Office of Publication *(Not printer) (Street, city, county, state, and ZIP+4®)*
ELSEVIER INC.
230 Park Avenue, Suite 800
New York, NY 10169

Contact Person: STEPHEN R. BUSHING
Telephone *(Include area code)*: 215-239-3688

8. Complete Mailing Address of Headquarters or General Business Office of Publisher *(Not printer)*
ELSEVIER INC.
230 Park Avenue, Suite 800
New York, NY 10169

9. Full Names and Complete Mailing Addresses of Publisher, Editor, and Managing Editor *(Do not leave blank)*

Publisher *(Name and complete mailing address)*
TAYLOR BALL, ELSEVIER INC.
1600 JOHN F KENNEDY BLVD. SUITE 1800
PHILADELPHIA, PA 19103-2899

Editor *(Name and complete mailing address)*
JESSICA MCCOOL, ELSEVIER INC.
1600 JOHN F KENNEDY BLVD. SUITE 1800
PHILADELPHIA, PA 19103-2899

Managing Editor *(Name and complete mailing address)*
PATRICK MANLEY, ELSEVIER INC.
1600 JOHN F KENNEDY BLVD. SUITE 1800
PHILADELPHIA, PA 19103-2899

10. Owner *(Do not leave blank. If the publication is owned by a corporation, give the name and address of the corporation immediately followed by the names and addresses of all stockholders owning or holding 1 percent or more of the total amount of stock. If not owned by a corporation, give the names and addresses of the individual owners. If owned by a partnership or other unincorporated firm, give its name and address as well as those of each individual owner. If the publication is published by a nonprofit organization, give its name and address.)*

Full Name	Complete Mailing Address
WHOLLY OWNED SUBSIDIARY OF REED/ELSEVIER, US HOLDINGS	1600 JOHN F KENNEDY BLVD. SUITE 1800 PHILADELPHIA, PA 19103-2899

11. Known Bondholders, Mortgagees, and Other Security Holders Owning or Holding 1 Percent or More of Total Amount of Bonds, Mortgages, or Other Securities. If none, check box ☐ None

Full Name	Complete Mailing Address
N/A	

12. Tax Status *(For completion by nonprofit organizations authorized to mail at nonprofit rates) (Check one)*
The purpose, function, and nonprofit status of this organization and the exempt status for federal income tax purposes:
☒ Has Not Changed During Preceding 12 Months
☐ Has Changed During Preceding 12 Months *(Publisher must submit explanation of change with this statement)*

13. Publication Title: CLINICS IN GERIATRIC MEDICINE
14. Issue Date for Circulation Data Below: AUGUST 2019

15. Extent and Nature of Circulation			Average No. Copies Each Issue During Preceding 12 Months	No. Copies of Single Issue Published Nearest to Filing Date
a. Total Number of Copies *(Net press run)*			138	170
b. Paid Circulation *(By Mail and Outside the Mail)*	(1)	Mailed Outside-County Paid Subscriptions Stated on PS Form 3541 (Include paid distribution above nominal rate, advertiser's proof copies, and exchange copies)	59	71
	(2)	Mailed In-County Paid Subscriptions Stated on PS Form 3541 *(Include paid distribution above nominal rate, advertiser's proof copies, and exchange copies)*	0	0
	(3)	Paid Distribution Outside the Mails Including Sales Through Dealers and Carriers, Street Vendors, Counter Sales, and Other Paid Distribution Outside USPS®	31	34
	(4)	Paid Distribution by Other Classes of Mail Through the USPS (e.g., First-Class Mail®)	0	0
c. Total Paid Distribution *[Sum of 15b (1), (2), (3), and (4)]*			90	105
d. Free or Nominal Rate Distribution *(By Mail and Outside the Mail)*	(1)	Free or Nominal Rate Outside-County Copies included on PS Form 3541	38	54
	(2)	Free or Nominal Rate In-County Copies Included on PS Form 3541	0	0
	(3)	Free or Nominal Rate Copies Mailed at Other Classes Through the USPS (e.g., First-Class Mail)	0	0
	(4)	Free or Nominal Rate Distribution Outside the Mail *(Carriers or other means)*	0	0
e. Total Free or Nominal Rate Distribution *(Sum of 15d (1), (2), (3) and (4))*			38	54
f. Total Distribution *(Sum of 15c and 15e)*			128	159
g. Copies not Distributed *(See Instructions to Publishers #4 (page #3))*			10	11
h. Total *(Sum of 15f and g)*			138	170
i. Percent Paid *(15c divided by 15f times 100)*			70.31%	66.04%

* If you are claiming electronic copies, go to line 16 on page 3. If you are not claiming electronic copies, skip to line 17 on page 3.

16. Electronic Copy Circulation	Average No. Copies Each Issue During Preceding 12 Months	No. Copies of Single Issue Published Nearest to Filing Date
a. Paid Electronic Copies		
b. Total Paid Print Copies (Line 15c) + Paid Electronic Copies (Line 16a)		
c. Total Print Distribution (Line 15f) + Paid Electronic Copies (Line 16a)		
d. Percent Paid (Both Print & Electronic Copies) (16b divided by 16c × 100)		

☒ **I certify that 50% of all my distributed copies (electronic and print) are paid above a nominal price.**

17. Publication of Statement of Ownership
☒ If the publication is a general publication, publication of this statement is required. Will be printed in the NOVEMBER 2019 issue of this publication. ☐ Publication not required.

18. Signature and Title of Editor, Publisher, Business Manager, or Owner
Stephen R. Bushing
STEPHEN R. BUSHING - INVENTORY DISTRIBUTION CONTROL MANAGER
Date: 9/18/2019

I certify that all information furnished on this form is true and complete. I understand that anyone who furnishes false or misleading information on this form or who omits material or information requested on the form may be subject to criminal sanctions (including fines and imprisonment) and/or civil sanctions (including civil penalties).

Printed and bound by CPI Group (UK) Ltd, Croydon, CR0 4YY

03/10/2024

01040483-0020